MW00619841

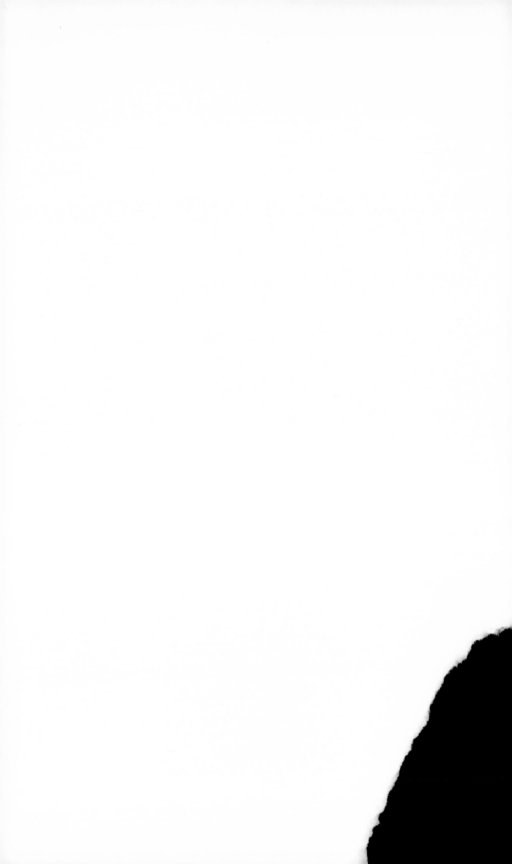

THE MOSS METHOD™

FIGHT CANCER NATURALLY

By Ralph W. Moss, Ph.D.

First edition 2024

For information about special discounts, subsidiary rights, or bulk purchases, contact: info@themossreport.com

Manufactured in the United States of America

Library of Congress Control Number: 2024906842
ISBN (hardback): 978-1-881025-78-8
ISBN (paperback): 978-1-881025-79-5
ISBN (ebook): 978-1-962471-16-9

Special thanks to:
Pat Downs Bright, MLS
Elizabeth Moss, MLS
Martha B. Moss
Isabelle Georges Aun, DBA
for their valuable contributions above and beyond the call of duty.

CONTENTS

PREFACE

Cancer, as I can testify, is a life-altering diagnosis. But what if there were steps you could take to reduce your risk of its occurrence or recurrence? In this book, I explore how dietary and lifestyle changes can empower you on your journey to stay healthy. It encapsulates the essence of what I have learned after half a century of research and a decade of dealing with a particularly aggressive form of prostate cancer.

The Moss Method is a comprehensive program to prevent cancer's appearance or return. Since it is primarily based around food and drink, with a minimum of supplements, its basic principles are accessible to almost everyone who wants to make better dietary choices and thereby reduce the risk of serious life-threatening diseases, such as cancer.

The Moss Method is not intended as a substitute for conventional medical care. It is not meant as a treatment plan at all, but as a helpful adjunct in the self-help realm. While conventional medicine plays a vital role in cancer treatment, The Moss Method focuses on complementary lifestyle changes that you can use to support your overall well-being.

This method has some unique features, but it is also firmly rooted in a robust body of scientific knowledge; it draws on a vast amount of data, including 700+ medical journal articles listed in the Bibliography. This literature spans more than half a century of work, including both recent discoveries and time-tested approaches, providing a solid foundation for the self-help strategies formulated in this book.

The Moss Method bridges the gap between the everyday concerns of those at risk of the disease and the latest discoveries in cancer research. Through clear insights into the science, combined with practical guidance, my aim is to empower the non-specialist with the most effective means of cancer prevention known to science.

The importance of avoiding cancer-causing chemicals (carcinogens) is well-documented, as my colleague, Samuel S. Epstein, MD (1926-2018), demonstrated in his seminal work, *The Politics of Cancer* (Epstein 1982, Roberts 2018). Although Sam and I worked closely for a time, my main focus has been on what individuals can do through the use of diet, functional foods (also called nutraceuticals), supplements, herbs, and lifestyle modification to combat cancer at the molecular level. Neither he nor I saw any contradiction between these two parallel tracks.

Cancer presents linguistic as well as medical challenges. Navigating the specialized terminology of researchers can often feel like entering a labyrinth that might require years to fully comprehend. The Moss Method, however, simplifies these complex concepts, providing clear and actionable information for people who have no prior familiarity with this complicated subject.

In fact, my objective throughout is to demystify science, to empower the lay reader to make good decisions based on reliable knowledge. I have done everything in my power to translate "Science-ese" into language that every reader who has had an average high school education can understand. Driven by this conviction, I will explain some very advanced medical science using clear, everyday language.

To aid in this process, I have minimized the use of technical terms. Where they are unavoidable, I have provided definitions in the text itself. Furthermore, to augment the reader's understanding of The Moss Method, I have included three glossaries at the book's conclusion. The first explains technical terms used in the book, the second clarifies some common abbreviations, and the third gives details on some of the scientists mentioned in this work.

Finally, I have included a bibliography of all cited works, where the underlining indicates a live link to free full texts, whenever possible. I have also minimally edited some of the quotations, trying to preserve the flavor of the original authors' words, while clarifying arcane terminology.

My goal is to clarify essential concepts while remaining true to the intent of the authors and thereby deepen one's understanding of this vital material. I strongly encourage you to use these resources to enhance your understanding and equip yourself to have informed discussions with your healthcare providers regarding this critical aspect of your health – preventing the occurrence or recurrence of cancer.

UNIFYING ELEMENTS

Cancer consists of well over 100 types, depending on the cell type and the tissue of origin. Despite this vast diversity of features, there are also unifying elements that are actionable for everyday people. This justifies talking about cancer as a single disease with many aspects. For instance, cancer in general can be described as having a dozen or so key "hallmarks," that are present in almost all types and cases. Thus, cancer in general is characterized by uncontrolled cell growth, invasiveness, and an ability to spread to other organs, or, as scientists say, to metastasize (Liskova 2019).

(The Hallmarks of Cancer are discussed in a later chapter.)

Another shared feature is the very beneficial role of substances known as plant chemicals (our substitution of the technical term, phytochemicals) in attacking numerous types of cancer. Just to take one example, curcumin, the natural yellow pigment in turmeric root, is active against lung (Tang 2021), breast (Kaya 2024), colon (Chen L 2013), pancreas (Al-Ishaq 2020), and numerous other types of cancer cells. The same can be said about EGCG (green tea), resveratrol (red wine), polyphenols (olive oil), and almost all the other plant chemicals discussed in this book.

I emphasize these shared features, since the tendency today is to regard cancer as an individualized, and therefore incredibly complex, phenomenon. Many people believe that a strategy of targeting mutated genes (for either treatment or prevention) is the ultimate goal. But I recently reviewed a paper in which a dozen urology researchers went looking for a putative kidney cancer gene. But what they found instead were *1,124 abnormal genes in just one kind of cancer* (Liu Y 2024). Kidney cancer is hardly alone in this regard. Most cancers present a staggering array of genetic abnormalities.

Incidentally, these same urologists looked for a drug that could counteract this array of mutations that they had detected in kidney cancer. They analyzed over 60 promising substances, including well-known forms of toxic chemo. But in the end, here was their conclusion:

> *"After consulting the current medical literature, we found that the most significant potential molecule was resveratrol" (ibid., edited)*

(Resveratrol is one of the anticancer elements in The Moss Method, and is fully discussed in its proper place.)

As a result, simplifying our discussion to focus on broad-acting strategies is both scientifically justified and also practical from the point of view of prevention. It is also easier to understand and is supported by numerous scientific studies. Of course, mainstream scientific research will continue to explore the great genetic diversity found in cancers. However, I believe that, over time, more oncologists will accept the fact that natural elements have a broad usefulness in many kinds of cancer. The purpose of The Moss Method is to bring these natural ways of controlling cancer to the fore, and to make knowledge of them more widely available to the average person who usually does not have any scientific or medical background.

Thus, the essence of The Moss Method is empowerment—to provide the knowledge to make informed decisions that are appropriate for your situation, based on the latest and most comprehensive findings. This is the core message of my life work, and of this fruit of decades of exploration, The Moss Method.

In this book, I shall not just talk in generalities, but shall point out how this knowledge relates to particular kinds of cancer. This is particularly so when it comes to the exciting breakthrough represented by the emerging science of cancer stem cells.

It is possible that in the future, doctors will analyze a person's own tumor for their unique genetic abnormalities and then prescribe an individualized array of foods and nutraceuticals to target their particularly important markers. We make a start towards that process in another chapter.

(This is outlined in <u>Plant Chemicals & Particular Kinds of CSCs</u>.)

But the most prudent course is to incorporate the anticancer nutraceuticals discussed in this book into your own comprehensive anticancer program.

CONVENTIONAL CANCER PREVENTION ADVICE

In establishing The Moss Method, it is essential, first of all, to acknowledge the conventional cancer prevention advice that has stood the test of time and scientific scrutiny. These recommendations form the bedrock of all public health guidelines around the world and offer a solid starting point for understanding how lifestyle choices impact cancer risk.

The Moss Method is not a substitute for sensible advice but is meant as a helpful addition for those who want to go further based on the growing understanding of the link between diet and cancer prevention. While The Moss Method emphasizes natural and alternative approaches, integrating it with conventional wisdom provides a holistic view that respects both traditional and contemporary perspectives on cancer prevention.

One of the most widely recognized pieces of advice is to *avoid tobacco in all its forms.* The link between smoking and various cancers, particularly lung cancer, is unequivocal. Tobacco is a potent carcinogen, and its avoidance is a primary strategy in reducing cancer risk. The devastating impact of tobacco on health is a well-documented fact that underscores the necessity of steering clear of smoking and other forms of tobacco, including second-hand smoke.

Maintaining a healthy weight is another cornerstone of cancer prevention. Obesity is a significant risk factor for several cancers, including breast, colorectal, and pancreatic cancers. The correlation between excess body weight and cancer is attributed to various mechanisms, including hormonal imbalances and chronic inflammation. Therefore, achieving and maintaining a healthy weight through balanced nutrition and regular physical activity is crucial. This approach not only helps in cancer prevention but also promotes overall health and well-being.

Diet plays a pivotal role in cancer prevention. A healthy diet rich in fruits, vegetables, and whole grains, while low in processed foods and red meats, especially highly processed and preserved meats, is associated with a lower risk of cancer. Fruits and vegetables are packed with vitamins, minerals, and antioxidants that protect against cellular damage. Whole grains provide fiber, which aids in digestion and can help prevent colorectal cancer. Conversely, limiting the intake of red and processed meats can reduce the risk of colorectal cancer, as these foods have been linked to carcinogenic processes in the body.

(Red meat is discussed in a separate section.)

Physical activity is another critical factor. Regular exercise helps maintain a healthy weight and has been shown to reduce the risk of various cancers, including of the breast, prostate, and colon. The benefits of physical activity extend beyond weight control; it also enhances immune function, improves hormone regulation, and reduces inflammation—all of which contribute to a lower cancer risk.

Sun protection is vital for preventing skin cancers. The harmful effects of ultraviolet (UV) radiation from the sun and tanning beds are well known. Using sunscreen, wearing protective clothing, and avoiding peak sun exposure times can significantly reduce the risk of skin cancer. These simple yet effective measures highlight the importance of protecting our skin from harmful UV rays.

Vaccinations offer a powerful tool in cancer prevention. Certain infections are known to cause cancer, and vaccines can help prevent these infections. The human papilloma virus (HPV) vaccine, for instance, can prevent cervical and other cancers. Similarly, the hepatitis B vaccine reduces the risk of liver cancer. These vaccines represent a significant advancement in public health, providing a proactive means to reduce cancer risk.

Regular medical check-ups and screenings are fundamental to early cancer detection. Routine screenings, such as mammograms, colonoscopies, and Pap tests, can detect cancers at an early stage when they are most treatable. Early detection through regular check-ups increases the chances of successful treatment and survival, underscoring the importance of staying vigilant about one's health.

So, obviously, The Moss Method is not intended to replace this conventional advice but to augment and extend it by incorporating the latest scientific findings, especially relating to plant chemicals and cancer. By combining the time-honored strategies of mainstream cancer prevention with cutting-edge research on natural products and lifestyle modifications, The Moss Method offers a comprehensive approach to cancer prevention.

This synergy between conventional wisdom and innovative natural approaches provides a robust framework for reducing cancer risk and promoting overall health.

This synthesis more generally underscores the importance of a balanced perspective that values the contributions of mainstream medical advice while exploring the promising potentials of natural and alternative strategies. By doing so, The Moss Method empowers individuals with a well-rounded set of tools to combat cancer more effectively.

FOLLOWING EINSTEIN'S PHILOSOPHY

As a science writer, I constantly strive to make complex research findings accessible to those without a specialized background in a topic. Achieving the right balance is crucial: oversimplifying can distort the truth, while too much detail can be overwhelming. This balance is particularly vital for explaining how cancer cells behave and react to the 20 natural plant chemicals central to The Moss Method.

For over five decades, my guiding principle has been a maxim attributed to Albert Einstein:

> *"Make everything as simple as possible, but not simpler."*

This statement underscores the art of making complex ideas accessible without oversimplifying them. This quotation formed the guiding philosophy of one of the great media pioneers of the 20th century, Henry R. Luce (1898-1967), founder of *Time, Life, Fortune,* and *Sports Illustrated* magazines. After quoting Einstein, he wrote that he strove to:

> *"...render an account that is plain and simple, yet does no violence to the complexity of the subject, so that the uninformed reader can understand us while the expert cannot fault us" (Luce 1962).*

This philosophy holds profound significance for me, particularly due to an unlikely personal connection to Einstein. In 1954, when I was ten, my older brother, Bob, corresponded with the great scientist. Their exchange of letters was sparked by negative statements Einstein had made about his own scientific career, after his younger colleague, J. Robert Oppenheimer, Ph.D., lost his security clearance—a situation later depicted in the 2023 Academy Award-winning film, *Oppenheimer*. In his response to my brother, Einstein referred to the life of his hero, the 17th-century philosopher Baruch Spinoza, who "refused a professorship at the University of

Heidelberg," as Einstein wrote to Bob, "preferring to earn his living as a lens grinder to maintain his independence."

This cherished letter became a cornerstone of my own development and profoundly shaped my approach to life, including the autonomous stance on cancer that my career has taken. It reinforced my belief in the value of independence. While independence doesn't automatically confirm the correctness of anyone's views, it does allow you to express your genuine opinions without being forced to yield to external pressures.

```
                                        December 11,1954


        Mr.Robert Moss
        214 West End Ave,
        Brooklyn N.Y,


        Dear Sir:
                I received your letter of December 10th.
        Baruch Spinoza was wholly devoted to the striving
        for truth and knowledge. But he refused a professor-
        ship at the university of Heidelberg and preferred to
        earn his living as a lens-grinder in order to keep his
        independence. One can well compare the present situation
        with that of Spinoza's time.
                                        Sincerely yours,

                                        A. Einstein.

                                        Albert Einstein.
```

Einstein's letter to my brother, Bob, dated December 11, 1954.

The idea for this book also gradually emerged from thousands of discussions with cancer patients and from my own decade-long battle with cancer. The need for such a guide became urgent in the early days of the COVID-19 pandemic. At the time I was still doing phone consultations for individual cancer patients and their caregivers. Often, I would discuss new drugs or clinics that I had visited where they might wish to go for treatment.

But, almost overnight, we were all sheltering at home as the pandemic raged around us. So, I had to drastically reorient my thinking to discuss what people could do for themselves, using the tools available to them at local food stores or through online marketplaces. It turned out that there was much that they could do that was harmless, and that made sense in the light of the basic biology of cancer.

The Moss Method is above all a practical guide. Although based on hundreds of scientific studies, all of which are referenced in our Bibliography, in the final analysis, it is a mosaic, where each individual piece contributes to a broader picture.

In this case, the final image is that we have the ability through our choice of food and lifestyle modifications to minimize the burden of cancer and maximize the odds of having a long and healthy life. A key to doing so is to integrate the principles of do-no-harm natural medicine with the latest scientific findings concerning cancer stem cells.

I hope that The Moss Method will prove helpful to you in your own quest for an answer to one of life's enduring mysteries: What is the root cause of cancer? And how can you use the tools at hand—such as food, herbs, plant chemicals, and lifestyle—to fight back against this often-devastating disease? I wish you success in your quest for a long and fruitful life, free from the shadow that cancer so often casts over our happiness.

–Ralph W. Moss, Ph.D.

HOUSEKEEPING NOTES

1. Abbreviated references such as this—(Smith 2024)—are provided in the text to explain the source of statements or quotations in the text. Full citations are contained in the Bibliography at the end of this work.
2. Unless otherwise noted, any bold or italic emphasis in a quotation is my addition and was not part of the original author's text.
3. When I ascribe a study to a particular individual, it is to be understood that usually this is just the first of the authors in question. Scientific work is almost always collaborative team work, and there are usually multiple authors to every study.
4. When I write (in parentheses) that a quotation has been "edited," it means that I have changed the wording for greater readability. Usually, these changes are minor, as I have taken care not to alter the meaning or intent of the authors.

5. For the sake of consistency, I have Americanized most UK spellings, such as substituting the word "tumor" for "tumour" or "randomized" for "randomised."

6. When I state that there is a certain number of articles on a topic in the U.S. government's PubMed database, that is the number of references that are returned by the program itself in response to a query. However, the number is an approximation and there is no guarantee that this is the exact number of references on that topic. To achieve a more exact number, I generally put the search term in parentheses, which limits references to those that contain the exact search term and not also related concepts.

7. Finally, the information provided in this book is for general educational purposes only. Neither the author nor the publisher makes warranties, expressed or implied, that this information is complete nor do they warrant the fitness of this information for any particular purpose. **This information is not intended as medical advice. We encourage all cancer patients to be under the care of licensed medical providers.**

INTRODUCTION

> *"Know your enemy and know yourself, and you need not fear the result of a hundred battles. If you know neither your enemy nor yourself, you will succumb in every battle."*
> —Sun Tzu, The Art of War (c. 500 BCE)

MY JOURNEY

A decade ago, I faced several personal health challenges that profoundly influenced my understanding and approach to health and disease, thereby shaping the development of *The Moss Method*. It began with a fall, followed by a painful bout of shingles, type 2 diabetes (T2D), and then a diagnosis of aggressive prostate cancer.

Shingles (a *Herpes zoster* viral infection) confined me to bed for several weeks, a period of inactivity that set the stage for T2D as well, since scientific evidence suggests a strong link between an inactive lifestyle and the risk of developing conditions like obesity and diabetes. Indeed, each two-hour daily session of TV watching is associated with an alarming 23% increase in obesity and a 14% increase in the risk of diabetes (Hu 2003).

A WAKE-UP CALL

My T2D diagnosis was a wake-up call. My afternoon glucose on that memorable day was 372 mg/dL (about triple the normal score). My hemoglobin A1C score at the time was 12.3%. Hemoglobin A1C is a standard blood test measuring the average blood glucose (sugar) level over the previous two to three months, often used to monitor diabetes control. A score of 12.3% also indicates severe diabetes.

My doctors recommended a variety of medications, such as metformin. However, they agreed to let me first try a lifestyle approach. Taking control of my health with diet and exercise, I reduced my A1C to 5.6% within a year, indicating reasonable blood glucose control. Ten years on, my A1C score remains in the prediabetes range, which I achieved without taking prescription drugs of any kind.

To be clear, I am not against taking prescription drugs on principle. For example, I recently took a course of antibiotics following a deer tick bite. However, I consider drugs a *last resort* for many health challenges and have managed to get by without

20

routinely needing any of them for my type 2 diabetes. About half of Americans in their 80s take five or more prescription drugs to manage their health conditions (Charlesworth 2015). Fortunately, I am among the rare older people who routinely take no medications. The Moss Method has proven to be sufficient to keep me in good health since my encounter with these serious diseases more than a decade ago. This astonishing transformation reinforced my belief in the power of lifestyle changes in managing health conditions, a vital part of The Moss Method.

PREVALENCE OF DIABETES

I wish to underline the seriousness of the "diabesity" epidemic. This is centered around the intake of huge amounts of sweetened beverages, but extends to the consumption of many fast foods as well. Most government statistics will put you to sleep, but this one is definitely a wake-up call. It is the <u>National Diabetes Statistics Report from the Centers for Disease Control and Prevention (the CDC).</u> As of 2024, here are some "fast facts" on diabetes in America:

- *Diabetes:* 38.4 million people have diabetes (11.6% of the U.S. population)
- *Prediabetes:* 97.6 million people aged 18 years or older have prediabetes (38.0% of the adult U.S. population)

Simply put, half (49.6%) of the U.S. population has either diabetes or prediabetes—an astonishing and frightening figure. Many of these people are either on powerful medications or are suffering the manifold negative consequences of the disease.

NEXT CAME PROSTATE CANCER

A year after the onset of my T2D, I navigated the challenges of prostate cancer, diagnosed through an experimental blood test, called ONCOblot, that was invented by two retired professors at Purdue University in Indiana (Morré 2016). Thus began my personal journey through the medical system, from the skepticism of my urologist about the test's results to the eventual diagnosis of two highly aggressive, life-threatening "Gleason 8" tumors in my prostate. I encountered various approaches and attitudes within the medical community, some quite negative, which deepened my understanding of patients' difficulties in navigating their treatment options. This was eye-opening. My experiences underscore the importance of integrating conventional medical treatment with a holistic approach to health, as advocated in The Moss Method.

(A holistic approach is a wide-ranging method that considers the whole person, including their physical, mental, and emotional health, rather than focusing only on specific symptoms or diseases.)

When it came to treating my prostate cancer, I opted for a rare, but Medicare-approved, procedure called *focal cryoablation*. This decision was influenced by a desire to avoid the more invasive and potentially life-altering side effects of mainstream treatments, such as radiation or surgery. I chose focal cryoablation after thoroughly researching the topic, reflecting The Moss Method's emphasis on informed decision-making and considering alternative, less invasive treatment options. By coincidence, I was scheduled to attend the 50ᵗʰ reunion of my New York University (NYU) undergraduate class that fall. But instead of attending that happy event I found myself a patient in the Langone NYU medical center, being treated for prostate cancer.

Through these experiences, I gained not just a deeper understanding of prostate cancer and its treatments but also an empathetic insight into what most patients endure. This personal journey with cancer, after decades of writing and consulting on the subject, added a crucial dimension to my work. It reinforced my commitment to a holistic, patient-centered approach in cancer care, the essence of The Moss Method.

As of this writing, after nearly ten years, there has not been any sign of a return of my prostate cancer. After the first year, I had a repeat biopsy, which was negative for recurrence. I have since followed a schedule of regular PSA blood and magnetic resonance imaging (MRI) tests. As of 2024, my repeat MRI showed no changes in the benign status of my prostate since the original cryoablation. Nor have I experienced any negative effects from the treatment itself.

ON THE EFFECTIVENESS OF FOCAL PROSTATE CRYOABLATION

Since this topic will be of intense interest to some of my readers, allow me a brief digression into the details of my treatment. How effective is focal prostate cryoablation? (*Focal* in this context means that only the tumors were destroyed, and not the whole gland, as occurs in most other prostate cancer treatments.) Let's explore some recent research to provide an educated guess. A 2022 study by my doctors at New York University (NYU) Langone included 27 men who underwent focal "cryo" for prostate cancer—the same treatment that I had for my condition.

Two years after treatment, there were cancer recurrences in seven instances: two recurrences occurred in areas of the gland that had been previously treated, and 5 appeared in untreated areas. This resulted in a two-year disease persistence or return rate of 25.9% (Chao 2018, Nazeemi 2022).

However, a recurrence does not necessarily indicate a dire outcome; many such tumors can be effectively *re-ablated* using the same cryo technique as before. More detailed data covering longer post-treatment periods are still needed to fully understand the safety and effectiveness of this therapy. But this study provides a preliminary estimate of the return rate within two years after prostate cryoablation; it is about one-quarter. Luckily for me, I am in the three-quarters of patients who have not had a recurrence (in my case for almost a decade).

In the years since my diagnosis, I have followed most of the dietary and lifestyle recommendations that I now present as The Moss Method. So in a sense I am the "pilot patient" of my own method for decreasing the return of the disease. The research basis for these methods, taken together, is huge. For instance, there are at present over 7,000 journal articles on curcumin + cancer alone. And curcumin is just one of the 20 plant elements for which substantial evidence exists of profound anticancer effects.

NECESSITY OF CLINICAL TRIALS

Before launching into a detailed discussion of The Moss Method, I want to address a question that is bound to be on the minds of many readers: If our new method is so effective, why hasn't it already been universally acknowledged and adopted in mainstream medicine?

The answer lies mainly in the rigorous standards required to validate new treatments in the medical field. In cancer treatment, questions cannot be settled by laboratory findings alone. If it were so, then cancer would have been cured many times over. While the foundation of almost all methods originates in the laboratory, their effectiveness must be established through robust and rigorous clinical data.

Randomized controlled trials (RCTs), often mentioned in medical research, are vital for testing new drug treatments. In these studies, participants are assigned by a computerized 'flip of a coin' to different groups to test a treatment's effects. By comparing results with a group that doesn't receive the treatment, scientists can determine if it really works, ensuring the study's findings are reliable and unbiased.

There are several dozen trials of plant chemicals, but proving the efficacy of dietary measures through randomized trials is exceptionally difficult. This challenge is not due to the researchers' lack of knowledge or good intentions but rather the complexity of dietary and lifestyle interventions. For example, the Mediterranean diet, widely recognized as beneficial, has limited clinical trial data specifically related to cancer. The PREDIMED study, one of the most influential trials, faced significant challenges and even required retraction and republishing due to protocol deviations.

Conducting clinical trials where diet or lifestyle is modified in a given population is a huge undertaking. The Moss Method, which involves a complex combination of foods, plant chemicals, and lifestyle modifications, would require extensive and sophisticated trials to convince the medical profession of its value in cancer prevention.

Most laypeople have no idea about the amount of money we are talking about. According to standard sources, it costs on average about US $2.2 *billion* to bring a new drug to market (Deloitte 2023). This can pay off big time for drug manufacturers. In fact, in 2023, annual sales of a single patented anticancer drug, pembrolizumab (Keytruda), reached US $25 *billion* (Reuters 2024). Yet the low cost of the substances highlighted in The Moss Method, from a purely economic point of view, does not justify any such expenditures. So in the United States at least, they are legally relegated to a lesser category of "dietary supplements." The Dietary Supplement Health and Education Act (DSHEA) of 1994 defined dietary supplements as products taken by mouth that contain a "dietary ingredient" intended to supplement the diet. Dietary ingredients may include vitamins, minerals, herbs or other botanicals, amino acids, and substances such as enzymes, organ tissues, gland extracts, and metabolites. They can be marketed, but any efficacy claims are severely limited by the Food and Drug Administration (FDA).

So there is in fact no incentive, or even a disincentive, for manufacturers of dietary supplements to perform high-cost randomized controlled trials (RCTs) of these items. In the U.S., at least, there is nothing to stop us as individuals from following the healthy dietary program outlined here. This approach is designed to be safe, offering little to lose and much to gain for most people concerned with cancer prevention. As Siddhartha Mukherjee, MD, eloquently put it, cancer is the "Emperor of All Maladies" (Mukherjee 2010). However, do not expect these elements to have the same level of proof that patented drugs have. Anyone demanding such proof is unaware of the realities of the health field in the 21st century.

REDUCTIONISM & ORGANICISM

Understanding the complexity of cancer requires a broad perspective. In analyzing the complex nature of cancer, we draw on two philosophical approaches: *reductionism* and *organicism*. While reductionism breaks down the disease into its smallest components, organicism emphasizes the interconnectedness of bodily systems. Together, these perspectives offer a holistic framework for addressing cancer through The Moss Method. We shall have occasion to visit this distinction in the coming chapters.

THREE GEARS

Cancer is a complex disease characterized by uncontrolled cell growth, invasiveness, and an ability to spread to other organs, which is the primary cause of cancer illness and death (Welch 2019). This description, however, barely scratches the surface. Cancer exhibits a dozen or so key characteristics, and the body of scientific knowledge surrounding it is constantly expanding. To date, over three million scientific articles have been published on this disease, with around 600 new ones emerging daily. Starting with the early insights of pioneers like Benjamin Rush, MD, a signer of the Declaration of Independence and Surgeon General of Washington's Continental Army, our collective understanding of cancer has evolved tremendously, especially in the last 250 years (Rush 1786).

Cancer is a critically important topic for many outside the medical profession. Approximately 40% of the population is expected to face internal cancers during their lifetime, and many others have already battled the disease and are seeking ways to prevent its recurrence (ACS 2024). Unlike many other approaches, The Moss Method is based entirely on plant chemicals (phytochemicals) and other natural products—a clean, traditional diet, special functional foods, select high-quality herbs and supplements, and lifestyle modifications. This method could also be called a "Do No Harm" approach, as it aims to prevent the onset or recurrence of cancer through natural and non-toxic means.

So let's delve into how specific dietary patterns, nutrients, and plant chemicals, such as turmeric, green tea, and garlic, can potentially lower cancer risk or impact the return of existing disease. This includes closely examining the scientific evidence behind the anti-cancer qualities of foods and supplements. Beyond diet, other lifestyle factors such as physical activity, sleep quality, and stress reduction play vital roles in cancer risk and overall well-being. We'll discuss actionable strategies to modify these aspects of your life in ways that can support cancer prevention and complement mainstream treatments.

The immune system's interaction with cancer is also pivotal. Enhancing immune function through natural means and understanding how to leverage it in the fight against cancer is another focus of The Moss Method. This discussion includes a look at how lifestyle choices can bolster your body's natural defenses. *I will also present evidence that plant chemicals can be essential to building immunity in the fight against cancer.*

INTEGRATING EVIDENCE-BASED STRATEGIES

While no single approach can guarantee cancer prevention, integrating evidence-based natural and conventional strategies offers the best path forward. The Moss Method is an informed, balanced approach to cancer prevention and care, emphasizing the importance of working with healthcare professionals. Indeed, this is the path I took in dealing with my aggressive type of prostate cancer.

I am sometimes called a "promoter" of complementary and alternative medicine (CAM). However, this term often carries a negative connotation. As you will see, I do not reject modern medicine, nor am I proposing The Moss Method as a substitute for what oncologists and other doctors offer. In fact, I expect readers to use mainstream medicine as their principal form of cancer treatment, as I myself did. In this book, except for one chapter, I avoid discussions of cancer treatment and focus instead on prevention, including the prevention of disease recurrence.

This approach aligns with empowering individuals to take proactive steps in managing their health. At the same time, many valuable treatments, from spruce tree needles in the 16th century to yoga and acupuncture in the 21st, have originated outside the medical establishment as Dr. Benjamin Rush concluded in his February 1786 lecture to the American Philosophical Society in Philadelphia:

> *"It was from the inventions and temerity of quacks that physicians have derived some of their most active and useful medicines" (Rush 1786).*

There is a profound truth here since, even in our lifetime, we have seen several health approaches once derided as quackery become integrated into conventional medicine. Recognizing that some unconventional treatments have later proven effective is not about "promoting" CAM or any other approach but about remaining open-minded to ideas that initially go against the grain. Ultimately, it helps us reach meaningful conclusions based on the best available scientific evidence.

(Please see the chapter on Cancer Treatment & The Moss Method.)

CANCER SURVIVORSHIP

Cancer survivorship is the period during and after cancer treatment in which a person deals with the physical, emotional, and practical aspects of having cancer. It includes managing long-term side effects, monitoring for recurrence, and addressing psychological and social issues.

The concept of cancer survivorship didn't exist when I entered the field in the 1970s. It only emerged about 20 years later as a consumer movement, primarily driven by patients and their close ones (Leigh 1994). It arose because a greater number of people were surviving their disease due to advances in treatment. Initially, it entered oncology indirectly through the work of nurses, who published in specialized journals not typically read by doctors. Today, cancer survivorship is a significant movement, with new research articles appearing daily. It even has dedicated medical journals, such as the *Journal of Cancer Survivorship: Research and Practice* (founded in 2007).

According to the American Cancer Society, there are currently over 18 million cancer survivors in the United States (ACS 2024), comprising around 5.4% of the total U.S. population and 21.5% of the population aged 65 and over. There are comparable numbers in most other countries.

The recognition of cancer survivorship represents significant progress, but there are still gaps. While many people diagnosed with cancer make changes to their tobacco and alcohol usage, one-third still have an elevated body mass index (BMI), and almost half do not meet recommended physical activity levels. The majority also have inadequate fruit and vegetable intake (Gregory 2023).

Many survivors live in a state of heightened awareness, anxiously checking for signs of recurrence. However, their response to the prospect of a recurrence is often confused and inadequate. Our main goal with this book is to help fill that gap by providing clear, actionable strategies to improve survivorship and reduce the risk of recurrence.

THE THREE GEAR LOGO & SUN TZU

My son, Benjamin Moss, a skilled designer who deeply understands the principles of The Moss Method, created the logo for this book. The logo features three interlocking gears, each representing a cornerstone of our approach: disordered metabolism, immune system dysfunction, and cancer stem cells (CSCs). These gears are surrounded by a corona of leaves, symbolizing the plants and herbs central to our methodology, emphasizing the power of the natural world in impacting serious diseases like cancer.

You may be wondering why I began this book with a quote from Sun Tzu's classic "Art of War". Recall his formula: "Know your enemy and know yourself, and you need not fear the result of a hundred battles." In contrast, our global "war on cancer" over the past 50 years has often reflected a one-dimensional approach, focused on attacking diseased cells directly without fully considering how our own biological and psychological makeup contributes to the conflict. This is why The Moss Method places significant emphasis on self-knowledge.

To understand the comprehensive approach of The Moss Method, we must delve into the three critical gears that drive its efficacy: disordered metabolism, a weakened immune system, and cancer stem cells (CSCs). These gears represent the interconnected processes that contribute to cancer development and progression.

The first two gears—"disordered metabolism" and "immune system dysfunction"—are designed to correct our own deficiencies. They enhance our understanding of what problems in our bodies and minds give cancer a foothold. The third gear delves into the intrinsic nature of cancer, drawing on cutting-edge research about cancer stem cells (CSCs) and integrating the ten classic "hallmarks of cancer." This comprehensive understanding embodies what Sun Tzu envisioned as his formula for success: to know yourself and your enemy thoroughly.

Armed with this profound knowledge, The Moss Method aims to advance us toward the ideal warrior that Sun Tzu described 2,500 years ago. By deeply understanding both our metabolism and the microbiome, as well as the fundamental nature of cancer, we equip ourselves to engage in countless battles, not merely to participate, but to prevail.

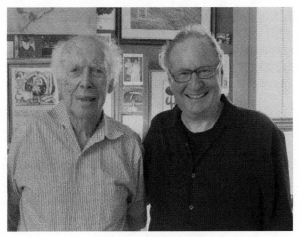

James D. Watson and Ralph W. Moss in Watson's office in Cold Spring Harbor, New York, July 2012.
On the wall above Watson's head is the world's first depiction of the DNA molecule.
Source: Author's collection, photo courtesy of David Wales.

GEAR #1: FAULTY METABOLISM

Faulty metabolism refers to how cancer cells use fuel differently from healthy cells, often consuming sugar at a higher-than-normal rate. This phenomenon was first discovered by Otto Warburg, MD, Ph.D., who found that cancer cells produce most of their energy through the fermentation of sugar, despite the presence of sufficient oxygen to support a more efficient process. Warburg's discoveries were so significant that he won the Nobel Prize in 1931 for his work in respiration.

Despite Warburg's groundbreaking findings, the focus on cancer metabolism diminished after the double helix structure of DNA was discovered by James Watson, Francis Crick, and their colleagues in the 1950s. This shift directed scientific attention towards molecular biology and genetics, sidelining Warburg's results. The decline in focus on Warburg's work also stemmed from the increasing emphasis on genetic mutations as drivers of cancer, facilitated by technological advancements in genetics.

However, the importance of metabolism in cancer revived, with researchers like Dean Burk (1904-1988) of the National Cancer Institute, Peter Pedersen, Ph.D., of Johns Hopkins University, and Thomas N. Seyfried Ph.D. of Boston College exploring and validating many of Warburg's theories.

Today, the resurgence of interest in Warburg's work is evident, with thousands of references to his theory in the PubMed database as od 2024. Cancer cells' ravenous appetite for sugar, or glucose, is a key indicator of their faulty metabolism. This metabolic quirk is so pronounced that it forms the basis of positron emission tomography (PET) scans, where radioactive glucose tracers are routinely used to detect malignant tumors.

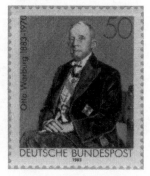

German postage stamp honoring Otto Warburg.
Source: Author's collection.

FAULTY ENERGY PROCESSING IN CANCER CELLS

Understanding how our cells produce energy is key to grasping why cancer cells behave differently than other cells. Cellular metabolism encompasses all chemical reactions within a cell that keep it alive, including breaking down nutrients to release energy, building new cell parts, and eliminating waste.

Cellular respiration converts energy from food into ATP, the cell's fuel supply. This process occurs in three stages: glycolysis in the cytoplasm, the citric acid cycle (Krebs cycle) in the mitochondria, and using oxygen in oxidative phosphorylation (OxPhos) to produce large amounts of ATP. This citric acid cycle acts as a critical engine in this process, while OxPhos ensures a high-energy yield.

But faulty cell metabolism is a major characteristic of cancer cells that aids their growth and survival. Cancer cells preferentially use glycolysis even when oxygen is sufficient, a phenomenon known as "aerobic glycolysis." This inefficient energy-related shift supports continuous growth and division, similar to a city using an inefficient but fast-producing power source. Cancer cells also alter how they use other food building blocks, like proteins and fats, tweaking their energy systems to grow without limits.

This point is crucial for understanding cancer, so let's dive deeper into how cancer cells behave differently:

- *Hungry for Sugar:* Cancer cells consume a lot of sugar (glucose) to fuel their rapid growth.
- *Producing Waste:* Like an inefficient power plant, cancer cells produce a lot of waste, specifically lactate (similar to lactic acid), which they must quickly expel due to its toxicity. Once outside the cell, this acidity breaks down neighboring tissue, making room for the tumor to grow, and keeps immune cells that could attack the cancer at bay.
- *Tough Survivors:* These changes help cancer cells thrive under difficult conditions, resist dying off, and sometimes dodge treatments.

Understanding these behaviors is like uncovering an enemy's strategy, giving researchers clues to develop better treatments that cut off cancer's fuel supply or use its waste production against it. Some applications of this knowledge are:

- *Targeting Weaknesses:* By pinpointing and attacking crucial enzymes or substances that cancer cells depend on, researchers can develop new treatments.

- *Tailored Treatments:* Personalizing therapy based on an individual's specific metabolic makeup can lead to more successful outcomes.
- *Lifestyle Impact:* Understanding how diet and lifestyle choices affect metabolic processes helps in preventing cancer and supporting treatment. This knowledge falls within the realm of non-toxic self-help, the focus of this book.

This exploration shows how understanding cancer at a metabolic level not only guides scientific advances in treatment but also empowers individuals with actionable knowledge for prevention and supportive care.

METABOLIC SYNDROME

Metabolic syndrome, characterized by high blood pressure, elevated blood sugar, and abnormal cholesterol levels, significantly increases the risks for heart disease, stroke, and type 2 diabetes (Ervin 2009). It is also ultimately related to the rise in certain forms of cancer. Recent surveys indicate a rapid rise in its prevalence, with a 2023 study in the *Postgraduate Medical Journal* showing an increase from 38% to 42% among American adults between 2012 and 2018, and elevated glucose levels rising from 49% to 65% (Liang 2023).

The authors of that study emphasize the need for lifestyle modifications to prevent metabolic syndrome and its associated risks (Liang 2023). The Moss Method manages those risks through lifestyle changes, including adopting a clean traditional diet and utilizing powerful plant chemicals, as explained in this book.

Chronic inflammation, a hallmark of metabolic syndrome, creates an environment conducive to cancer. Additionally, hormonal imbalances and damage from excess oxygen further contribute to cancer's onset and growth. Lifestyle factors such as a fast food or junk food diet and physical inactivity are also independently associated with increased cancer risk.

The intimate connection between damaged metabolism and type 2 diabetes (T2D) further emphasizes the role of metabolic health in cancer risk. Type 2 diabetes is characterized by insulin resistance, leading to high blood sugar levels. These elevated levels are linked to an increased risk of overweight and obesity, which are then associated, among others, with colorectal, breast, and pancreatic cancer. Cancer is often the final result of a decades-long problem stemming from a poor diet, particularly characterized by the overconsumption of sugar and junk food in general. This fact, grounded in an abundance of rigorous scientific research, underscores the central importance of diet in managing cancer risk and aligns with the holistic, evidence-based philosophy of The Moss Method.

The PREDIMED Trial

Although this book primarily focuses on cancer, it is essential to further explore the relationship between diet and rising rates of prediabetes and type 2 diabetes (T2D). The landmark PREDIMED trial, published in the prestigious *Annals of Internal Medicine*, demonstrated a significant reduction in diabetes incidence among participants who adhered to a clean traditional diet supplemented with either extra-virgin olive oil (EVOO) or mixed nuts. After a median follow-up of four years, the incidence of new-onset diabetes was reduced by 40% in the clean traditional diet plus EVOO group, and 18% in the group that received a daily supply of mixed nuts (Salas-Salvadó 2014). When these two intervention groups were combined, the incidence of diabetes was reduced by about half compared to the control group (Salas-Salvadó 2011).

You should not assume, however, that all the benefits against diabetes are attributable to one or two "magic ingredients," in this case EVOO or mixed nuts. A meta-analysis, which combines results from multiple scientific studies, examined the effect of adherence to a traditional diet on type 2 diabetes risk. The main findings were consistent: a clean traditional diet (in this case the Mediterranean diet) helped protect against type 2 diabetes, with risk reductions ranging from 12% to 83% depending on the degree of adherence to the doctors' dietary recommendations. This meta-analysis, conducted by researchers at the University of Vienna, reviewed studies involving 122,000 people. It found that those adhering to this clean traditional diet had a 19% lower risk of developing type 2 diabetes (Schwingshackl 2015).

The Moss Method builds on rigorous findings such as these by combining an overall clean traditional diet with an emphasis on particular plant chemicals, such as those found in EVOO (Salas-Salvadó 2015). By integrating a variety of health-promoting foods ingredients, I aim to create a balanced, nutrient-dense diet that supports metabolic health and reduces the risk of chronic diseases, including both diabetes and cancer.

CRITIQUE OF THE MEDITERRANEAN DIET

Because the Mediterranean Diet formed the basis of the PREDIMED clinical trial, and many other studies, you may assume that I strongly advocate this diet as the backbone of The Moss Method. However, this would be a mistake. While the

Mediterranean Diet is generally beneficial, it can be problematic for people with diabetes or prediabetes due to its high carbohydrate content. For instance, the influential *U.S. News and World Report* is not alone in considering the Mediterranean Diet the "No. 1 Best Diet Overall," describing its excellence with statements like:

- "There are nearly unlimited fresh fruits and vegetables on the Mediterranean diet.
- "Fill your pantry with quinoa, barley, farro, freekeh, and other whole grains.
- "Plenty of beans, lentils, and peas will add protein, fiber, vitamins, and minerals to your meals" (Hinzey 2024).

In my experience, this type of "healthy" diet can help drive blood sugar levels to undesirable levels. People without diabetes may handle this many carbs, with their blood sugar returning to normal within an hour or two. However, for about half the U.S. population, this rise in glucose will linger and may be reflected in abnormally high blood glucose levels, including one's fasting glucose level the next morning.

Consider a typical 60-year-old American woman who weighs 170 pounds. Each gram of carbs she consumes will raise her blood sugar by about three milligrams. Although fiber and fat may help reduce this impact, the basic effect of dietary carbs on blood sugar remains significant.

For example, if she follows standard dietary advice and eats three servings of fruit per day—an apple, a banana, and a bowl of fruit salad with yogurt—she'll ingest about 70 grams of carbs. This could increase her blood glucose by approximately 210 points, showing the challenge of processing these sugars. Moreover, the common advice to consume three to six servings of whole grains and starchy vegetables daily will also add a substantial carb load. For instance:

- One cup of cooked quinoa contains about 34 grams of net carbs.
- One cup of cooked oatmeal has around 24 grams of net carbs.
- A medium-baked potato provides about 57 grams of net carbs.

These foods, while healthy in moderation, could contribute another 115 grams of carbs to her diet. Every gram of carbohydrate in the diet must somehow be "covered" by the pancreas gland's production of insulin. In the long-run, the resulting high insulin levels (called hyperinsulinemia) is itself a serious health risk factor (Giovannucci 2010).

While the general outlines are clear, each person's response to dietary carbs is somewhat different based on their individual circumstances. So readers are encouraged to monitor their own responses to dietary changes (blood glucose monitors are available without a prescription) and to consult healthcare professionals to tailor recommendations to their individual needs and health goals.

ROLE OF A CLEAN, TRADITIONAL DIET

A "clean traditional diet" refers to a modern-day adaptation of the natural, minimally processed diets consumed by various cultures worldwide before the introduction of fast or junk food diets. This approach emphasizes whole, unprocessed foods such as fruits, vegetables, whole grains, nuts, seeds, and legumes. It incorporates healthy fats from sources like olive oil, avocados, and fatty fish, and lean proteins from poultry, fish, eggs, and plant-based options like legumes and tofu. The diet focuses on complex carbohydrates from whole grains and starchy vegetables while avoiding refined sugars, processed foods, and artificial additives. Fermented foods, which offer probiotic benefits, play a significant role, and traditional cooking methods like steaming, grilling, and fermenting are preferred to preserve nutritional integrity.

This type of diet also encourages the use of a wide variety of seasonal and locally sourced produce, extensive use of herbs and spices for their health benefits, and balanced meals with appropriate portions of macronutrients. Traditional meals tend to be social events. By adopting these principles, individuals can enjoy a nutrient-dense, health-promoting dietary pattern that supports overall well-being and reflects the nutritional wisdom of diverse cultures around the world.

The shift from discussing dietary influences on cancer to examining how cancer alters basic energy-related processes reveals the complex interplay between what we consume and how our cells use these resources. This understanding of metabolism's impact on cancer cells highlights the importance of energy-related health in cancer prevention.

Consider the role of a clean traditional diet in this scenario. Most cancer cells thrive in a high-glucose environment. Such diets help stabilize blood sugar and insulin levels. It is reasonable to believe that a diet low in refined sugars and processed carbs could create a more healthful environment for normal cellular growth.

Moreover, their antioxidants and anti-inflammatory compounds help counteract cell damage from oxygen and inflammation, altering energy-related processes to the advantage of normal cells. Addressing these factors might disrupt cancer cells' energy-related manipulation.

Understanding individual metabolism can guide more effective disease prevention and treatment, including lifestyle choices that address the energy-related underpinnings of diseases like cancer. While the relationship between diet, metabolism, and cancer is an ongoing area of research, adopting a holistic approach is likely to prove helpful.

The Moss Method builds on the platform of a clean traditional diet in several ways. While accepting the basic idea of the Mediterranean diet, I am not parochial in my approach. Why limit ourselves to the healthful ingredients of one particular region? Let's also incorporate key foods and plant chemicals that originate outside a single geographic area. When it comes to cancer prevention, we can use any help we can get. This includes weak plant estrogens (such as genistein), healing mushrooms (beta-glucans), probiotics (kefir and yogurt), radish and broccoli sprouts (sulforaphane and sulforaphene), turmeric powder (curcumin), and green tea (EGCG and other antioxidants). All of these are important and well established, scientifically, but all originate outside the Mediterranean basin.

Followers of The Moss Method, therefore, have numerous time-tested and non-toxic options for addressing poorly regulated metabolism. Aside from what physicians might prescribe, you can alter your diet, and in doing so, significantly impact your metabolism.

(See our chapter on Healing Recipes for sample menus and dishes that support our approach to metabolism.)

CONCLUDING THOUGHTS

By understanding and targeting damaged metabolism, we can take significant steps toward preventing and managing cancer. The Moss Method provides an international perspective that integrates dietary strategies, lifestyle modifications, and the use of natural compounds to support metabolic health. This holistic approach, which emphasizes the synergy between diet and lifestyle, not only helps in combating cancer but also enhances overall well-being, empowering individuals with actionable knowledge for a healthier life.

LIFESTYLE STRATEGIES

Various lifestyle strategies can help optimize health and metabolism. For example, in addition to what we eat, the timing of our meals is also crucial. Intermittent fasting involves skipping meals at specific times to improve health and potentially extend lifespan. Another approach, time-restricted eating, concentrates all daily meals within a certain number of hours each day. Routine exercise, tailored to one's age and health condition, helps maintain or improve well-being, while calorie restriction limits daily intake to promote health and longevity without causing malnutrition. Lastly, ketogenic diets focus on consuming high-fat, low-carb foods to encourage the body to burn fat for energy, supporting weight loss and other health benefits.

Each of these methods provides non-medical, self-help ways to adjust cellular metabolism. These practices impose energy-related stress on cancer cells, potentially disrupting their energy supply and offering non-toxic means of blocking cancer growth.

These strategies are not new but have gained renewed interest due to recent serious research. For example, a systematic review of 15 clinical trials emphasized the importance of prescribing physical exercise programs as adjuvant therapy for cancer patients (Rodríguez-Cañamero 2022, edited).

ROLE OF PIONEERS

I want to take a moment to honor the pioneers of this method, some of whom I had the honor to know personally. Kanematsu Sugiura, D.Sc. (1890-1979), together with Stanley Benedict, Ph.D. (1884-1936), pioneered studies of fasting in animals in the 1920s (Sugiura 1926). Sugiura, who made innumerable contributions to cancer research over his long career and had a profound impact on my life, was particularly interested in the intersection of diet and cancer.

In 1974, Sugiura told me how he and Benedict had experimented with calorie restriction as an anticancer tool—fifty years before we spoke (ibid.). This dietary regimen reduced caloric intake without causing malnutrition or a reduction in essential nutrients. However, his efforts were blocked by conservative surgeons who were afraid of "starving" their patients, even though no starvation was being suggested, just a reduction in calories.

(See my discussion of Dr. Sugiura's life and work in my book, Doctored Results.)

In the 50 years since that conversation, I have tried to build on the foundation of what I learned from this pioneering figure of cancer research. This is part of the origin of The Moss Method.

In the 1940s and 1950s, Albert Tannenbaum (1901-1980) and Herbert Silverstone (1913-1956) of Michael Reese Hospital in Chicago conducted important studies on fasting and cancer. They wrote that "the diet and the nutritional state of the host [i.e. a person or lab animal] influence the formation and growth of tumors" (Tannenbaum 1950, Tannenbaum 1953). This observation, revolutionary at the time, seems obvious today.

However, for the next 50 or so years, there were virtually no follow-up studies on the topic. Now, new research articles on intermittent fasting appear about once per week.

Intermittent Fasting & Cancer: A Scientific Overview

According to a survey by the International Food Information Council Foundation, intermittent fasting (IF) was the most popular diet of 2022. Judging from Google Trends, it remains highly popular at this writing.

Patients with cancer often seek advice from their doctors about fasting's helpful effects for cancer prevention (Clifton 2021). This is a good idea, as the information about this topic is constantly evolving and many scientific questions remain.

The Marinac Study of TRE (2016)

The Marinac Study, published in the top-drawer journal *JAMA Oncology*, provided compelling evidence of the benefits of time-restricted eating (TRE). It involved women with early-stage breast cancer but may be relevant to other cancers as well. Conducted by researchers at the University of California, San Diego (UCSD) Moores Cancer Center, it involved over 2,400 women, aged between 27 and 70, who had been diagnosed with breast cancer. Part of the larger Women's Healthy Eating and Living study between 1995 to 2007, it looked into whether the length of nightly fasting influenced the return rate of breast cancer, the emergence of new breast cancer cases, and death rates.

By analyzing the recorded details of what people ate and tracking the health outcomes of these women over an average of 7.3 years for cancer recurrence and 11.4 years for deaths, researchers found that fasting fewer than 13 hours per night was associated with a 36% higher risk of breast cancer returning. Moreover, extending nightly fasting by two hours was linked with improved blood sugar control and longer sleep.

This groundbreaking study suggested that extending the period of nightly fasting could offer a straightforward, non-drug strategy to lower the risk of breast cancer's return. The benefits observed in blood sugar control and sleep quality may have played critical roles in connecting TRE with fewer breast cancer recurrences (Marinac 2016).

The Fasting Mimicking Diet Study (2020)

The U.S. government website, ClinicalTrials.gov, currently lists 40 studies on intermittent fasting and cancer. About twelve of these are presently looking for participants. Even though 16 studies have finished, none have posted their results yet. Of these, only the DIRECT study from 2019 at Leiden University Medical Center in the Netherlands was randomized.

This study looked at how a Fasting Mimicking Diet (FMD) affects cancer treatment and found encouraging outcomes (de Groot 2020). It included 131 women with stage II or III breast cancer who did not have diabetes and had a body mass index (BMI) of over 18 (meaning they were not underweight). They were split into two groups: one used the FMD for three days before and during chemo, while the other group ate their usual diet. The results showed that the FMD group was three times more likely to see their tumors shrink and over four times more likely to lose nearly all tumor cells, which is a significant success in treatment. Also, the FMD group had less genetic damage from chemo in their white blood cells. Importantly, these patients managed without dexamethasone, or "dex," a common chemo drug that can affect mood and sleep negatively.

These results show that the Fasting Mimicking Diet (FMD) has two main benefits: it helps protect against some of chemo's side effects and increases its effectiveness. This supports more research into fasting and FMD as additional options for cancer treatment. However, the initial response to the DIRECT study was disappointing because the diet did not lessen other negative effects of chemo, which was the main goal of the study. Following the FMD was also difficult (2020).

The strategy to target the energy usage of cancer cells looks promising, yet putting it into practice has been challenging for nearly a hundred years. While we are developing treatments that interrupt these energy processes, including some drugs and dietary supplements, the real challenge is not just in targeting these processes correctly but also in making sure patients can stick to such demanding treatment plans.

The Moss Method does not involve prolonged water or dry fasting or even the Fasting Mimicking Diet. We consider these approaches better managed under medical supervision due to the challenges in maintaining patient compliance.

However, the method does support time-restricted eating, a form of intermittent fasting, as a healthy practice for many. This approach is backed by research, feels doable for most people, and generally yields positive results.

University of Rochester Study (2021)

A ten-hour eating window trial at the University of Rochester studied its effects on fatigue among cancer survivors. The study involved 21 participants (most had breast cancer), on average 1.6 years post-treatment. They adhered to a 10-hour eating period each day for two weeks. The trial showed high completion and adherence rates, with only two minor side effects, suggesting it was safe.

Results presented at an annual meeting of the American Society of Clinical Oncology (ASCO) indicated significant increases in health scores and reductions in overall fatigue and its intensity on an objective scale. These improvements were statistically significant, indicating better overall well-being (Kleckner 2021).

University of Chicago Study (2023)

A study published in an American Medical Association (AMA) journal by University of Illinois Chicago scientists examined whether an 8-hour eating window was more effective for weight control than traditional calorie reduction, particularly in people with type 2 diabetes and obesity.

This six-month trial involved adults following three plans: an 8-hour eating window (12 pm to 8 pm) without calorie counting, reducing daily calories by 25%, or no dietary changes. The 8-hour window group lost 3.6% of their weight and saw significant improvements in blood sugar control, with HbA1c levels dropping by about 0.91%. No serious health issues were noted with this eating pattern (Pavlou 2023).

The response from the cancer treatment community to these studies has been minimal. Notably, the DeVita textbook, often taken as an authoritative reference, contains no references to these dietary strategies in either its 2019 or 2024 editions.

JNCI Monograph (2023)

A comprehensive 19-page monograph on intermittent fasting in the *Journal of the National Cancer Institute (JNCI)* emphasizes caution. It notes,

> *"An outstanding concern regarding the use of intermittent fasting among cancer patients is that fasting often results in caloric restriction, which can put patients already prone to malnutrition, wasting syndrome, or loss of muscle mass at risk"* (Kalam 2023, edited).

The Moss Method does not incorporate prolonged fasting or the Fasting Mimicking Diet as part of its program, as these approaches are better managed under medical supervision. However, we do support time-restricted eating, a form of intermittent fasting, as a viable practice for most readers. This approach is research-backed, manageable for most people, and generally yields positive results.

DURING WHAT TIME OF DAY SHOULD ONE FAST?

A logical question is, during what hours should one perform time-restricted eating (TRE)? Should you restrict eating to the early or the later part of the day? There are many opinions on the internet regarding this, but few are based on scientific evidence. Fortunately, a 2022 randomized clinical trial from a leading hospital in Beijing, published in Nature Communications, addressed this question (Xie 2022).

This five-week study compared different time-restricted eating schedules. Early time-restricted eating, where participants ate only between 6 AM and 3 PM, proved to be more effective than midday TRE, which had an eating window from 11 AM to 8 PM. Researchers found that those who ate earlier in the day were better able to use insulin effectively, which helps control blood sugar levels. This group also had lower insulin resistance, meaning their bodies were better at managing blood sugar compared to those who ate later. Additionally, the early eaters saw a significant drop in their fasting blood sugar levels.

Participants following the early eating plan not only lost more weight—about 3.5 pounds on average—but also reduced their body fat more than those who ate later in the day. They also had less inflammation, a sign of better overall health. These findings suggest that eating earlier could be more beneficial and might help improve various health factors, including blood sugar levels, weight loss, and inflammation.

CELLULAR & MOLECULAR PROCESSES

The potential anticancer effects of intermittent fasting (IF) and TRE are attributable to several cellular and molecular processes. Fasting exerts stress on cells, leading to a process of natural selection where cancer cells, less adaptable to stress than normal ones, may be more susceptible to programmed cell death. This is partly due to reduced levels of insulin and insulin-like growth factor (IGF-1), which play crucial roles in cell growth and metabolism (Lee 2010).

Fasting induces an energy-related switch from glucose-based to ketone-based metabolism, reducing glucose availability to cancer cells. Since many cancer cells heavily rely on glucose for energy, this switch could potentially inhibit their growth

(Brandhorst 2015). Moreover, fasting can stimulate the immune system, enhancing the body's ability to recognize and destroy cancer cells (Cheng 2014). Additionally, fasting promotes autophagy, a normal process by which cells remove damaged components, thus maintaining cellular health (Pietrocola 2015).

The Sun Meta-Analysis (2024)

A significant meta-analysis published in March 2024 in an online offshoot of *The Lancet* concluded that intermittent fasting may have beneficial effects on various health outcomes for adults with overweight or obesity (Sun ML 2024). This study, involving nearly 20,000 participants, found improvements in waist size, body fat, cholesterol levels, and insulin sensitivity. Despite these positive findings, the study received limited public attention, highlighting the need for greater awareness and further research.

A Bombshell at the AHA Meeting (2024)

Conversely, a study presented at an American Heart Association (AHA) meeting suggested a 91% increase in the risk of dying from heart disease among people following an intermittent eating pattern (Chen 2024). This study has still not been published in a peer-reviewed journal, but received significant media attention. It challenged the assumption that intermittent fasting is universally beneficial. But critics quickly pointed out methodological flaws, such as relying on limited self-reported dietary data, which could confound the results (Callahan 2024).

Another clue to the negative results was that participants in the Chen study tended to be younger and less educated than average, to have lower income and less access to food, and be more likely to smoke than the other participants. In other words, they seemed to come from a lower socioeconomic stratum and be more prone to food insecurity, which the U.S. government defines as limited or uncertain access to adequate food (USDA 2023).

Joann Carson, Ph.D., told *U.S. News & World Report* that economic constraints rather than health choices might have determined the participants' eating patterns (Johnson SR 2024). Put bluntly, they delayed eating because they were poor, not because they were trying to optimize their health. Given that food insecurity is firmly linked to an increased risk of heart disease and can reduce lifespan by up to 4.5 years, its omission from the study raised questions about the validity of this study for the broader population (Vercammen 2019, Ma 2024).

LOOKING FORWARD

The intersection of diet, health, and socioeconomic factors is complex, underscoring the need for broad research and personalized dietary advice. But unless some new data emerges to support conclusions (and that's highly unlikely), I think it is safe to ignore this "health scare" and base your behavior on a large amount of clinical data, summarized in Dr. Sun's broad review, of the health effects of intermittent fasting. The balance of evidence supports the health benefit of intermittent fasting in otherwise healthy people. I myself have practiced intermittent fasting for about ten years, routinely allowing at least 13 hours of non-eating per day, and sometimes more. Barring some unforeseen new developments, I intend to keep doing so.

THE KETO DIET

Ketogenic (keto) diets in the context of cancer have been a subject of growing interest in both scientific and clinical treatment circles. A keto diet is marked by high fat, moderate protein, and very low carb intake. This diet alters the body's metabolism, forcing it to burn fats rather than carbs as a primary energy source, ultimately leading to the production of ketones.

The keto diet is thought to exert anticancer effects by reducing the availability of glucose, which many cancer cells rely on for growth. Cancer cells often show altered metabolism, known as the Warburg effect, marked by a preference for fermentation even in the presence of oxygen (Warburg 1930, Warburg 1956). In other words, ketone bodies (chemicals produced during the state of ketosis) might stop cancer's growth through multiple processes, including reducing inflammation and cell damage from excess oxygen (Poff 2013).

Animal Studies

Animal and test tube studies give support to the idea of harnessing ketosis to fight cancer. For instance, scientists at the University of Wuerzburg, Germany, examined the impact of a keto diet on cancer growth in mice. Twenty-four female mice injected with stomach cancer cells were divided into two groups, one fed a keto diet and the other a standard diet. The scientists then observed tumor growth and survival time until the tumors had reached 600 to 700 cubic millimeters in volume.

Mice on the keto diet experienced delayed tumor growth, taking an average of 34 days to reach the targeted tumor volume, compared to 23 days for the standard diet group. Notably, tumors in the keto diet group also developed larger dead areas, with fewer blood vessels. Further studies were suggested to explore the diet's impact on cancer growth and spread (Otto 2008). This, and other studies suggest a possible healing role for ketosis but need to be interpreted with caution as human physiology can differ from animal models.

Clinical Trials of Keto Diet

Clinical trials on keto diets and cancer are limited but growing. At present, there are over 500 clinical articles on the topic in PubMed with new ones appearing every few days. Some studies suggest that keto diets might be safe and practical for cancer patients (Schmidt 2011, Fine 2012).

For instance, a pilot study from Germany of 16 advanced cancer patients with no remaining conventional treatment options explored the practicality and effects of a keto diet, which is low in carbs (under 70 grams per day) but rich in fats and proteins. Participants reported improvements in emotional well-being and less insomnia. The diet was well-tolerated, with minor side effects like constipation and fatigue, and no changes in cholesterol or blood lipids, suggesting possible benefits for quality of life in advanced cancer patients (Schmidt 2011).

The Cohen Trial (2018)

Another clinical trial examined the effects of a keto diet in patients with ovarian and endometrial cancer, showing its possible role for improved quality of life and reduction in insulin levels. Researchers at the University of Alabama at Birmingham compared the effects of a keto diet (KD) with the American Cancer Society's (ACS) high-fiber, low-fat diet.

After 12 weeks, the KD group showed a more pronounced reduction in fat mass, with a 21% decrease in visceral fat compared to only 5% in the ACS diet group. Additionally, the KD group had lower fasting blood insulin levels. The results suggest that KD may not only aid in fat loss but also improve energy-related factors potentially related to cancer growth. According to the authors, this indicates its possible benefit for women with these cancers (Cohen 2018).

SECOND THOUGHTS & CAUTIONS

- It is important to consider that the keto diet might not be suitable for all cancer types or patients. For example, patients with certain energy-related disorders or those undergoing specific cancer treatments may not be ideal candidates for this diet.

- The lack of nutrients is a concern with any restrictive diet, and close monitoring by healthcare professionals is essential.

- More randomized controlled trials are needed to establish the effectiveness and safety of keto diets in cancer patients. Research is also exploring the possible cooperative effects of combining keto diets with chemo, radiation, and targeted therapies (drugs designed to home in on unique molecular features on cancer cells).

- Such dietary interventions should always be done under the guidance of healthcare professionals, especially in the context of cancer.

A METABOLIC SUPPLEMENT: BERBERINE

Berberine, a plant chemical found in goldenseal and barberry, is widely recognized for its role in managing blood sugar levels, improving cholesterol profiles, and attacking cancer stem cells (CSCs), particularly in colorectal and breast cancer (Zhao Z 2021, Ma 2013).

The optimal dosage of berberine can vary depending on individual needs. In supplement form, it is commonly recommended to take between 500 to 1,000 mg daily, divided into multiple doses. While berberine can be found in small amounts in some foods, supplements are usually the only practical way to achieve beneficial amounts. Higher doses should only be taken under the supervision of a healthcare professional.

Berberine offers a wide range of potential health benefits. It is one of the best-researched herbs and is the subject of over 8,000 PubMed papers, with almost 2,000 focused on glucose control or cancer. New journal articles on berberine appear at a rate of almost two per day.

Unfortunately, there are few randomized trials of berberine in the context of cancer. In one study evaluating berberine's ability to prevent the recurrence of colorectal adenomas (benign tumors), 553 individuals received berberine, while a similar number received a placebo. After two years, adenomas recurred in 36% of the berberine group compared to 47% in the placebo group, without serious side effects.

This suggests berberine's potential as a preventive treatment following the surgical removal of polyps (Chen YX 2020).

Diabetes & Cholesterol

Berberine's positive effects on diabetes and cholesterol are well documented. In Shanghai, China, 116 patients with type 2 diabetes (T2D) and elevated cholesterol were randomly assigned to receive either 1,000 mg of berberine or a placebo for three months. The primary outcomes were changes in plasma glucose and serum lipid (fat) concentrations.

Initially, their fasting blood sugar levels were higher than normal at 126 mg/dL, indicating struggles in managing blood sugar. After taking berberine, this number dropped to a healthy 101 mg/dL. When these individuals were given a glucose drink to see how well their body could handle a sudden increase in sugar, their blood levels reduced from 216 to 160 mg/dL after taking berberine, which was much better than the placebo group.

Additionally, their A1C levels, representing average blood glucose over the past three months, decreased from 7.5 to 6.6, indicating long-term improvement. These results suggest that berberine could be helpful for naturally improving blood sugar control.

In the same study, cholesterol levels also improved, with notable reductions in triglycerides, total cholesterol, and LDL cholesterol. However, mild to moderate constipation did occur in a few participants in the berberine group (Zhang Y 2008).

PRACTICAL TIPS

Practical tips for using berberine include selecting high-quality supplements from reputable brands to ensure safety and effectiveness. It is also essential to exercise caution regarding possible interactions with diabetes drugs and blood thinners. One of the top-selling brands, sourced from the roots of the Indian barberry bush, suggests a dose of two 500 mg capsules taken once per day with a meal. However, it might be better to divide the dose and take one capsule with breakfast and the second one with dinner, as berberine is an alkaloid, a type of chemical that can be hard on the digestive system.

Consistency is key when it comes to taking berberine. Routine and sustained use is essential for experiencing its full range of benefits. Some individuals may choose to cycle their use of berberine under the guidance of a medical professional. Be aware of possible drug interactions, particularly with blood thinners, diabetes drugs, and drugs that suppress the immune system.

Beyond supplements, natural sources of berberine, such as *Berberis* berries and goldenseal root, can be explored, though the concentrations of the key chemical are relatively low. Additionally, discuss the potential combination of berberine and turmeric with your healthcare provider, as turmeric/curcumin may enhance its effectiveness.

(See our discussion of turmeric/curcumin.)

GEAR #2: WEAKENED IMMUNE SYSTEM

Cancer was once thought to start from a weakness of the immune system, based on the "immune surveillance theory" of Sir MacFarlane Burnet (1899-1985). This Nobel laureate suggested that the immune system identifies and destroys abnormal cancerous cells (Betts 2007). Burnet's theory was publicly endorsed by my former boss at MSKCC, Lewis Thomas, MD, and held sway for several decades (Thomas 1959). However, the Burnet-Thomas theory proved simplistic. One obvious problem was that cancer patients often, initially, had adequate numbers of white blood cells (WBCs), the main measure of immunity. Cancer's relationship to the immune system turned out to be more complex. Starting in the mid-1990s, scientists like James P. Allison, Ph.D., showed that cancer cells produce chemicals that prevent a successful immune response (Leach 1996).

Almost 30 years later, the 2018 Nobel Prize was awarded to Allison and Tasuku Honjo, MD, Ph.D., of Japan for their discovery of immune checkpoint inhibitors. Immune checkpoint inhibitors help the immune system recognize and attack cancer cells by blocking their use of natural checkpoints to hinder the activity of white blood cells. This discovery has led to such drugs as Yervoy (ipilimumab) and Keytruda (pembrolizumab), now the top-selling cancer drug in the world. In the process, immunotherapy became what, in the 1970's, many of us dreamed of, the "fourth modality" of cancer treatment, after surgery, radiation, and chemotherapy (Bell 2016).

However, the immune system's role in fighting cancer is not limited to these advanced therapies. A healthy immune system can help prevent the development and progression of cancer through various mechanisms. This includes identifying and destroying emerging cancer cells, promoting apoptosis (programmed cell death), and inhibiting angiogenesis (the formation of new blood vessels that supply tumors).

ENHANCING IMMUNE FUNCTION

In this book, I focus on prevention rather than mainstream cancer immunotherapy. It is important to highlight that certain natural substances can function as non-toxic immune checkpoint blockers, potentially without causing systemic damage, unlike mainstream drugs. These findings, though currently limited to laboratory studies, suggest that natural agents could be harnessed as a non-toxic way to free the immune system to attack cancer more effectively.

Patients could employ these substances at home with little trouble, supported by a sympathetic physician. I have even suggested a unique "immune checkpoint blockade" dietary menu plan to specifically address this aspect of cancer with nutrition. For example, curcumin, a compound found in turmeric, has been shown to modulate the immune response and inhibit the growth of various cancer cells (Aggarwal 2007). Similarly, resveratrol, a compound found in grapes and red wine, has been shown to enhance immune function and inhibit cancer cell growth (Cao 2009).

Green tea (EGCG) is another powerful substance with immune-boosting properties. Studies have shown that EGCG can enhance the function of T cells, which are critical for the immune system's response to cancer (Kawai 2003). Additionally, mushrooms such as reishi and maitake contain compounds that have been shown to enhance immune function and inhibit cancer growth (Jin 2013).

LIFESTYLE CHOICES TO SUPPORT IMMUNE

Beyond specific natural substances, lifestyle choices play a crucial role in maintaining and enhancing immune function. Physical activity, for instance, has been shown to bolster immune defenses. Regular moderate exercise can enhance the circulation of immune cells, making the immune system more efficient at identifying and targeting cancer cells (Nieman 1994). Exercise also helps reduce inflammation, a known risk factor for cancer, and can improve overall immune competence.

Sleep quality also has a significant impact on immune function. Poor sleep can weaken the immune response, while good sleep strengthens it. Research indicates that sleep deprivation can lead to a decrease in the production of protective cytokines, which are essential for a robust immune response (Irwin 2015). Therefore, ensuring adequate and quality sleep is a vital component of maintaining a strong immune system.

Stress management is another critical factor. Chronic stress can suppress the immune system, making the body more susceptible to cancer. Techniques such as mindfulness meditation, yoga, and other stress-reducing practices can improve immune function and overall well-being (Black 2016). Stress reduction can lead to lower levels of cortisol, a hormone that, when chronically elevated, can inhibit immune function.

HOLISTIC IMMUNE SUPPORT

Enhancing immune function through natural means and lifestyle choices is a pivotal aspect of The Moss Method. By focusing on prevention and leveraging the body's natural defenses, individuals can take proactive steps in managing their health and reducing their cancer risk. This holistic approach aligns with the philosophy of using evidence-based strategies to support the body's ability to fight cancer.

The Sen Paper (2018)

I want to highlight a pivotal study from the M.D. Anderson Cancer Center in Houston, Texas—repeatedly ranked as the top U.S. cancer center in the annual U.S. News & World Report survey. M.D. Anderson is also where James P. Allison, Ph.D., conducts his Nobel Prize-winning research, which paved the way for the creation of immune checkpoint inhibitors (ICI) drugs.

In this significant study, led by Allison's colleague, Shiraj Sen, MD, Ph.D., more than a dozen researchers aimed to refine the selection of patients for ICI clinical trials by developing a scoring system. They used sophisticated statistical techniques to identify which health indicators most strongly influenced patient survival. From 172 patients with metastatic cancer who were enrolled in early-stage trials, they identified seven key predictors of a clinical response (Sen 2018).

This is important because immune checkpoint inhibitors like Keytruda do not directly kill cancer cells. Instead, they are sometimes remarkably effective at enabling the patients' own immune systems to combat cancer; you could call them immune-liberating agents. But often the response to these drugs is unpredictable and even idiosyncratic (peculiar to the individual).

Knowing in advance who is likely to respond would be a big plus for practitioners and patients alike. Of the seven influential factors that were evaluated, the "absolute lymphocyte count" proved to be particularly important. A relatively low number of lymphocytes was linked to shorter survival times. Specifically, patients with lymphocyte counts below 1,800 cells per microliter of blood faced a risk of death **3.3 times higher** than those with robust counts.

This finding underscored the vital role of lymphocytes, especially in treatments that harness the immune system to fight cancer.

Though this study focused on patients with advanced cancer undergoing immunotherapy, its implications for prevention are equally profound. Lymphocytes are essential for everyone, not just cancer patients, serving as a cornerstone of our native anticancer defenses. Since the drugs in question only work by activating the immune system, logically speaking, this study indicates that you need a robust number of immune cells for the system to work at all.

The problem is that most labs deem any lymphocyte count above 1,000 as normal. This is indicated in the so-called reference range that is typically included in your bloodwork. For adults, the reference range for lymphocyte counts ususally lies between 1,000 and 4,800 lymphocytes per microliter (µL) of whole blood. (This can vary by laboratory.) A lymphocyte count within this range is considered indicative of a healthy or at least an adequate immune system. However, the M.D. Anderson researchers showed that at least 1,800 lymphocytes per microliter were necessary for an *optimal* immune response, at least when used with ICIs, and probably more generally (Ibid.)

To maintain a robust immune system, particularly for cancer prevention, regular CBC-with-differential tests are therefore recommended. This test offers a detailed count of each type of blood cell and is the most straightforward, cost-effective method to assess immune competence. Consult with your doctor to interpret these results and take appropriate actions based on your immune status.

(On a personal note, it is a source of frustration for me that since the CBC panel that is part of my annual physical wellness visit doesn't specify the various types of white blood cells, but gives a single figure for them as a totality. If you find yourself in the same situation, you could order your own blood tests, including the CBC with differential, which provides a detailed count of different types of blood cells.

I do this through an online service, Life Extension Foundation (of which I am a scientific advisor). The web page for their testing service is https://www.lifeextension.com/sales/lab-tests.)

NOTE ON IMMUNE-RELATED ADVERSE EVENTS

One caveat is that patients with a very high lymphocyte count may be more prone to immune-related adverse events (irAEs) characteristic of immune checkpoint inhibitor therapy (Diehl 2017). Although this book is not intended as self-help for cancer patients currently under mainstream treatment, if you fall into that category, please consult with your oncologist before undertaking any program to enhance your immune system.

HEALING MUSHROOMS

"An accumulating body of evidence suggests that intake of dietary mushrooms can protect against breast cancer."
—*Arizona State University scientists (Martin 2010, edited)*

There is no magic formula for raising the immune system, particularly the lymphocytes. There are some powerful prescription drugs that can do this. But among non-prescription and nutritional methods, the most powerful is the so-called healing mushrooms. The exact number of species of fungi worldwide remains unknown, but estimates range from 1.5 million to an astonishing 10 million. It is a vast kingdom with many undiscovered or unexamined varieties. But half a dozen stand out for their well-documented health benefits.

Prominent examples of healing mushrooms include shitake, maitake, reishi, turkey tail, and lion's mane. Several of these (shiitake, maitake, and lion's mane) are often for sale in the supermarket produce section, while also being of interest for their possible role in immune support, inflammation reduction, and anticancer qualities.

Many mushrooms that are classified as edible are also considered medicinal due to their possible health benefits. The world of medicinal mushrooms is divided between those advocating the use of the fruiting bodies (the visible, above-ground portion of the mushroom) and those who recommend the usually invisible root system, called the mycelium.

This is a huge topic of intense competition and debate. I incline towards the fruiting body "school," for the simple reason that the majority of the research (not to mention the folk usage) on medicinal mushrooms has taken place with hot water extracts of fruiting bodies. This includes the studies of turkey tail that led to Asian governmental approval in the 1970s and 1980s. Of the 11 studies on mushrooms and cancer in clinicaltrials.gov, only one of these is self-identified as a study of mycelia.

SHITAKE & CANCER

Asian people have long used shiitake mushrooms (Lentinula edodes) in traditional medicine, and recent scientific studies have started to unravel their possible health benefits, particularly regarding the immune system and cancer. Shiitake is renowned for its lentinan, a compound studied for its immune-boosting qualities and blocking tumor growth (Ng 2002). Lentinan's immune-altering effects have earned approval from the Japanese equivalent of the FDA as a supplemental therapy for cancer (Kobori 2007). Additionally, shiitake mushrooms have been shown to stop tumor growth (Cheng JH 2016).

Polysaccharide-K (PSK), extracted from *Trametes versicolor* (formerly classified as *Coriolus versicolor*, a.k.a. turkey tail), was the first fungus extract to be approved as a cancer treatment. This happened in Japan in 1977. It was followed by lentinan (from shiitake mushrooms), also in Japan, in 1985, and by schizophyllan (SPG), a kind of beta-glucan, from the fungus *Schizophyllum commune* in the following year. Meanwhile, PSP (like PSK, a polysaccharide peptide from turkey tail) was approved in China in 1983.

Shiitake mushrooms in particular are rich in healthful chemicals like lentinan, beta-glucans, and other compounds that improve immune function. They can stimulate the body's natural defenses by boosting the activity of various cells in the immune system, such as macrophages and natural killer (NK) cells, which play a crucial role in identifying and destroying cancer cells.

TURKEY TAIL (TRAMETES VERSICOLOR), PSK & CANCER

Turkey tail mushrooms (*Trametes versicolor*, formerly called *Coriolus versicolor*) are of particular interest for cancer prevention because they contain a healthful chemical called polysaccharide K (PSK, also known as Krestin). There are over 1,000 articles indexed in PubMed on this topic, including some clinical trials.

Trametes versicolor is a mushroom of the Basidiomycetes class. It is used in traditional Chinese medicine (TCM) as a tonic. Studies also suggest that it has immune-stimulating and anticancer qualities. Polysaccharide-K (PSK), a proprietary product derived from Trametes, is an approved form of cancer treatment in Japan. Other turkey tail extracts such as PSP and VPS are available as dietary supplements.

The Memorial Sloan-Kettering Cancer Center (MSKCC) website states that PSK appears to improve survival rates in patients with gastric (stomach) and colorectal cancers. It may also benefit people with cancer of the esopagus. A study of turkey tail mushrooms suggests benefits in patients with advanced non-small cell lung cancer (NSCLC) as well. According to a study at Harvard Medical School, Boston, PSP acts as a prebiotic and helps adjust the human intestinal microbiome (Pallav 2014).

Studies of turkey tail extracts alone or in combination with other botanical substances have suggested positive effects on the immune system. However, data on their effects on breast or liver cancer or leukemia have been mixed. A meta-analysis (a.k.a. study of studies) reported reduced risk of death with added use of turkey tail across a variety of cancers, but MSKCC warns that confirmatory studies are needed. They add that Trametes extracts are generally well tolerated but minor side effects have been reported. Also, many over-the-counter products are not standardized, making it difficult to compare brands.

Since 1977, a turkey tail extract has been approved as an adjunct cancer treatment in Japan. It was once ranked 19th on the list of the world's most commercially successful drugs with annual sales of $255 million. It has since been described as:

> *"...one of the most commonly used healing mushroom extracts with a long history as an additive in cancer therapy in Asia, especially in Japan" (Sun 2012).*

Kanagawa Clinical Trial (1999)

The Kanagawa Clinical Trial was the first study on the effects of lentinan, a beta-glucan from shiitake mushrooms, in patients with advanced stomach (gastric) cancer. The median survival in the lentinan-added group was **297 days vs. 199 days** in the chemo-alone group, for a gain of almost four months. The one-year survival rate in the lentinan-added group was **49.1% versus 0%** in the chemo-alone group. The quality of life, including appetite and sleep quality, was also improved with the administration of lentinan (Nakano 1999). These results were substantially repeated a dozen years later at Nagoya Memorial Hospital, also in Japan (Ina 2011).

University of Florida Study (2015)

There was a randomized controlled trial at the University of Florida, Gainesville, on the effect of daily intake of shiitake mushrooms on human immunity (Dai 2015). Fifty-two healthy males and females aged 21-41 participated in a 4-week study, consuming 5 or 10 grams of mushrooms daily. Eating shiitake mushrooms boosted the number and effectiveness of two important types of immune cells in the body, enhancing the body's ability to defend itself against diseases. Gamma-delta T cells increased by 60%, and the number of natural killer T cells doubled. There was also improved gut immunity and some key markers of inflammation went down. These results were all highly statistically significant, i.e., not likely due to chance (Dai 2015).

Taken together, these studies from the Journal of the American College of Nutrition provided a glimpse into the intriguing role of shiitake mushrooms in immunology and cancer science, emphasizing the importance of further research in these areas.

CHAGA & CANCER

On the other hand, some healing mushrooms are neither tasty nor safe to eat. Some of these contain toxins or require specific preparation methods to be safe for eating. For example, chaga (*Inonotus obliquus*), which is an odd kind of fungal tree growth, not a conventional mushroom, is known for its healthful qualities. But it is typically powdered or chunked and then consumed as a tea or extracts rather than eaten directly, due to its tough texture and some potentially harmful compounds when taken raw.

Chaga is found on birch trees in cold northern climates, notably in Russia, Northern Europe, and in parts of North America. This dark, hardened, and cracked growth has been used in most of the circumpolar regions for its healing qualities. Historically, it has been harvested and used in teas and powders by local populations, particularly in Siberia and Eastern Europe, for its health benefits.

The Nobel laureate Aleksander Solzhenitsyn, in his novel *Cancer Ward* (1966), discussed the alleged benefits of chaga on his own cancer. This description helped to popularize the mushroom in the West and sparked interest in its possible healthful qualities. This unusual fungus has been used as a folk remedy for various ailments, ranging from GI issues to tuberculosis (Hu Y 2017, Szychowski 2020).

Chaga contains powerful antioxidants. In one laboratory study, cells treated with Chaga extract showed a 40% reduction in DNA fragmentation (a good thing) compared to non-treated cells (Park YK 2004).

At present, there are about 300 PubMed-indexed journal articles on chaga. About one new one appears each week, a steady stream of research on the topic. However, unlike shiitake and maitake, there are no clinical trials in PubMed on this unusual fungus. While experimental studies suggest that chaga mushrooms may have anticancer and immune-boosting qualities, more clinical research should be conducted on human subjects. The existing test tube and animal studies provide a basis for possible benefits. Still, they are not sufficient to conclusively recommend chaga as a treatment for cancer or immune disorders. Clinical trials would be necessary to validate these findings and to determine the safety, effectiveness, and appropriate usage of chaga in humans.

You probably will have to buy chaga from online suppliers or in a health food store or coop if you live below the 44th parallel north. On a personal note, when my family lived in seaside Maine (just above 44° N) while traipsing in the snow one winter day, we came across a large chaga growing on a storm-battered birch tree. We took it home, ground it up, and used it as a source of chaga tea.

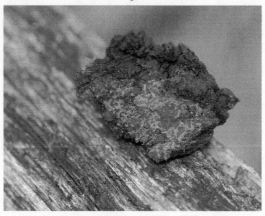

Chaga (Inonotus obliquus) a parasitic fungus that primarily grows on birch trees.
Source: Wikimedia Commons

BETA-GLUCANS

Beta-glucans are naturally occurring polysaccharides found primarily in the cell walls of bacteria, fungi (including mushrooms), yeasts, algae, and plants such as oats and barley. They are recognized for their ability to modulate the immune system, making them of great interest both in medical research and as dietary supplements.

Beta-glucans act as immunomodulators. They help strengthen the immune system by enhancing the functions of macrophages and natural killer cells, crucial for the innate immune response. Beta-glucans also stimulate the activity of other immune cells, such as dendritic cells and neutrophils, which can help defend against harmful germs and potentially reduce infection risk. Additionally, research has explored their role in cancer therapy, as they may help prime the immune system to recognize and destroy tumor cells more effectively.

There is significant research interest in beta-glucans, with over 6,000 journal articles on the topic, about 1,600 of which concern their role in immunity. Several hundred articles specifically address their anticancer effects, though few include human clinical data (Liu 2023). Generally, for cancer prevention, complex mushroom extracts are preferable to purified chemical beta-glucans.

There is a considerable degree of overlap between culinary and medicinal mushrooms, and also among the various species. One common element is the presence of a class of chemicals called **beta-glucans.** These are naturally occurring polysaccharides, found in the cell walls of bacteria, fungi, yeasts, algae, and even some common cereals such as oats and barley. Beta-glucans are recognized for their modulation of the immune system, making them of great interest both in medical research and as dietary supplements.

Beta-glucans help strengthen the immune system by enhancing the functions of specific cells called macrophages and natural killer (NK) cells, which are crucial for the innate immune response. Beta-glucans also stimulate the activity of other immune cells, such as dendritic cells (DC) and neutrophil. This enhanced activity can help the body defend against harmful germs and potentially reduce the risk of infections. Additionally, research has explored their role in cancer therapy, as they may help prime the immune system to recognize and destroy tumor cells more effectively.

There is a surprisingly large amount of research on beta-glucans. It has been the subject of over 6,000 journal articles, about 1,600 of which concern its impact on immunity. There are several hundred articles specifically on its anticancer effects, but few of these include human clinical data (Liu 2023).

Healing mushrooms are the visible type of fungi that have been used for centuries in various cultures for their perceived health benefits and healing abilities. While the effectiveness of some claims requires further scientific validation, these fascinating fungi continue to spark interest due to their various bioactive compounds with possible health applications. They figure prominently in many traditional cultures across the globe, from the circumpolar regions to the tropics.

A company in Calgary, Canada, *Real Mushrooms,* produces a variety of powders and capsules containing organic extracts of healing mushrooms, including lion's mane, cordyceps-M, tremella, turkey tail, reishi, maitake, shiitake, and chaga. The last five of these are included in their *Five Defenders* product. Here are the five ingredients listed in order of the extent of research on cancer (indicated in brackets, as of June 2024):

- Reishi (*Ganoderma lingzhi*) [1,544 articles, 395 on cancer]
- Turkey tail (*Trametes versicolor*) [1,200 PubMed articles, 172 on cancer]
- Maitake (*Grifola frondosa*) [564 articles, 154 on cancer]
- Shiitake (*Lentinus edodes*) [1,169 PubMed articles, 130 on cancer]
- Chaga (*Inonotus obliquus*) [362 articles, 102 on cancer]

A pleasant and convenient way to consume these is in the form of a chocolate bar, which they produce. Each bar contains cacao and two grams of their *Five Defenders* mixture. Two such chocolate squares are equal to one capsule of the powdered product. This is a rather sinful way to get one's mushrooms, with excellent taste and a reasonable price.

WHY A MUSHROOM COMBINATION?

Mushrooms are probably among mankind's oldest medicines. Given the fact that some species can be deadly, I will assume that one of humanity's first specialized skills has been telling the difference between the delicious and the deadly strains.

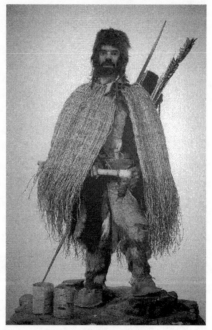

An artistic representation of Ötzi, the Ice Man, who knew a thing or two about fungi.
Source: Wikimedia Commons.

One hint in this direction is Ötzi, the so-called IceMan. He lived nearly 5,500 years ago and his mummified corpse was discovered in 1991 in the Ötztal Alps between Italy and Austria. Ötzi currently is housed in the South Tyrol Museum of Archaeology in Bolzano, Italy. It is very interesting that in his leather pouch were the following items:

- *Birch Polypore (Piptoporus betulinus):* This fungus, found on birch trees, has medicinal properties. It is known for its antimicrobial effects and was likely used by Ötzi for its antibiotic properties and as a natural laxative.

- *Tinder Fungus* (*Fomes fomentarius*): Also known as hoof fungus, this type of fungus was used primarily for starting fires due to its flammability when dry. It is also known for its antiseptic properties.

The discovery of mushrooms on his person underscores early humans' understanding of their natural surroundings and their ability to harness their resources for survival and health. To put things in perspective, the profession of oncology is 60 years old (the largest oncology organization, ASCO, was founded in 1964), while the science of mushrooms is at least one hundred times as old.

SYNERGY AMONG MUSHROOMS

Most research attention has focused on individual mushroom species. However, in line with our emphasis on synergy, we are focusing on whether a *mixture* of mushrooms provides a better overall anticancer effect. As a general rule, one can safely say (to quote Croatian mycologists, or mushroom specialists) that

> *"...the cytotoxic effect of healing mushroom blends is stronger than that of single mushroom species extracts" (Durgo 2013, edited).*

(See the section on The Power of Synergy among natural compounds.)

Below is a bar graph from a Croatian study showing the cancer-arresting qualities of several individual mushroom extracts vs. a mixture of five such extracts—shiitake, maitake, reishi, blazei, and oyster mushrooms.

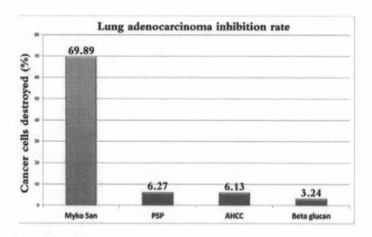

This European study shows the extraordinary degree of synergy in a mixed mushroom formula called Myko San vs. individual mushroom derivatives PSP, AHCC, and Beta Glucan. Source: Myko San website.

BATTLE BETWEEN THE IMMUNE SYSTEM & CANCER

While the immune system eliminates many possible threats, some cancerous cells evolve strategies to evade detection. They can render themselves invisible to immune cells. In addition, certain tumors can suppress the immune system, creating a protective microenvironment that acts as a shield against the immune system's attacks.

The tumor microenvironment is a dynamic area around a tumor, which interacts with the tumor to influence its growth and spread. It is an object of increasing scientific attention. In the 1980s, articles on this topic appeared at a rate of about one per year. However, at this writing, there are 14,000 such papers in PubMed, with over 1,000 of them focused on the microenvironment's relationship to cancer stem cells (CSCs).

To be clear, while not malignant in itself, the tumor microenvironment includes various cell types and molecules, which can act as collaborators, influencing the growth and spread of the cancer. It includes blood vessels, immune cells, signaling molecules, and fibroblasts, which help build and repair the body's connective tissues. All of these can interact with the tumor to influence its growth and spread.

NATURAL IMMUNE BOOSTERS

"An accumulating body of evidence suggests that intake of dietary mushrooms can protect against breast cancer" (Martin 2010, edited).

There is no magic formula for boosting the immune system, particularly lymphocytes. However, among non-prescription and nutritional ways, healing mushrooms stand out. It is advisable to seek out organic extracts of fruiting bodies (not the mycelium). Many mushrooms are both edible and medicinal due to their potential health benefits. Prominent examples include shiitake, maitake, reishi, turkey tail, and lion's mane. Fresh shiitake, maitake, and lion's mane are often available in supermarket produce sections. These mushrooms are enjoyed in culinary dishes while also being studied for their possible roles in immune support, inflammation reduction, and anticancer properties.

Most medicinal mushrooms are edible; white button mushrooms are the standard type found in supermarkets globally. Some healing mushrooms, however, are not palatable or safe to eat raw. For example, chaga is typically consumed as tea or extract rather than eaten directly due to its tough texture and potentially harmful compounds when raw.

If you live below the 44th parallel north, you may need to buy these mushrooms from suppliers. On a personal note, when living in seaside Maine (just above 44º), I came across a large chaga growing on a birch tree and used it as a tea.

There are so many mushroom species that it can be overwhelming. Estimates range from 1.5 million to 10 million species of fungi worldwide, making it a vast kingdom with many undiscovered varieties.

NATURAL IMMUNE CHECKPOINT BLOCKERS

A major focus of immunity research today is the development of immune checkpoint inhibitor (ICI). This is a form of immunotherapy that has progressed significantly in the past two decades. When I was at MSKCC, three of my top bosses–Lloyd J. Old, Robert A. Good, and Lewis Thomas–were immunologists. Naturally, many of the articles that I wrote for *Center News* were on the topic of immunotherapy research. That reflected their wishes, but also my own strong incliniation towards the idea of using the body's own resources to fight cancer. However, it took decades before these early beginnings bore fruit. This development finally earned Profs. James P. Allison and Tasuku Honjo the 2018 Nobel Prizes for Physiology or Medicine and led to top-selling new drugs like Keytruda (pembrolizumab) and Yervoy (ipilimumab).

Our focus in this book is obviously not on new cancer treatments. However, I musy point out a recent development that may have profound implications for the future. And that is the discovery that some of the natural agents that appear in our extended discussion of plant chemicals also function as natural immune checkpoint inhibitors. This fact has not received nearly the attention it deserves.

South Korean scientists have summarized the situation in a highly technical paper. I will paraphrase their main points: Even though immune checkpoint inhibitors can be effective in treating cancer, they don't work for everyone. As a result, researchers are actively looking for other immune checkpoint proteins that could serve as new targets for cancer therapy. Natural compounds, especially those found in medicinal or dietary plants, have been studied for their potential to fight tumors in various lab animal studies. Some plant-based chemicals can help fight cancer by regulating the immune system. They do this by either blocking the interactions between proteins involved in immune checkpoint signaling or by changing how these proteins are expressed or how the function (Chun 2022).

A 2024 review in *Frontiers in Immunology* identified two dozen natural agents that target the same immune checkpoint as Keytruda and Opdivo, namely PD-L1 (Zhou Y 2024)

Again, this book is not about treatment, and so we cannot get into details. But here is a very abbreviated summary:

- *Apigenin:* Found in dried parsley, it enhances immune cell attack on melanoma, reducing PD-L1 and making cancer cells more vulnerable (Xu L 2018).
- *Berberine:* Reduces inflammation and helps immune cells penetrate tumors by disrupting PD-L1 (Liu Y 2020).
- *Bilberry Extract:* Enhances PD-L1 antibody treatments by increasing beneficial gut bacteria (Wang L 2020).
- *Curcumin/Turmeric:* Reduces levels of immune suppressors like PD-L1, making cancer cells more vulnerable (Liu L 2021).
- *EGCG:* Blocks 70% of immune checkpoints in non-small cell lung cancer cells, similar to Keytruda (Rawangkan 2018).
- *Luteolin:* Acts as an immune checkpoint inhibitor, enhancing the immune system's ability to attack cancer cells (Jiang ZB 2021).

- *Silibinin (Silymarin):* Lowers PD-L1 levels, aiding in overcoming resistance to treatment (Sellam 2020).

There are at present over 60 papers in PubMed on using natural products as immune checkpoints. Broadly speaking, this highlights a shift towards including diet and lifestyle in cancer treatment. Bear in mind that these are all laboratory studies in either the test tube or lab rodents. But the results so far are both consistent and powerful. One should bear in mind that not so long ago Keytruda, Yervoy and other blockbuster immune drugs were also confined to laboratory studies, with little prospect of clinical development.

(For substantiation, please see my video interview with James P. Allison, PhD., as well as my grandson, Jacob Moss's, award winning documentary, Immunotherapy: The Battle Within.)

The Moss Method promotes lifestyles that support overall health and directly target cancer at a crucial molecular level. It could be that one of the ways that our Primary and Secondary Plant Chemicals work is by functioning as immune checkpoint blockers.

CHRONIC INFLAMMATION

Chronic inflammation has been linked to various stages of tumor development, including its initiation, growth, progression, invasion, and metastasis. This connection underscores the dual role the immune system can play in cancer. While acute inflammation can help fight and kill cancer cells, chronic inflammation has been described as the seedbed of cancer.

The concept that chronic inflammation plays a role in cancer dates back to the 19th century when Rudolf Virchow, MD (1821-1902), a prominent German pathologist, first observed white blood cells infiltrating cancerous tissues. Virchow's observation suggested a link between inflammation and cancer, proposing that the body's immune response to chronic irritation could be involved in tumor development. PubMed contains a very old article on the topic stating:

> *"It has long been known that chronic inflammations are common precursors of cancer. The association of cancer with gall-stones, gastric ulcer, and leucoplaia [white patches ed.] of the tongue are familiar examples" (Anonymous 1909).*

However, it wasn't until the late 20th and early 21st centuries that the mechanisms behind this observation were deeply explored, primarily through advancements in molecular biology. Research during this time revealed how chronic inflammation contributes to cancer. Persistent inflammation creates an environment that promotes cancer cell survival and growth. Immune cells produce substances, such as cytokines and chemokines, that activate pathways encouraging tumor development. Chronic inflammation can also induce genetic changes that transform normal cells into cancerous ones.

Scientists have studied specific pathways, such as nuclear factor kappa beta (NF-κB) and STAT3, which are often active in chronic inflammation. These pathways help cancer cells avoid death, grow faster, and develop new blood vessels, all of which support cancer progression. This understanding has led to new strategies for cancer prevention and treatment, including the use of anti-inflammatory drugs. For example, aspirin has shown potential in reducing the risk of certain cancers, such as colorectal cancer, by blocking inflammatory pathways.

Virchow's early observations paved the way for over a century of research, leading to the modern view that chronic inflammation is a key factor in cancer development and progression.

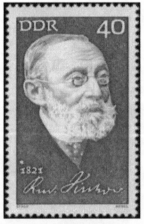

Rudolph Virchow, MD (1821-1902) German DDR postage stamp.
Source: Author's collection

Chronic inflammation is a prolonged and persistent form of inflammation lasting several months or even years. It is akin to a smoldering fire in the body. Unlike acute inflammation, which is a rapid and often beneficial response to injury or infection, chronic inflammation represents a lingering, low-level degree of irritation. This long-term inflammation often results from unresolved acute inflammation, persistent infections, autoimmune diseases, or exposure to irritants such as tobacco smoke.

Chronic inflammation can sometimes be "silent," with no noticeable symptoms and only detectable through blood tests. Signs of chronic inflammation are usually less obvious than those of acute inflammation and can include fatigue, low-grade fever, and abdominal and joint pain. Blood markers, such as C-reactive protein (CRP), tumor necrosis factor (TNF), and interleukin 6 (IL-6), are often elevated during chronic inflammation. They are linked to various chronic diseases, including cancer.

Because chronic inflammation often lacks immediate, overt symptoms, it can quietly contribute to the development and growth of various diseases, including cancer, as discussed earlier. Recognizing and managing chronic inflammation is essential for disease prevention and treatment.

Clean, traditional diets, renowned for their rich blend of healthy oils, fruits, vegetables, whole grains, and fish, offer dietary patterns that may reduce chronic inflammation. These diets are high in natural antioxidants and anti-inflammatory compounds, such as omega-3 fatty acids from fish and antioxidants in olive oil and red wine. These nutrients lower pro-inflammatory markers that are often elevated in chronic inflammation. By incorporating the principles of a clean, traditional diet, individuals can harness the power of nutrition to support their body's natural anti-inflammatory processes.

The Moss Method integrates a broad approach to cancer care, emphasizing the importance of personalized, evidence-based treatment plans that include diet and lifestyle modifications. This method aligns well with the principles of a clean, traditional diet, advocating for a holistic approach to cancer. By combining the anti-inflammatory benefits of a traditional diet with the focus of The Moss Method on individualized care, patients can create a cooperative strategy aimed at reducing inflammation-driven cancer risks. This method helps you change what you eat right away and supports lasting changes in how you live, making it easier to maintain a healthier lifestyle for overall well-being.

In this way, The Moss Method offers a set of powerful tools to combat the subtle effects of chronic inflammation. For an individual grappling with cancer, chronic inflammation not only paves the way for tumor initiation but also aids in its growth and spread. Moreover, chronic inflammation can destabilize the genetic material of tumors, making them harder to treat and more likely to recur (Coussens 2002, Mantovani 2008).

As we explore the many aspects of cancer prevention and management, it is crucial to recognize how cell damage from free radicals and singlet oxygen, key factors that can impact both the onset and growth of cancer, plays a role. Free radicals and singlet oxygen are highly reactive substances that can damage cells in our body. Free radicals are unstable because they have an uneven number of electrons, making them likely to react with other molecules. Singlet oxygen, while not a free radical, is also very reactive due to its unique structure. Both of these can lead to oxidative stress, a condition that occurs when there is excessive cell damage from these substances, potentially causing inflammation and diseases like cancer and heart disease. The body uses antioxidants, substances found in fruits and vegetables, to protect against this damage by neutralizing these reactive molecules.

Gear #3: Cancer Stem Cells (CSCs)

"The cancer stem cell might be the ultimate determinant of relapse. Is it possible that our quest to treat cancer has stalled because we haven't even found the right kind of cell?"
—Siddhartha Mukherjee, MD, author of The Emperor of All Maladies *(2010).*

"A diet-caused shift from disruption to control of cancer stem cells (CSCs) could have a profound influence on cancer relapses and therefore is of immense societal importance."
—National Cancer Institute (NCI) scientists (Kim 2012, edited)

"Investigations have revealed groups of highly tumor-forming cancer cells in essentially every solid cancer type. Cancer stem cells represent a very small subpopulation of cancers. Methods for attacking CSCs could have impressive effects on cancer elimination."
—Thomas E. Carey, Ph.D., DeVita Cancer Textbook, 11th edition (2019, edited).

Cancer stem cells (CSCs) are widely recognized as the most malignant part of a tumor population. These cells are the drivers behind tumor occurrence, recurrence, and spread—the features that typically define the danger of cancer.

Although little known by the public, many cancer researchers now recognize the profound importance of cancer stem cells (CSCs) in understanding and targeting the disease. CSCs are a special type of cells, unique in their ability to self-renew and to differentiate into various "daughter" cells. They also possess a remarkable ability to expel cell toxins, thereby contributing to 'multiple drug resistance' (MDR) in tumors. In some sense, they are a hybrid between a normal stem cell (of the type that renews damaged or aging tissues) and what we think of as an ordinary cancer cell.

Because the concept is so little known to the public, I must underline the fact that recognition of the key role of CSCs has been going on for a very long time and has engaged a great many researchers around the world. Researchers at Case Western Reserve University aptly describe CSCs as:

> *"...the roots of cancer, the seeds of its spread, and the source of therapy resistance."* CSCs generate one non-CSC daughter cell in their reproduction process while producing an identical CSC, perpetuating cancer (Adorno-Cruz 2015, edited).

Emphasizing their significance, scientists at Tufts University Medical School, Boston, have observed:

> *"Cancer stem cells play an important role when it comes to cancer aggressiveness, spread, recurrence, resistance to chemo, and overall survival" in several common types of cancer (Habib 2013, edited)*

(Overall survival refers to the length of time from the start of a particular treatment, such as a medication or therapy, until death from any cause.)

CSCs stand at the apex of the cancer cell hierarchy. Their rarity within tumors is sometimes as low as one in a thousand among the total cancer cells (Hart 2008), making them almost indiscernible among the many cell types in a tumor. Yet they are a crucial driving force behind it.

Jim Moselhy, Ph.D., of the University of Louisville elucidated the growth process of CSCs:

> *"The process is governed by a group of distinct cells with stem-like character termed cancer stem cells (CSCs). CSCs possess qualities of self-renewal and survival processes. The viewpoint of cancer as fundamentally a stem cell disease represents an important shift" in the medical model (Moselhy 2015, edited).*

The American Association for Cancer Research (AACR) defined CSCs during a 2006 workshop as cells within a tumor that possess the ability to self-renew and to cause the diversity seen within the tumor (Clarke 2006). These cells encapsulate what is most feared about cancer: their role in constant self-renewal and in resistance to conventional therapies makes them dangerous foes in both the prevention and treatment of cancer.

Today, CSCs are recognized as the most malignant part of a tumor population, driving tumor occurrence, recurrence, and spread. They possess the ability to self-renew and to cause the diversity seen within the tumor (Clarke 2006). These cells encapsulate what is most feared about cancer: their role in constant self-renewal and resistance to conventional therapies makes them dangerous foes in both the prevention and treatment of cancer.

TARGETING CSCs WITH NATURAL AGENTS

What is of particular importance to *The Moss Method*, however, is the merger of the field of cancer stem cells with the plant chemical approach. In 2008, the first plant chemical research on CSCs was published by National Cancer Institute (NCI) scientists. They stated,

> *"The benefit of many plant chemicals is that they are well tolerated and are found in many food products that can be added to one's diet. Furthermore, plant chemicals could be taken on a long-term basis to either prevent primary tumor formation or its return" (Kawasaki 2008, edited).*

This is, in fact, one of the core principles of The Moss Method.

In 2010-2011, researchers at the University of Michigan (where CSCs in solid tumors were discovered) explored several natural compounds, including curcumin and sulforaphane, against breast CSCs (Li Y 2010, Li Y 2011). A senior author on this research was Max Wicha, MD, Founding Director Emeritus of the U of M's Rogel Cancer Center.

In 2016, scientists in the anatomy department of the University of Kansas, after noting the "great impact" that the discovery of CSCs has had, proposed the use of natural chemicals in the treatment of breast cancer. I'll summarize their rather technical comments:

> *"Plant chemicals have gained a lot of attention due to their safety and their ability to target various cancer cells, including CSCs. The plant-based chemicals that impact these cells include curcumin, resveratrol, tea polyphenols,*

sulforaphane, genistein, vitamin E, quercetin, and several others. These plant chemicals might "serve as novel therapeutic agents for breast cancer treatment and future leads for drug development" (Dandawate 2016, edited).

In 2018, researchers at Temple University, Philadelphia, and Rutgers, the State University of New Jersey, published a lengthy review in the prestigious *Cancer Letters* in which they made four points:

- Cancer stem cells (CSCs) are the culprits for cancer drug resistance and cancer relapse.
- Dietary phytochemicals (curcumin, resveratrol, EGCG, and genistein) target CSCs.
- Repositioned drugs (such as metformin) target CSCs.
- Plant chemical-drug combinations targeting CSCs may exhibit synergistic effects (Chan MM 2018).

This too, is very close to the core message of The Moss Method, although our focus is obviously on prevention, rather than treatment. But the idea of combining *Generally Recognized as Safe* (GRAS) foods and supplements with repurposed FDA-approved medications is a very good one, which hasn't received the attention it deserves.

In the following year, scientists in Bratislava, Slovakia, provided a comprehensive review of plant chemicals and CSCs.

"Dietary plant chemicals have a significant impact on CSCs which may be applied in cancer prevention and treatment." (Liskova 2019, edited).

There is now evidence from over 100 journal articles (too numerous to summarize here) that natural products represent non-toxic ways to kill CSCs. I use the military terminology reluctantly since the effect of natural agents on CSCs is often more subtle than their outright destruction. For instance, certain plant pigments, including quercetin, can halt the Warburg effect, a defective cellular process, thus minimizing toxicity (Suolinna 1974). Natural compounds like curcumin (Shanmugam 2013), resveratrol (Shankar 2011), green tea/EGCG (Kawai 2003) and medicinal mushrooms (Jin 2013) have all been shown to diminish CSCs in non-aggressive and therefore non-toxic ways.

REDIFFERENTIATION: A PROMISING APPROACH

This is more than a dream. One promising approach to targeting CSCs in a non-aggressive way is through redifferentiation. This means inducing cancer cells, particularly CSCs, to revert to a less malignant state, thereby regaining some normal cellular functions. Redifferentiation therapy has shown promise in treating various cancers, including thyroid cancer, using agents such as all-trans retinoic acid (ATRA).

ATRA, a vitamin A derivative, has demonstrated the ability to make cancer cells behave more normally, enhancing their responsiveness to conventional treatments or promoting apoptosis (programmed cell death). For instance, in metastatic thyroid cancer, redifferentiation therapy has significantly improved radioactive iodine (RAI) uptake, leading to clinical improvements in a substantial percentage of patients (Rothenberg 2015).

Further affirming this approach, a French study observed that a combination of drugs increased radioactive iodine uptake from 5% initially to 65% within a month and an impressive 95% by the end of treatment. This was accompanied by clinical improvements, with 38% of previously desperate patients then showing partial responses after six months (LaSolle 2023).

Although translating these successes to other cancers involves overcoming significant complexities, there are explorations of similar strategies in at least half a dozen other kinds of cancer:

- *Acute promyelocytic leukemia:* This type of leukemia has seen significant advancements with redifferentiation therapy, primarily using all-trans retinoic acid (ATRA) to induce differentiation and remission in patients (Warrell 1991).

- *Brain cancer, glioblastoma:* This type of brain tumor is another focus for redifferentiation therapy, exploring how cell differentiation pathways can be manipulated to treat these highly aggressive tumors (Dhermain 2014).

- *Breast cancer:* Research into redifferentiation therapy for breast cancer focuses on reversing the epithelial-mesenchymal transition (EMT), a key process in cancer metastasis, to manage cancer progression and resistance (Polyak and Weinberg 2009, Hitchcock 2022).

- *Colorectal cancer:* Approaches in colorectal cancer include restoring the function of key tumor suppressor genes like the adenomatous polyposis coli (APC) to promote redifferentiation and potentially reverse malignancy (Dow 2015, Faqar-uz-Zaman 2020).

71

- *Esophageal Squamous Cell Carcinoma (ESCC):* Redifferentiation therapy for ESCC includes using drugs that target the EGFR pathway and enhances the effectiveness of chemoradiation with minimal side effects. Another approach involves using a drug that targets the HER2 pathway, which, when combined with chemo, can help reduce tumor size and improve survival rates (Yang Y 2020, Wang L 2024).

- *Nasopharyngeal carcinoma (NPC):* Studies have demonstrated the potential for redifferentiation therapy in NPC, particularly using ATRA to influence epigenetic mechanisms and promote the re-differentiation of poorly differentiated NPC cells (Yan M 2014).

At present, there are 30 studies on the use of ATRA in cancer at ClinicalTrials.gov that are looking for participants, 11 of which are based in the U.S. So it is still an area of active investigation.

Moreover, research from South Korea suggests that elements featured in *The Moss Method*, such as genistein, quercetin, and resveratrol, can induce redifferentiation in thyroid cancer cells. These agents interact with specific cellular features that control cell growth and differentiation, thereby reducing traits associated with aggressive cancer behavior (Kang 2011).

In conclusion, by integrating strategies to target CSCs through natural agents and promoting redifferentiation, The Moss Method provides a comprehensive and holistic approach to cancer prevention and care. This method emphasizes the importance of understanding and targeting the root causes of cancer, leveraging natural and evidence-based strategies to manage cancer more effectively.

THE HISTORICAL CONTEXT & DISCOVERY OF THE CSC

The concept of cancer stem cells (CSCs) is not exactly new. In the mid-19th century, renowned European pathologists Robert Remak (1815-1865), Rudolph Virchow (1821-1902), and Julius Cohnheim (1839-1884) brilliantly theorized about the existence of cells within tumors that could initiate and sustain cancer growth (Virchow 1858). Early experimental evidence came from studies of teratomas, peculiar tumors containing various tissue types, suggesting their origin from primitive embryonic cells with the potential to develop into different tissues.

In 1961, James Till and Ernst McCulloch at the University of Toronto identified normal stem cells in the blood-forming system, laying the groundwork for future CSC discoveries (Till 1961, McCulloch 1971). The first CSC was identified in human acute myeloid leukemia (AML) by Lapidot and Dick in 1994 (Lapidot 1994). This discovery was followed by the identification of CSCs in solid tumors such as breast cancer by Michael Clarke's team (Al-Hajj 2003) and in brain tumors by Sheila K. Singh (Singh 2004).

The following timeline traces the key landmarks of the development of the CSC concept, especially in relation to plant chemicals:

1961: James Till and Ernst McCulloch at the University of Toronto discovered stem cells in the hematopoietic system, setting the stage for future CSC discoveries (Till 1961, Mcculloch 1971).

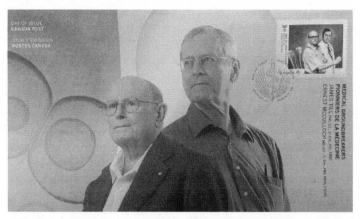

Canadian first day cover and stamp paid homage to James Till and Ernest McCulloch, discoverers of the stem cell. Source: Author's collection.

- *1980s:* While the term "cancer stem cell" wasn't coined until the early 2000s, Janet Rowley (1925-2013), Lewis Cantley, and others performed research laying the groundwork for the concept by identifying subpopulations within tumors.

- *1994:* First cancer stem cell (CSC): Tsvee Lapidot, Ph.D., working in Professor John E. Dick's University of Toronto lab, identified the first human acute myeloid leukemia (AML) initiating cells, marking the first identification of CSCs (Lapidot 1994)

- *2001:* A paper in *Nature* revealed the nature of stem cells in cancer, propelling CSC research into the mainstream (Reya 2001).

- *2003:* First solid tumor CSC: Michael Clarke's team at the University of Michigan (now at Stanford University) pinpointed the first CSCs in a solid tumor, breast cancer (Al-Hajj 2003).

- *2004:* Discovery of Brain Tumor CSCs: Sheila K. Singh, MD, Ph.D., also at the University of Toronto, identified CSCs in brain tumors, particularly glioblastoma, broadening the CSC concept to neurological malignancies (Singh 2004).

- *2007:* Identification of Colorectal CSCs: Katherine A. O'Brien, MD, of Toronto and Lucia Ricci-Vitiani, MD, of Rome, working independently, identified CSCs in colorectal cancer, advancing the understanding of tumor hierarchy and potential targets in colorectal tumors (O'Brien 2007, Ricci-Vitiani 2007).

- *2008:* First plant chemical research on CSCs: National Cancer Institute (NCI) scientists published the first paper to discuss mechanisms by which plant chemicals might target CSCs. They stated, "The benefit of many plant chemicals is that they are well tolerated and are found in many food products that can be added to one's diet. Furthermore, plant chemicals could be taken on a long-term basis to either prevent primary tumor formation or its return" (Kawasaki 2008, edited). This is a core principle of *The Moss Method*.

- *2010-2011*: Researchers at the University of Michigan investigated several natural compounds, including curcumin and sulforaphane, against breast cancer stem cells (Li Y 2010, Li Y 2011). A senior author on this research was Max Wicha, MD, Director of the Forbes Institute for Cancer Discovery and Founding Director Emeritus of the Rogel Cancer Center of the University of Michigan.

- *2012:* CSCs Identified in Melanoma: Elsa Quintana, Pharm. D, Ph.D., at the University of Michigan, demonstrated the presence of CSCs in melanoma, challenging earlier models of cancer organization and highlighting new therapeutic targets (Quintana 2012).

- *2016:* Lucy Laplane publishes the first book for non-specialists on CSCs, Cancer Stem Cells: Philosophy and Therapies (Harvard University Press). She raises the issue of whether stem cells are physical entities or just cells exhibiting a quality called "stemness." That issue is still not resolved.

- *2019:* Scientists in Bratislava provide comprehensive review of plant chemicals and CSCs. "Dietary plant chemicals have a significant impact on CSCs which may be applied in cancer prevention and treatment." (Liskova 2019, edited).

- *2021:* Annual publications on CSCs reach almost 2,000, or five per calendar day, reflecting continuing scientific interest and understanding of their role in cancer dynamics.

- *2024:* The total number of entries on "cancer stem cells "in the PubMed database approaches 20,000.

This timeline underscores the steady progress in understanding cancer stem cells (CSCs) and their pivotal role in cancer research. From the pioneering identification of blood system stem cells in 1961 to the recognition of CSCs in various cancers, and the exploration of plant-based therapies, each milestone has progressively shaped our approach to cancer treatment and prevention. There has also been a steady drumbeat of interest in the use of plant chemicals as a non-toxic way of hitting multiple targets on the otherwise elusive CSCs. The greatest obstacle to that development is a regulatory system that is designed for strongly patentable pharmaceuticals, rather than low-cost, non-toxic food elements.

Earlier, I quoted Sun Tzu (544-496 BCE) in his classic *Art of War*, where he said:

> *"If you know the enemy and know yourself, you need not fear the result of a hundred battles.... If you know neither the enemy nor yourself, you will succumb in every battle."*

In the realm of cancer, modern advances in immunotherapy and metabolic research have significantly enhanced our understanding of our own biological responses — in other words "'knowing ourselves." The discovery of cancer stem cells marks a similar advance in "knowing the enemy," providing us with crucial insights into the very origins of cancer.

TARGETING CANCER STEM CELLS WITH A CLEAN, TRADITIONAL DIET

As indicated in a 2024 article by the hematologist Francesca Andreazzoli, MD (discussed below), the idea that diet can impact CSCs is also gaining scientific support. A traditional dietary program, such as the Mediterranean diet, rich in specific plant chemicals, can stop these highly malignant cells. Antioxidants in fruits and vegetables, like berries and spinach, can disrupt CSCs' growth and networks to proliferate. The healthy fats in olive oil and fish, containing compounds that challenge the survival processes of CSCs, also play a crucial role.

A clean, traditional diet's emphasis on whole, unprocessed foods translates to lower use of sugars and processed carbs, which are the preferred energy sources for CSCs. Depriving these cells of their favorite fuel might make them more susceptible to treatments like chemo and radiation.

We have found no prior articles stating clearly that a clean, traditional diet with a combination of nutraceuticals and supplements is likely to be effective at attacking the most dangerous portion of cancer yet discovered, the cancer stem cells.

LIFESTYLE FACTORS & STRESS REDUCTION

Our approach is not just about the food. The stress-reducing aspects of the Mediterranean lifestyle could also be important. Stress hormones create an environment conducive to CSC survival. The community-oriented, outdoor, and mindful lifestyle typical in Mediterranean cultures reduces stress, potentially weakening CSCs' dominance.

HOLISTIC APPROACHES & THE MOSS METHOD

Conventional cancer treatments like surgery, radiation, and chemo are powerful tools. However, recent research has brought increasing attention to holistic approaches that focus beyond the tumor itself, exploring the underlying factors that may contribute to cancer development. In a sense, this is a form of the old "seed and soil" debate of the late 19th century. A London surgeon, Stephen Paget (1855-1926), formulated the "seed and soil" hypothesis in the 1880s (Paget 1889). It had long been noted that certain cancers had a proclivity to spread to particular organs, such as pancreatic cancer to the liver, or prostate cancer to the bone.

According to Paget's theory, metastatic spread was not a random process but required a suitable environment in a distant organ. This gave rise to a more general theory of the cooperation between tumor cells, called the 'seeds,' and a target organ, called the 'soil' (Ghannam 2022)

The "seed" is the malignant cell per se. However, the "soil" is what we now call the "tumor microenvironment," meaning the normal cells and chemicals that surround the tumor cell, and, by extension, the health and integrity of the whole organism.

This perspective meshes well with the theory of cancer stem cells (CSCs). These specialized cells, likened to seeds of cancer, possess the ability to self-renew and drive tumor growth. But, broadening our perspective, and understanding the environmental and lifestyle factors that influence CSC formation and behavior presents another avenue for advancing cancer prevention and treatment strategies.

Take folate, for example. Studies suggest it can affect how genes behave in cancer cells, possibly by affecting a process called DNA methylation. This could play a role in turning on or off CSCs. Understanding how natural remedies impact these important factors could lead to new ways to prevent and treat cancer.

The Moss Method also exemplifies this holistic philosophy. It advocates personalized lifestyle modifications centered around diet, exercise, and stress reduction, aiming to optimize overall health and well-being (the "soil") while potentially impacting CSC dynamics ("the seed"). This aligns seamlessly with the emerging research on CSCs and natural treatments, offering a promising avenue for empowering individuals to actively participate in their cancer journey.

Preliminary findings are encouraging, revealing the significance of exploring the interplay between lifestyle choices and the underlying complexities of cancer development. While mainstream cancer treatments remain essential, embracing the possibility of holistic approaches alongside individual empowerment efforts, as exemplified by The Moss Method, offers an opportunity to revolutionize cancer care. By addressing factors that may influence the very core of tumor formation, we pave the way for a future in which prevention and sustainable management will take center stage alongside curative efforts.

CONVENTIONAL CANCER DRUGS & TARGETED THERAPIES

The development of traditional anti-cancer drugs like imatinib (Gleevec), trastuzumab (Herceptin), and erlotinib (Tarceva) has been a big step forward. Together, they ushered in the present stage of "targeted therapies" of cancer. It is rare, nowadays, for a patient to be treated exclusively with conventional, toxic chemotherapy. More often, targeted drugs—such as tyrosine kinase inhibitors (TKIs) and nanoparticle albumin-bound drugs play an increasingly important role in treatment. These are the so-called "nibs and nabs" of cancer drug treatment (named after their final syllables).

However, cancer treatment today is rarely straightforward, with many targets and complex communication routes among cells. Targeted therapies aim to interfere with specific chemicals involved in tumor growth. But cancer's complexity, with its numerous changes and networks, often makes attacking single molecules limited in its effectiveness.

Current treatments and their limitations show the need for holistic, patient-centric approaches, such as those outlined here in The Moss Method.

A clean, traditional diet, key nutraceutical elements, and a healthy lifestyle provide a broad non-toxic strategy against CSCs. Targeting their markers using natural plant chemicals, The Moss Method leverages this understanding to equip patients with a powerful tool in their fight against cancer, preventing its first appearance, and potentially making any remission more long-lasting.

Readers might wonder why such a discovery as cancer stem cells (CSCs) has yet to be a common topic of discussion, even when talking to oncologists. The primary reason is that, for a mainstream physician, and for society as a whole, this information needs to be actionable to justify spending valuable time on an explanation. It will become actionable if and when a drug attacking CSCs receives FDA or EMA approval, a process that will require rigorous clinical trials published in major medical journals, which are subject to extensive peer-review and discussion at meetings of the American Society of Clinical Oncology (ASCO) or the American Association for Cancer Research (AACR). Such treatments then have a good chance of becoming an integral part of mainstream medicine. But there are numerous obstacles to overcome before that happens.

It is a source of hope that this is exactly what happened with the field of cancer immunotherapy, and in particular with immune checkpoint blockers. The basics of cancer immunotherapy were established over 100 years ago. Starting in the late 19th century, a New York Surgeon, William B. Coley, MD, began treating cancer with what we would now consider immunological means. When I began working at Memorial Sloan-Kettering Cancer Center 50 years ago three of the four top administrators and thought leaders were cancer immunologists. Yet it wasn't until 2011 (with the FDA's approval of Yervoy) that the broad public began to wake up to the enormous potential of using the immune system against many forms of this disease.

Meanwhile, some plant chemistry researchers have enthusiastically embraced the treatment of CSCs. It is somewhat ironic that this once-neglected area now appears to hold the key to arguably the most pivotal development in cancer understanding over the past 50 years.

We now have substantial knowledge of the primary CSC markers for most forms of cancer and the plant chemicals that attack cells bearing these markers.

While our understanding of CSC behavior and the best use of plant chemicals is still under examination, it is sufficient to make a start. For instance, there are currently 225 PubMed articles on the use of plant pigments for CSCs. These are substances found in many plants and have demonstrated antioxidant effects.

The emerging focus on cancer stem cells (CSCs) and their central role in the growth, spread, and resistance to treatment of cancer reveals a pivotal shift in our approach to understanding and combating this complex disease. As research continues to uncover the ways through which CSCs operate and how they can be targeted, we stand on the brink of a new era in cancer treatment. This promises to translate into more effective therapies that could improve patient outcomes. This illustrates the critical importance of ongoing research and the need for public and professional awareness about the role of CSCs in cancer.

A CULTURAL HERITAGE

The United Nations Educational, Scientific and Cultural Organization (UNESCO) has recognized one particular traditional eating pattern, the Mediterranean diet, as part of the Intangible Cultural Heritage of Humanity. This badge of recognition spans several countries, revealing its transnational importance. UNESCO's citation gives an expansive definition of the Mediterranean Diet:

> *"A set of skills, knowledge, rituals, symbols, and traditions involving crops, harvesting, fishing, animal husbandry, conservation, cooking, and particularly the sharing and eating of food. Eating together is foundational to the cultural identity and continuity of communities in the Mediterranean basin" (UNESCO 2003, edited).*

This citation recognizes that the Mediterranean Diet is more than just food. It includes community rituals, traditional knowledge, and techniques passed down through generations. UNESCO has recognized that the Mediterranean Diet is a lifestyle honed over thousands of years.

While we explore the chemical ingredients in foods and their role in cancer prevention, we must remember that a clean, traditional diet is more than a sum of its parts.

CLEAN, TRADITIONAL DIETS & THEIR ROLE IN CANCER PREVENTION

All over the world, people recognize clean, traditional diets for their possible role in cancer prevention. For example, the EPIC study was a massive research effort exploring the relationship between diet, nutritional status, lifestyle, environmental factors, cancer incidence, and other chronic diseases. Its Greek segment revealed reductions in overall cancer deaths, including colorectal, breast, and gastric cancers (Trichopoulou 2005).

Scientists at the University of Athens conducted the Greek cohort of over 25,000 individuals. They found that closer adherence to the traditional Greek diet is associated with substantially reducing overall cancer risk, proving that even modest dietary changes yielded health benefits (Benetou 2008). As a result, for every two-point increase in adherence to the diet, there was a 12% decrease in cancer risk, with women experiencing a more pronounced protective effect. This study showed a cumulative protective effect, suggesting a unique synergy within this dietary pattern contributing to its anticancer qualities.

These findings suggest a traditional diet could boost the effects of established cancer treatments. While broad clinical trials are still limited, the evidence firmly positions this traditional diet as a strategic part of cancer care. This agreement of ancient dietary wisdom with modern cancer research presents a detailed approach to cancer prevention and treatment.

EXPERIMENTAL EVIDENCE OF ANTICANCER EFFECTS

Experimental evidence sheds light on how traditional diets contribute to cancer prevention at a molecular level. Individual items of The Moss Method have been examined in controlled settings, revealing possible ways for cancer prevention and control.

Olive oil, a Mediterranean staple that has spread around the globe, contains key ingredients such as hydroxytyrosol and oleuropein, which hinder cancer cell growth (Hassan 2014). *(Hydroxytyrosol is in fact a breakdown product of oleuropein, created in the course of digestion.)*

According to PubMed, the former is the subject of ~2,000 journal articles, while oleuropein has ~1,500 such references! Together, they account for 2,875 articles, with new ones appearing at a rate of six per week. This testifies to a considerable amount of scientific interest. Why the excitement? These compounds can reduce cell damage from oxygen, change genes associated with cancer growth, and cause normal cell death in cancer.)

An important factor for The Moss Method is that these two compounds, when taken in the form of EVOO, slow the absorption of glucose after a meal (Carnevale 2018). This is of potentially great benefit in terms of prediabetes and diabetes. This traditional diet also contains dietary fiber, antioxidants, and plant chemicals from fruits, vegetables, and whole grains. These ingredients reduce inflammation and oxidative damage (Giacosa 2013). Pigments in fruits, vegetables, and red wine have been studied for their possible role to stop tumor growth and spread (Wang 2014).

(By spread, we mean what scientists call "metastasis." This is the process by which cancer cells migrate from the original tumor to other body parts, forming new growths.)

Fish, another critical dietary element, provides omega-3 fatty acids that show anti-inflammatory qualities and potentially reduce cancer risk (Cockbain 2014).

Beyond its cancer prevention potential, the Mediterranean diet, marked by a relatively high use of fatty fish, addresses a broad spectrum of health concerns. It reduces the risk of neurodegenerative diseases, control of energy-related disorders, weight control, improvement of bone health, and reduced risk of depression. These benefits arise from the diet's rich content of omega-3 fatty acids, antioxidants (polyphenols), and nutrients like calcium, vitamin D, and magnesium (Scarmeas 2009, Salas-Salvado 2008a, Benetou 2013, Sanchez-Villegas 2009).

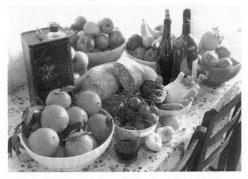

Elements of the Mediterranean Diet. Source: Wikimedia Commons

THE HALLMARKS OF CANCER: A CRITICAL OVERVIEW

Well-informed readers may be surprised that I have not strictly adhered to the classic description of cancer that most scientists now embrace. This is the perspective detailed in a series of articles that two professors, Douglas Hanahan, Ph.D. and Robert Weinberg, Ph.D., produced between 2000 and 2022, commonly referred to as 'Hanahan and Weinberg' or, more familiarly, "H&W."

As even their critics concede, H&W's framework has "dominated the discourse" on the causation of cancer among researchers in recent times. The foundational principles of their theory define cancer as a cell-based, genetic disease whereby DNA alterations cause uncontrolled cell proliferation. Over the years, H&W have provided support for what is called the "somatic mutation theory of cancer" (SMT). This has been succinctly described by the theory's defenders:

> *"According to the somatic mutation theory (SMT), cancer begins with a genetic change in a single cell that passes it on to its progeny, thereby generating a clone of malignant cells" (Vaux 2011).*

However, this traditional 20th-century view has now been challenged by other significant scientific developments. There are powerful critiques of the somatic mutation theory in the writings of Thomas N. Seyfried, Ph.D., a professor of biology at Boston College (Seyfried 2010, Seyfried 2014, Seyfried 2021). Seyfried's thinking is encapsulated in over 200 PubMed-listed articles and in a popular book, *Cancer as a Metabolic Disease* (2012). We might call this the "neo-Warburgian theory" in that it updates and provides experimental proof of the ideas initially proposed by Otto Warburg in the period 1923-1970.

Another important critique has been that of Carlos Sonnenschein, MD, and Ana M. Soto, MD, who are long-time scientific coworkers at the Tufts University School of Medicine, Boston. Sonnenschein and Soto's thinking is found in over 160 PubMed articles and is summarized in their little-known but fascinating book, *The Society of Cells* (1998). As they explained in a series of YouTube videos, this was the culmination of a train of thought that went back to 1970.

When it came out, there was a very favorable review of their book in the *New England Journal of Medicine*:

"Sonnenschein and Soto argue persuasively that healthy, well-nourished cells, unless constrained by inhibitory factors or signals, will undergo mitosis [cellular division]. According to their view, cells do not remain quiescent of their own accord...free-living cells will divide if they are given the opportunity" (Prehn 1999).

Other than this one review, however, the book received very little attention and has long been out of print. However, in my opinion, it has been unfairly neglected. Its interlocking main points are as follows:

- The default state of all normal cells is proliferation (growth in number), not peaceful non-division (or "quiescence").

- Cancers, like normal tissues, exist in a matrix of other cells, hormones, and other chemical signals. They are not found outside the laboratory in a single aberrant state. They form, to quote the title of their book, a "society of cells."

- Cancer does not typically arise from a mutation in a single "wayward cell" (Richards 1972) or as Robert A. Weinberg (the "W" of "H&W") put it in the title of his popular book, "One Renegade Cell" (Weinberg 1999). Rather it originates from the disruption of the whole society of cells, the matrix that affects an entire tissue or organ that eventually causes cancer in the whole colony.

I am not prepared to make a full-scale evaluation of these competing theories of cancer's origins, nor would it be appropriate for a work for non-specialist readers. However, I believe that both the Seyfried and the Sonnenschein/Soto critiques have compelled a reexamination of the underlying assumptions of the Hanahan and Weinberg articles.

Interestingly, H&W, over the years, have ceded much ground to the point of view of these critics, without mentioning them by name. They now acknowledge "deregulating cellular metabolism" as a key hallmark, which in my opinion is a nod in the direction of Warburg and Seyfried. Similarly, they now include among the hallmarks the tumor microenvironment (TME), which Hanahan says "is now widely appreciated to play an integral role in tumor formation and malignant progression" (2022). And what is this if not a belated recognition of what Sonnenschein and Soto were saying decades earlier? We could add to this their recognition of the role of a defective immune system—a clear affirmation of the train of thought leading from

William B. Coley, MD (1862-1936), to Lloyd J. Old, MD (1933-2011), and then to Old's protégé, the 2018 Nobel laureate, James P. Allison, Ph.D.

(See my grandson, Jacob Moss's, award-winning documentary on this tradition, Immunotherapy: The Battle Within.)

So by focusing on H&W in this section, I do not mean to imply that I necessarily agree with their overall view of the cancer problem. I just want to show that, even if you agree with their perspective (as many oncologists do), The Moss Method still makes perfect sense as a means of cancer prevention.

Critiques of the somatic mutation theory (SMT), such as those by Seyfried and Soto/Sonnenschein, underscore the need for a much broader perspective on cancer. By combining reductionist insights—like identifying specific markers on CSCs—with organicist strategies that emphasize the body's overall health and immune system, The Moss Method offers a unique system-wide approach to targeting these elusive cells.

THE ORIGIN OF THE H&W HALLMARKS

It is not surprising that H&W (especially in early versions of the hallmarks) centered their description of cancer around DNA changes. This view has had to be modified with the inclusion of changes to the tumor microenvironment, the immune system, and metabolism, all of which are taking them far afield of where they began the hallmark series over two decades ago.

Hanahan now also includes a key element of the metabolic theory among his hallmarks:

"Deregulating cellular metabolism and avoiding immune destruction were [previously] segregated as "emerging hallmarks," but now, eleven years later, it is evident that they, much like the original six, can be considered core hallmarks of cancer" (Hanahan 2022).

Another key element is recognition of the gut microbiome as a regulator of the body's response to the tumor: Here is a paraphrase of a key sentence from the paper:

"An exciting new area in biomedicine is exploring the wide variety of microorganisms, known as the microbiota, that live in our body tissues exposed to

So in the 21st century, we see a new paradigm of cancer emerging that encompasses not just the "somatic mutation theory," but key elements of the various conflicting theories that have long challenged the status quo.

I critiqued the somatic cell theory in my 2020 book *Cancer, Incorporated*. This critique explores the limitations and evolving nature of cancer theories, advocating for a broader perspective that includes the role of cancer stem cells as central to understanding and treating cancer effectively.

FURTHER INSIGHTS ON CSCs

There is only one glancing mention of cancer stem cells in Hanahan's 2022 updated version of the hallmarks. To paraphrase this influential article:

"The tumor microenvironment (TME) is composed of various populations of cancer cells and cancer stem cells along with a number of other cell types. This is now widely appreciated to play an integral role in tumor formation and cancer's progression" (Hanahan 2022, edited)

In my opinion, this is damning by faint praise. It fails to acknowledge that the emergence of the CSC concept challenges conventional oncology, including its treatment. That is because, all too often, conventional therapeutics kill run-of-the-mill cancer cells but fail to kill CSCs. This makes CSCs by far the most important component of the tumor. Therefore, the "hallmarks" of non-CSCs are of much less importance than these uniquely dangerous entities.

In the 4th century BCE, the Greek philosopher Aristotle said "we do not have knowledge of a thing until we have grasped its why, that is to say, its cause" (Physics 194 B17-20). According to the *Stanford Encyclopedia of Philosophy*, "For Aristotle, a firm grasp of what a cause is, and how many kinds of causes there are, is essential for a successful investigation of the world around us" (Falcon 2023).

Many eminent scientists, such as John Dick, Ph.D., of the University of Toronto, Michael F. Clarke, MD, of Stanford University, and Max Wicha, MD, of the University of Michigan, have proposed a complete upending of the usual hierarchy of the cancer cell populations. In their view, there are many remote causes of cancer, but only one cause which is ultimately responsible for the numerous characteristics of cancer; that is the CSC.

And if this is so—and I believe it is—then H&W's ten hallmarks will need serious revision. The key task is then to understand the origin and behavior of the main cause—the cancer stem cell—which also becomes the central target for future therapeutics. There is a vigorous worldwide effort underway to find such agents. According to a review article:

> *"Methods of targeting CSCs include nano-drug delivery systems, mitochondria targeting, hyperthermia, immunotherapy, and tumor microenvironment (TME) targeting. However, this field remains in its infancy, and considerable research will be required to produce mature products that can contribute to curing cancer" (Du FY 2019, edited).*

So far, the FDA has approved a handful of drugs to target one particular marker on CSCs. These are vismodegib (Erivedge) and sonidegib (Odomzo) for advanced skin cancers, and glasdegib (Daurismo) for a type of leukemia. Others are in the pipeline. But so far these drugs have been plagued by problems of resistance and toxicity. This in turn is bringing natural medicine to the fore, since as patented drug solutions prove difficult, non-toxic plant chemicals show a robust ability to simultaneously target and counteract many of the markers of CSCs.

A decade earlier Hanahan had enthusiastically acknowledged the significance of CSCs. In an article with Lisa M. Coussens, MD, Ph.D., of the Oregon Health and Science University, they described CSCs as crucial to cancer's origin, despite the body's defenses, spread to other body parts, and persistence after seemingly successful treatment (Hanahan 2012). Here's how they put it:

> *"It has become evident in the past decade that most if not all malignancies contain a subpopulation of cancer cells with stem-like properties—cancer stem cells (CSCs)—that are instrumental in the manifestation of cancer, affecting initiation, persistence in the face of barriers to proliferation, metastases, and the ability to rebound from cancer therapies" (Hanahan 2012, edited)*

But, despite this apparent endorsement, the hallmarks of cancer that he proposed in 2022 did not reflect his earlier understanding of CSCs' central role. In April 2024, I addressed an email to Professor Hanahan, which read in part:

"What I am having difficulty understanding is why the existence of cancer stem cells, or at least the quality of stemness, does not figure in your latest iteration of the hallmarks (in Cancer Discovery 2022). You seemed to be edging towards the inclusion of CSCs in your Cancer Cell article of 2012 with L.M. Coussens. Do you feel I am misguided in including CSCs as a potential target for phytochemicals (per the work of Wicha and others)?"

Unfortunately, I never received a reply.

In light of these misgivings, the reader may wonder why I am devoting so much attention to H&W's hallmarks. We must recognize that their work has influenced generations of cancer scientists and medical students, and continues to affect the field profoundly. It's not that Hanahan and Weinberg's hallmarks are incorrect; rather, their list doesn't fully incorporate newer findings that support alternative perspectives, including those proposed in The Moss Method.

The root cause of their problem is that they still adhere to the dominant somatic mutation theory (SMT) of cancer. Their original hallmarks were based on the assumption that cancer originates in a single renegade cell (to quote the title of one of Weinberg's books). To be sure, by including the tumor microenvironment in the hallmarks, they acknowledge that the other members of the "society of cancer" (to quote Sonnenschein and Soto's book title) have equal, if not greater, status with the malignant cell. They have also brought in metabolism and immunotherapy—two of the "gears" of The Moss Method. But for reasons of their own they fail to address, much less include, CSCs among the hallmarks. This is a serious deficiency in their decades-long project.

WHAT YOU NEED TO KNOW ABOUT THE HALLMARKS OF CANCER

I have explained the reasons for my refusal to fully base The Moss Method on Hanahan and Weinberg's of cancer, the way others in the field have done. For instance, they form the framework for the otherwise excellent Halifax Project recommendations (Block 2015). Nevertheless, in the following section, I will set aside my differences and demonstrate how The Moss Method also addresses this popular framework for understanding the main features of the disease.

I do this to facilitate communication with the myriad of people who still believe that H&W represent the "last word" in understanding the nature of cancer. I also hope that this will help in discussions between my readers and their healthcare providers who are likely to embrace H&W's framework in understanding the nature and treatment of cancer.

Here then is a brief overview of the ten hallmarks of cancer as I have "translated" them into lay language.

#1 - UNCONTROLLED GROWTH

Cancer is characterized by its relentless and unchecked growth, similar to cars that ignore red lights, continuously multiplying without the usual cellular stop signals. In certain cancers, such as lung cancer, specific genetic errors constantly tell the cells to keep growing. Most scientists believe that cells are normally in a quiescent state, and that cancer represents a departure from this universal state of peace. (See *The Society of Cells* {1998} for a trenchant critique of this point of view.)

When it comes to excess growth, we emphasize the use of nutraceuticals for prevention. Nutraceuticals, like green tea, turmeric, and soybeans, are packed with beneficial compounds—in this case, EGCG, curcumin, and genistein. These substances help curb the rampant growth of cancer cells through natural dietary means, playing a crucial role in preventing both the onset and return of cancer. This method leverages the natural qualities of these compounds to manage and restrain cancer's aggressive behavior without resorting to drugs.

#2 - IGNORING GROWTH CHECKS

Cancer cells often ignore the body's natural ways that normally pause or stop their growth, similar to a car that's lost its brakes, which leads to unchecked cell division and tumor growth. A crucial player in these growth checks is the protein p53, which normally works to detect and fix DNA damage or to initiate cell death if the damage is irreparable. However, in many cancers, the gene responsible for producing p53 is mutated, allowing defective cells to keep multiplying.

The Moss Method places a strong emphasis on supporting the body's natural growth control processes. While certain drugs target these processes by trying to fix or replace the functions of p53, The Moss Method advocates the use of natural substances to achieve similar outcomes. For example, compounds found in cabbage can help restore p53 function, and other substances like berberine, resveratrol, soy isoflavones, and elements in extra virgin olive oil can boost the body's ability to maintain growth controls. These natural agents, rich in anticancer qualities, complement rather than replace medical treatments, showcasing The Moss Method's strategy of utilizing smart dietary choices for effective cancer prevention.

#3 - HIDING FROM THE IMMUNE SYSTEM

Cancer cells can become "invisible" to the body's immune system, akin to a stealthy intruder bypassing a home's security. Normally, our immune system, particularly the white blood cells, detects and destroys such threats. But cancer cells have evolved ways to escape this detection, effectively sneaking past our immune surveillance.

Immune checkpoint blockers, a significant advancement since 2011, have revolutionized cancer treatment by restoring the immune system's ability to recognize and destroy cancer cells. These drugs, such as ipilimumab (Yervoy) and pembrolizumab (Keytruda), target proteins like PD-L1, which cancer cells use to turn off immune responses.

Reflecting my longstanding interest in the immune aspects of cancer, The Moss Method emphasizes natural compounds that may influence these immune checkpoints. This is a promising but little recognized idea. Ingredients like beta-glucans in certain mushrooms, healing compounds in extra virgin olive oil, probiotics, and omega-3 fatty acids can bolster the immune system's natural fight against cancer. This approach, focusing on diet and natural substances, supports and extends beyond conventional medical treatments, reinforcing the body's defenses against cancer in a holistic and non-toxic manner.

#4 - IMMORTAL CELLS

Cancer cells defy the natural limits of cell reproduction known as the Hayflick limit, which caps the number of times a human cell can divide. This limit involves the progressive shortening of telomeres, the protective end caps of chromosomes that are crucial for maintaining genetic stability during cell division (Hayflick 1965).

While the scientific community has developed drugs to counteract this trait of immortality in cancer cells, natural dietary elements also show promise. Diets rich in specific compounds can stop such unchecked growth and offer possible anti-cancer benefits. These compounds include curcumin from turmeric (Anand 2007), EGCG from green tea (Naasani 2003), and resveratrol from grapes and berries (Baur 2006a).

The Moss Method promotes integrating these natural compounds with conventional scientific advances, exemplifying our approach to addressing the challenge of immortality in cancer cells. By combining scientific knowledge with natural dietary strategies, this method seeks to harness the full spectrum of anticancer tools, balancing traditional remedies with modern medical interventions.

#5 - INFLAMMATION BENEFITS FROM TUMORS

Inflammation serves both as a protector against and a promoter of cancer, presenting a complex challenge in cancer prevention. Acute inflammation can act as a defensive response to precancerous conditions, but chronic inflammation often becomes a fertile ground for cancer development. This prolonged inflammatory state can cause silent tissue damage and foster tumor growth, typically characterized by excessive production of inflammatory chemicals and the activation of tumor-supportive networks.

In response to these challenges, treatments have been developed, including FDA-approved anti-inflammatory drugs, for example, tofacitinib (Xeljanz), which target these cancer-promoting inflammatory processes.

Additionally, natural interventions such as omega-3 fatty acids and curcumin, as well as components of a clean traditional diet, are increasingly recognized for their possible role to reduce the inflammation that can promote tumors. These natural solutions are part of a broader strategy to combat cancer effectively.

Understanding the nuanced role of inflammation in cancer continues to be a critical area of research, showing the need for a multifaceted approach that incorporates both natural dietary strategies and scientific advancements. The Moss Method advocates for this comprehensive approach, utilizing natural dietary options to address the pro-tumoral effects of chronic inflammation alongside conventional therapies.

#6 - SPREADING TO NEW AREAS

The spread of a tumor represents a critical and aggressive stage of cancer, characterized by cancer cells breaking away from their original location to form new tumors in distant body parts. This process is particularly daunting as it often resists standard treatments and involves cancer cells migrating through the bloodstream or lymphatic system, helped by molecular changes.

Conventional medical treatments target specific aspects of growth and tumor spread, including networks involved in prostate and breast cancers and secondary tumors in the bones. These treatments are designed to stop the networks that allow cancer cells to invade new areas and establish secondary tumors.

Parallel to these medical interventions, natural dietary strategies provide a complementary approach to combating cancer's spread. Compounds such as ellagic acid found in berries, sulforaphane in cruciferous vegetables, and antioxidants in foods like olive oil, garlic, onions, legumes, nuts, tomatoes, and red grapes (notably rich in resveratrol) are researched for their abilities to hinder cancer cell invasion and migration.

The Moss Method leverages these insights, incorporating a diet rich in anti-metastatic compounds into a comprehensive cancer management strategy. This approach not only addresses the immediate challenges of cancer's spread but also enhances overall cancer care by integrating beneficial dietary choices that support the body's natural defenses against cancer spread. This combined approach underscores the possible role of combined natural and conventional strategies to manage the complex issue of cancer migration effectively.

#7 - MAKING THEIR OWN BLOOD SUPPLY

A pivotal element in cancer's growth is the formation (and recruitment) of blood vessels, by which tumors supply themselves with nutrients and oxygen and dispose of waste. Normally, this process occurs during wound healing or growth phases in healthy adults. Cancer cells, however, hijack this process, turning it on permanently to support their uncontrolled growth—similar to an unchecked expansion of a city's road network.

In response, medical science has developed therapies specifically aimed at disrupting this vascular lifeline. These therapies stop the growth factors that cancer cells use to construct their own blood vessels, effectively cutting off the resources needed for their survival.

Additionally, certain natural compounds have shown promise in controlling blood vessel formation. Antioxidants in extra virgin olive oil, resveratrol in red grapes and wine, and lycopene in tomatoes are all studied for their effects on new blood vessel formation. These substances offer a natural means to suppress the tumor's ability to expand its blood supply.

By integrating targeted therapies with these natural compounds, we can effectively limit the growth and spread of cancer by starving it of the necessary resources it needs to thrive. This strategic approach forms a crucial part of comprehensive cancer treatment plans, including those proposed by The Moss Method, which uses the combined effects of scientific advancements and natural dietary interventions to combat cancer.

#8 - GENETIC ERRORS PILE UP

At the core of cancer's vicious cycle is genetic instability and changes, which can be likened to a continually changing blueprint of life. This genetic anarchy, characterized by frequent and random DNA alterations, fuels cancer's growth, ability to adapt, and diversity. Such continuous evolution allows cancer cells to quickly adapt, making them dangerous opponents to the standard treatments that often fall behind in effectiveness.

The Moss Method shows the critical role of lifestyle choices in reducing the risks of cancer. A diet abundant in antioxidants and nutrients, staples of a traditional diet, forms a primary line of defense against the DNA damage that propels cancer's advance. Foods such as berries, cruciferous vegetables, nuts, and olive oil are rich in compounds that aid in DNA repair and maintenance. Moreover, physical activity is essential as it reduces oxidative damage to DNA and boosts the body's natural repair methods.

This dietary strategy, rich in antioxidants and anti-inflammatory qualities, offers a robust defense against the genetic instability that marks cancer. Integrating these natural dietary elements with conventional medical treatments provides a comprehensive approach to cancer prevention and control, underscoring The Moss Method's holistic view in managing this complex disease.

#9 - AVOIDING PROGRAMMED CELL DEATH

Programmed cell death is a process where cells are programmed to die off as part of a normal cycle. This is different from sudden cell death due to injury, which is known as necrosis. Within our bodies, normal cell death is vital for maintaining health and preventing cancer. It is something that occurs at a rate of about two billion times per hour in the average healthy person's cells.

Cancer cells, however, are like malfunctioning computers that refuse to turn off, often due to changes in proteins like p53 that allow damaged cells to proliferate unchecked.

To combat this, medical science has developed drugs such as venetoclax (Venclexta) that specifically target proteins that cancer cells use to avoid dying. These interventions are critical in promoting the dying off of cancer cells.

The Moss Method emphasizes the significant role of diet in combating cancer's evasion of programmed cell death. A traditional diet, rich in antioxidants and nutrients, incorporates natural compounds such as curcumin (from turmeric), quercetin (from apples and onions), sulforaphane (from cruciferous vegetables), and various antioxidants (found in fruits, vegetables, and olive oil). These substances have shown promise in triggering the programmed cell death of cancer cells, thereby supporting the body's efforts to halt cancer growth.

Incorporating a traditional diet complements drug interventions and is a core component of The Moss Method. This approach not only enhances the effectiveness of targeted therapies but also leverages the natural anticancer qualities of dietary choices to form a comprehensive strategy against cancer's resistance to cell death. This combined approach underscores the importance of integrating natural dietary elements into a broader anti-cancer strategy.

#10 - CHANGING ENERGY USE

A variety of drugs have been created to target the unique energy-related characteristics of cancer cells, such as metformin, which interrupts the peculiar ways cancer cells process energy. Similarly, the effects of natural compounds like berberine and resveratrol on cancer metabolism are currently under investigation, showing promise in disrupting cancer cell energy production.

The Moss Method strongly advocates for the influence of diet and lifestyle on cancer metabolism. It reveals the importance of a traditional diet, which is rich in nutrients from sources like fatty fish, fermented dairy products, fruits, vegetables, whole grains, and olive oil. This diet alters how cells generate and use energy, creating conditions that are less conducive to cancer growth.

Additionally, lifestyle interventions such as routine physical activity, fasting, caloric restriction, keto diets, and time-restricted eating are emphasized for their possible role of placing energy-related stress on cancer cells. These practices challenge the cancer cells' energy management and can help to curb their growth.

By integrating these dietary and lifestyle measures, The Moss Method offers a comprehensive approach to modify the energy-related landscape in which cancer cells operate. This holistic strategy not only aims to disrupt cancer's energy-related dependencies but also deepens our overall understanding of cancer, opening the door to new and effective approaches to prevention and management. This proactive approach emphasizes creating an internal environment that is inhospitable to cancer, thereby enhancing the body's natural resistance to the disease.

THE FOOD MATRIX

The Food Matrix is another key concept in The Moss Method. It explains how various nutrients and other parts of one's food interact with each other. This interaction can change how nutrients work in our bod affecting how well we can absorb them, and how beneficial they are for our health. This is not unique to turmeric and curcumin.

It refers to the complex structure and composition of foods, encompassing not just the individual nutrients they contain but also how these nutrients are organized and interact within the food. This matrix can influence the nutritional value of a food, its digestibility, the availability of its nutrients, as well as the food's impact on health beyond the effects of its nutrients.

In essence, the food matrix comprises all the ingredients of food—vitamins, minerals, plant chemicals, fibers, fats, proteins, and carbs—and their physical and chemical interactions within the food's structure. This concept is important to The Moss Method because it suggests that the health effects of a food cannot be fully understood just by looking at its nutrient content in isolation; the structure and interactions within the food can alter how its nutrients are absorbed and used by the body.

SOME EXAMPLES OF THE FOOD MATRIX

The food matrix of whole fruits includes their fiber, which slows down the absorption of sugar and helps adjust blood glucose levels. In contrast, fruit juices, even if made from the same amount of fruit, lack this fibrous material, leading to faster absorption of sugars and potentially more pronounced impacts on blood sugar levels.

Another example is the matrix of dairy products, which includes a complex structure of water, fat, proteins (like casein and whey), minerals (like calcium), and vitamins, all of which influence the digestibility of these nutrients and their impact on health. Because of this, the calcium found in the matrix of cheese may be absorbed differently than calcium from supplements.

Similarly, the matrix of fermented foods is altered by the action of beneficial bacteria, which can transform nutrients into more bioavailable forms and produce new beneficial compounds. For example, the fermentation process in yogurt affects the structure of milk proteins and produces probiotics, influencing digestive health and nutrient absorption.

The concept of food matrix challenges the reductionist approach of evaluating foods solely based on their nutrient composition. It underscores the importance of considering the whole food, its structure, and the synergy between its ingredients when judging its nutritional value and impact on health. This holistic approach aligns with the increasing recognition of whole foods and dietary patterns over individual nutrients in promoting health and preventing disease. This concept tells us that we can't just look at nutrients on their own; we need to consider them as part of the whole food. The food matrix also plays a role in how food tastes and feels when we eat it, showing how complex and important the makeup of our food is.

Although little known to the public, the concept of the food matrix has come to the fore in scientific thinking in recent years. It suggests that the impact of whole foods cannot be fully understood by analyzing their ingredients in isolation. The matrix effect underscores the complexity of dietary impacts on health, advocating for a holistic approach to nutrition and diet planning.

(See our discussion of The Power of Synergy, a key concept in The Moss Method.)

CAN NATURAL AGENTS FIGHT CANCER?

It might seem overly optimistic to suggest that natural products be part of cancer therapy, especially in preventing cancer from coming back in survivors. I often hear that it is too soon to use such items and that we should wait for large randomized controlled trials (RCT) to be completed. RCTs are large research studies performed that evaluate medical, surgical, or behavioral interventions rigorously. However, such studies are designed to test purified drugs.

(See my books Cancer, Incorporated, The Cancer Industry, *and* Doctored Results, *for a full exploration of the difficulties of fairly evaluating natural methods of treating cancer.)*

These drugs not uncommonly originate as natural products. Anticancer drugs made from plants, marine life, and microorganisms are used daily, though sometimes their natural origin is overlooked. Examples in oncology include arsenic trioxide, bleomycin, dactinomycin, docetaxel, etoposide, irinotecan, L-asparaginase, paclitaxel, teniposide, vinblastine, and vincristine. In fact, one study showed that 68% of all the anticancer drugs introduced between 1940 and 2014 were based on natural products (Patridge 2016). Drugs derived from natural substances have not only been crucial in treating various cancers but serve as a foundation for developing new treatments and helping the discovery of new drugs. Modern oncology is still heavily reliant on these and other naturally derived agents for its drug arsenal.

95

However, it is one thing to isolate, modify, and patent a chemical first found in nature (such as vincristine from the periwinkle plant) and quite another to promote an unpatented and relatively unmodified plant chemical.

WHERE ARE YOUR CLINICAL TRIALS?

In discussions about natural cancer treatments, this question often arises: "Where are your clinical trials?" Critics note the relative scarcity of large, randomized, multi-center trials (RCTs) to validate these treatments and sometimes assume there is no human, clinical data to support this approach–only lab studies in cell lines or rodents.

This criticism often overlooks the complexities associated with diet and lifestyle clinical trials. For instance, despite its accolades the Mediterranean Diet also lacks strong clinical trial validation, and is mainly supported by lower levels of proof (Mogg 2024). Yet this non-RCT data is strong enough to convince millions of people to follow this healthy eating plan.

The challenges in executing RCTs are many. I speak from experience, since one of the main purposes for helping to found the U.S. government's Office of Alternative Medicine (now the National Center for Complementary and Integrative Health) was to arrange clinical trials of controversial non-toxic approaches to cancer. But doing so proved extremely difficult, and some of us on the advisory board felt like we were hopelessly entangled in red tape as we pursued that goal.

(My most extensive discussion of this period in print was in the 1996 preface to my book, The Cancer Industry. This book is available on Amazon or through The Moss Report website.)

Medical politics aside, setting up randomized controlled trials (RCTs) requires extensive collaboration and often stumbles due to not enrolling enough participants. In fact, about 80% of trials don't meet their participant recruitment goals and nearly half of research sites end up enrolling few if any patients at all (Earls 2012). Additionally, proponents of natural compounds seldom get FDA approval because such methods can't be patented, which contributes to their low success rate— historically, only 1.7% to 8.3% of these trials have succeeded in gaining regulatory approval (Wong CH 2019).

Yet, despite numerous hurdles, some clinical trials on plant chemicals have in fact occurred, often demonstrating very promising outcomes. Admittedly, these tend to be smaller studies with relatively few participants. But this is a function of the basic economics of drug development. Here are brief descriptions of some from around the world, arranged by country and date. All were published in peer-reviewed scientific journals in the English language.

1. **Japan**: Lentinan from shiitake mushrooms increased survival in advanced stomach cancer patients by approximately 100 days; one-year survival was 49.1% vs. 0% in the control group, an extraordinary result (Nakano 1999).

2. **South Korea:** A mushroom extract enhanced Natural Killer (NK) cell activity and reduced side effects in patients with gynecological cancers (Ahn 2004).

3. **Italy:** Green tea decreased high-grade prostate cancer incidence from 30% to 3% over one year, a study published in the top-drawer journal, *Cancer Research* (Bettuzzi 2006). This remarkable result was never pursued through larger trials.

4. **Oregon, U.S.:** A high-dose vitamin D formulation used with the standard chemotherapy drug docetaxel showed promising results by reducing cancer markers and improving survival rates (Beer 2007).

5. **Sweden:** A randomized trial from the famed Karolinska Institute, Sweden, to investigate the impact of a synbiotic mixture (i.e., a combination of prebiotics and probiotics) on colon cancer. Results indicated a reduction in cell growth and an improved immune response, suggesting protective effects against colon cancer development (Rafter 2007).

6. **Japan:** The mushroom extract lentinan extended survival in stomach cancer patients to 689 days versus 565 days with chemotherapy alone (Ina 2011).

7. **Australia:** In an RCT published in the *American Journal of Hematology*, curcumin decreased signs of multiple myeloma growth (Golombick 2012).

8. **Minnesota, U.S.:** At the Mayo Clinic, 42 chronic leukemia patients received a green tea extract twice daily for up to 6 months. About one-third (31%) had their lymphocyte counts decrease. For those with swollen lymph nodes, 69% had at least a 50% reduction in their size. In all, 69% had a therapeutic response over six months of treatment (Shanafelt 2013).

9. **New York, U.S.:** In a study from the University of Florida, Gainesville, daily intake of shiitake mushrooms boosted immunity and decreased inflammation (Dai 2015), and EGCG reduced cancer markers in breast cancer patients (Crew 2015).

10. **Michigan, U.S.:** In an RCT from Wayne State University, EGCG and another supplement, I3C, improved outcomes in ovarian cancer patients (Kiselev 2018).

11. **United Kingdom:** Just two grams per day of curcumin showed remarkable results in a colorectal cancer trial, more than *doubling survival* over FOLFOX, the classic chemo regimen alone (Howells 2019). This promising *Journal of Nutrition* article was never followed up by a larger RCT.

12. **New York, U.S.:** Positive results from Mt. Sinai Hospital of a soy protein, genistein, with standard chemo for colorectal cancer (Pintova 2019).

13. **India:** Green tea and curcumin treatments enhanced response in precancerous mouth conditions (Neetha 2020).

14. **China:** Maitake mushroom D fraction alleviated side effects of chemotherapy. The frequency of severe adverse events were fewer than in the placebo group. (Hu Q 2022).

15. **Indonesia:** Myeloma patients received either standard treatment with 8 grams of curcumin for 28 days or a placebo. The overall remission rate was 75% with curcumin added vs. 33.3% without it. It also decreased four markers of inflammation (Santosa 2022).

16. **Italy:** The PROVIDENCE study examining the impact of vitamin D supplements on patients with advanced cancer undergoing immunotherapy. The group receiving vitamin D3 showed a remarkable improvement in their survival chances, *with a 45% reduction in the risk of death compared to those who didn't receive supplements* (Bersanelli 2023).

17. **Greece:** In a study from four university hospitals, melatonin improved cancer-related fatigue in breast cancer patients adhering to a Mediterranean diet: "Only patients receiving melatonin improved cancer-related fatigue compared to baseline" (Nimee 2024).

18. **Italy:** In a large randomized trial, published in *Clinical Cancer Research* and involving 27 authors across Italy, strict adherence to a combined macrobiotic and Mediterranean diet resulted in a 41% reduction in breast cancer recurrences (Berrino 2024).

This sample of studies illustrates the possible value of natural compounds in enhancing cancer prevention and treatment and in patient quality of life using the same methodology as rigorous drug trials. We shall discuss some of these trials at greater length in this book. One limitation of many of these peer-reviewed reports is the relatively small number of participants in the trials. Another is the obscurity of some of the journals in which they are published. Nonetheless, I think it should be obvious that numerous sign posts point to the efficacy of plant chemicals in improving the outcome of mainstream therapies.

(For further details, see the chapter on Cancer Treatment & The Moss Method)

Yet, despite great promise, it has proven to be difficult, if not impossible, to proceed to full-scale randomized controlled trials (RCTs) for most of the natural methods that we discuss in this book. It is sometimes suggested that the lack of RCTs is the fault of the proponents of these methods. But the whole testing system is geared to accommodate drug manufacturers, who can look forward to a "pot of gold" at the end of the arduous testing rainbow.

Massive outlays are only possible under a strong patent system, which guarantees a legal monopoly for a specific number of years. But natural agents, by their nature, cannot be patented, as Johns Hopkins University found out in 2001 when their broccoli sprout patent was ruled invalid (IATP 2001).

So nutraceutical developers lack the economic incentive to perform extremely costly clinical trials. The difficulty of doing so has proven too much for even determined proponents of such methods. What is surprising is that any such trials have been done at all.

There is even a technical term for this problem in the field of drug development: it is called the "valley of death" of natural agents. This is the chasm between positive but relatively small studies and the "Grand Canyon" that looms into view when you attempt to proceed to full-scale trials (IOM 2001, U.S. House of Representatives 2005).

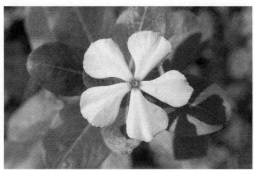

Madagascar periwinkle (Catharanthus roseus, formerly known as Vinca rosea).
Vinca alkaloids in its leaves are the source of two anticancer drugs, vincristine and vinblastine.
Picture courtesy of Wikimedia Commons

WHAT IS THE MOSS METHOD?

> *"The scientific connection between food and health has been well documented for many decades,* with substantial and increasingly robust evidence showing that a healthy lifestyle—including following a healthy dietary pattern— can help people achieve and **maintain good health and reduce the risk of chronic diseases throughout all stages of their lifespan."**
> —Dietary Guidelines for Americans 2020-2025 (USDA 2020)

Many books and articles suggest using foods, food supplements, over-the-counter or off-label drugs, exercise, and mind-body approaches for cancer prevention. But, to my knowledge, **The Moss Method is the first broad, integrative approach to prevention based on widely accepted principles of cancer research, including the targeting of cancer stem cells.** Based on substantial scientific research, and using easily accessible foods with safe supplements as a backup, I focus on specific goals that patients and others can influence, such as chronic inflammation, elevated blood glucose, and the interlocking state of the gut microbiome and the immune system.

At a time when dietary advice is seemingly everywhere, the challenge is to find reliable guidance. **The Moss Method is not just a list of impossible-to-fulfill recommendations but a practical approach, using methods shown to work in numerous scientific studies. It has been shaped by a half-century of in-depth investigation of historical and modern nutritional shifts and hundreds of research findings meticulously listed in a comprehensive bibliography including, whenever possible, links to free full-text journal articles.**

The Moss Method adapts age-old principles to today's scientific landscape. It employs a strategic combination of lifestyle modifications and natural agents to address cancer at its roots. This method reflects a deep respect for historical insights into health and wellness, such as the avoidance of tobacco, but also embraces the latest advances in understanding cancer's biology and the development of targeted therapies.

It is a practical, scientifically informed approach that blends holistic health practices with current understandings of cancer biology. It provides an alternative for individuals seeking proactive health strategies, and reduced cancer risk. By focusing on lifestyle changes and natural agents, this method

aims to broadly attack cancerous changes, aligning with the shift towards targeted therapies and personalized treatment plans.

(Targeted therapies are cancer treatments designed to specifically attack and interfere with molecules involved in tumor growth, such as proteins on the surface of cancer cells.)

Now that we've discussed the essential nature of the large family of diseases known as cancer, it is time to turn our attention to specific ways of combating it. The general understanding today is light years ahead of where it was 50 years ago. Chemotherapy (chemo) was then the only medical treatment, and it was only applicable to a few relatively rare cancers.

The idea of "targeted therapies" was just a twinkle in the eye of a few pioneers, such as Judah Folkman, MD, of Children's Hospital Boston (Folkman 1992). He suggested the idea of blocking the growth of cancer cells rather than poisoning them (along with the rest of the body).

You can think of cancer cells as weeds in a garden: traditional chemo acts like a powerful but indiscriminate weed killer, affecting both the weeds and the surrounding flowers. Targeted therapies, on the other hand, are like having a tool that only destroys the weeds, leaving the flowers unharmed.

These relatively new therapies are designed to zero in on specific markers or functions unique to cancer cells—such as proteins or genes that are different from those in healthy cells—and attack those cells without affecting normal, healthy parts of the body. This precision not only makes the treatment more effective but also reduces side effects, making the patient's journey through cancer care much more manageable.

This approach has become central in oncology because it represents a shift towards personalized medicine, where treatments are tailored to the individual traits of each patient's cancer. For many kinds of cancer, the inclusion of targeted drugs has become a seamless part of their regimen. It's all "chemo," although the targeted drugs are quite different, in both their positive and negative effects, from the traditional drugs that mow down both the weeds and the flowers.

Recognizing the diversity among cancers, understanding the specific biology of a patient's cancer is crucial for oncologists to select the most effective, tailored treatment. With incremental advancements in the molecular understanding of various cancers, the array of available targeted therapies has expanded, offering new hope and options for patients.

This precision and personalization marked an evolution in cancer treatment, promising a future where cancer care is not only more effective but also less taxing on

101

the patient's body. Believe me, none of this existed when the "war on cancer" was launched in the early 1970s. It would have been considered pure science fiction at the time, although today it dominates most new drug development in the cancer field.

Reflecting on the evolution of cancer treatment, my time at Memorial Sloan-Kettering Cancer Center (MSKCC) in New York City during this pivotal period provided me with invaluable firsthand insight into the groundbreaking work of several pioneers in innovative approaches.

Among the many influential figures were Lewis Thomas, MD, president of MSKCC (and author of the prize-winning book, Lives of a Cell), who championed the theory that the immune system patrols the body to detect and eliminate cancer; Robert A. Good, MD, Ph.D., president of Sloan-Kettering Institute; and Lloyd K. Old, MD, who is rightly considered the father of modern cancer immunotherapy (Smyth 2012). Another senior colleague, Kanematsu Sugiura, D.Sc., had been exploring the intersection of diet and cancer since the 1920s.

Dr. Good's pioneering work, including one of the first procedures to replace damaged bone marrow with healthy bone marrow stem cells, highlighted the transformative potential of innovative approaches. He also co-authored studies with former colleagues from the University of Minnesota on the influence of diet on survival in mice. Together they showed that dietary manipulations could have profound effects on immune functions, including the prolongation of survival in some animals' (Fernandes 1976).

THE EVOLUTION OF MAINSTREAM ONCOLOGY

Moving from the historical context to the present, we now understand that two million Americans (and a similar proportion of people around the world) are slated to develop cancer each year unless we take proactive prevention measures, such as are outlined in this book.

Historically, scientists believed that little could be done to prevent cancer. Any effort to alter the environment for cancer prevention was dismissed as 'alternative medicine' or outright quackery—the realm of fraudsters. During the 1960s and 1970s, the American Cancer Society (ACS) even maintained a list of 'forbidden' approaches to cancer (whose deficiencies were detailed in my first book, *The Cancer Industry*). As one example out of many, I recall the visit to MSKCC of the missionary doctor, Dr. Denis Burkitt, after whom Burkitt lymphoma is named. Burkitt believed that the high-fiber diet of sub-Saharan Africans protected them from colorectal cancer. As Burkitt tried to present his views he was heckled from the audience by some of the surgeons—an unforgettable sight. Today, of course, it is commonplace to recognize the beneficial role of dietary fiber, including in the "care and feeding" of the microbiome. At the time, though, any discussion of bowel movements was considered gross, and advocating a high-fiber diet was dismissed as quackery.

Supporting this proactive approach, the American Cancer Society (ACS) now offers compelling statistics:

> *"A substantial proportion of cancers could be prevented, including all cancers caused by tobacco use and other unhealthy behaviors. Excluding non-melanoma skin cancer, at least 42% of newly diagnosed cancers in the United States – about 840,000 cases in 2024 – are potentially avoidable, including the 19% of cancers caused by smoking and at least 18% caused by a combination of excess body weight, use of alcohol, poor nutrition, and physical inactivity"* (ACS 2024, edited).

But times do change, even if too slowly for some of us. While writing this book, an ad popped up on my phone bearing the following message: "When Fighting Cancer, the American Cancer Society Goes Holistic."

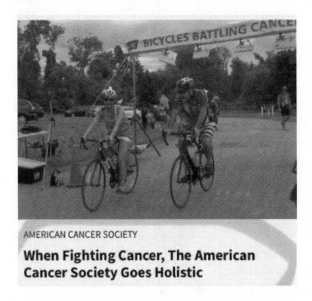

AMERICAN CANCER SOCIETY

When Fighting Cancer, The American Cancer Society Goes Holistic

In addition, according to the ACS,

"More than 18 million Americans with a history of invasive cancer are alive, most of whom were diagnosed many years ago and have no current evidence of the disease" (ACS 2024, edited).

Considering these statistics and the evolving understanding of cancer prevention, The Moss Method is designed not only for primary cancer prevention but also to assist the millions of individuals in the U.S. and worldwide who have been diagnosed with cancer and are striving to prevent a recurrence.

What distinguishes The Moss Method is its drug-free approach, eschewing prescription, experimental, over-the-counter, or repurposed drugs entirely. When it comes to cancer, in my opinion drugs should only be used under the direction of licensed healthcare professionals. Our approach is solely concerned with valid and harmless self-help aspects of cancer.

A "clean, traditional diet" is an approach that emphasizes whole, minimally processed, mainly organic foods and ingredients as they were consumed historically, focusing on nutritional quality and purity. In line with ancient Greek and Roman use of the term diet, it also refers to an active lifestyle that typically accompanies such a health food regimen. I follow the strategy often attributed to the founder of Western medical science, Hippocrates (c. 450 BCE), "Let food be thy medicine and medicine be thy food."

So The Moss Method involves no unique items nor secret remedies. It is composed of various ingredients–a clean, traditional diet; specific nutraceuticals; exercise and mind-body techniques such as forest bathing; and a selection of food supplements chosen for their lack of side effects. However, I believe that, taken together, these represent the most rational and effective way to activate the self-help realm against the occurrence and recurrence of the disease.

UNDERSTANDING THE RISE OF CANCER: A DISEASE OF CIVILIZATION

The efficacy of The Moss Method is underscored by the historical context of cancer's rise. Cancer incidence has increased dramatically over the past few centuries, and it is often described as a "disease of civilization." This notion suggests that industrialization and the adoption of an ultra-processed diet have been accompanied by a rise in cancer incidence in many countries. Scientists are increasingly linking these two broad trends.

Numerous reports from knowledgeable travelers have shown that cancer was virtually unknown before the introduction of Western ways, indicating a connection between modern diet and lifestyles, and the increasing incidence and death from cancer. For example, considerable evidence suggests that until the 20th century, cancer was exceedingly rare in sub-Saharan Africa. The famed explorer, David Livingstone, MD, during his travels in equatorial Africa, rarely saw cancer among the native populations. On one of his African voyages, he noted that he had seen zero cancer cases. He remarked:

"Many diseases common in England are here unknown" (Rijpma 2015: 248).

Similarly, the Nobel Peace Prize laureate, Albert Schweitzer, MD, who founded the missionary hospital in Lambaréné (Gabon 2024), said that he examined 2,000 persons in his first nine months in sub-Saharan Africa. He wrote:

"On my arrival in Gabon in 1913, I was astonished to encounter no case of cancer. I cannot, of course, say positively that there was no cancer at all. But, like other frontier doctors, I can only say that, if any existed, they must have been quite rare. This absence of cancer seemed to me due to the difference in nutrition of the natives compared to the Europeans'" (Berglas 1957).

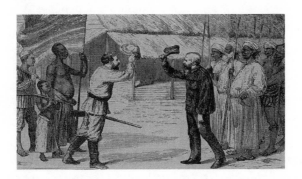

Journalist Henry Stanley greeting David Livingstone, MD, November 10, 1871 in Africa with the famous line, "Dr. Livingstone, I presume." Source: Wikimedia Commons

The Moss Method involves no unique items nor secret remedies. It is composed of various ingredients–a clean, traditional diet; specific nutraceuticals; exercise and mind-body techniques such as forest bathing; and a selection of food supplements chosen for their lack of side effects. None of this will come as a shock to people familiar with the world of natural medicine. However, I do believe that, taken together, they represent the most rational and effective way to activate the self-help realm against the occurrence and recurrence of the disease.

In sharp contrast, 'Fast Food Culture' is the name given to the global spread of ultra-processed foods by giant multinational corporations. It is largely blamed for many chronic diseases of modern life. There is a growing consensus that the pervasiveness of sugar, white flour, and salt in contemporary foods is driving an increase in non-communicable diseases, including cancer.

The Moss Method does not advocate a return to the long-list hunter-gatherer way of living. We also understand that the diet before the mid-1960s, when ultra-processed foods started its rapid rise, was far from perfect. But it contained more whole foods that helped preserve health. It also contained far fewer caloric sweeteners, a category that includes the various forms of sugar, including high-fructose corn syrup.

According to the CDC, the average American's intake of added sugars is 17 teaspoons per day. According to the same source,

"The high intake of added sugars from foods or beverages increases the risk of obesity, hypertension, dyslipidemia, and cardiovascular disease" (Lee SH 2023).

On a personal note, when I was growing up in Brooklyn in the 1950s, a standard Coca-Cola bottle was 6.5 ounces. This was widely recognized as the classic serving size for a bottle of Coke. Today, a 16.9 ounce bottle is considered a more standard size for an individual and the larger 20 ounce bottle has also become very popular for individual consumption. As a result, many kids today are drinking *three times as much soda* in one sitting than I did in my youth. (To be clear, I don't currently drink any sweetened beverages at all and my daily intake of added sugar is minuscule.)

A critical balance has been lost for most people over several generations. We advocate specific dietary practices that were prevalent just a few generations ago. But our method also goes beyond diet, encompassing lifestyle elements supporting physical and emotional well-being. This, too, has its roots in ancient medicine, for one of Hippocrates' most famous works concerned *Airs, Waters, and Places*, that is to say

106

the role of the environment on health. "These things one ought to consider most attentively," Hippocrates wrote (Bashford 2012). In modern terms, this implies an avoidance of cancer-causing substances, particularly tobacco and alcohol, as well as pesticides and other synthetic substances.

> *"Our total environment has become progressively permeated with industrial carcinogens in air, food, water and the workplace," as Professor Samuel S. Epstein, MD, and I wrote in a* Chicago Tribune *opinion article (op-ed) (Epstein 1991).*

Intuitively, mental and emotional health is essential, although scientific documentation of this connection is elusive. However, we will discuss the Roseto Effect, a study showing the role of friendship and community in preventing chronic diseases afflicting modern societies, including cancer (Wolf 1989).

(See the extended discussion of The Roseto Effect.)

The Moss Method shines a light on cancer's faulty metabolism, as well as the gut microbiome's role in either preventing or promoting cancer. It portrays cancer as, in part, a disease of the metabolism and advocates non-drug dietary strategies such as intermittent fasting, low-carb, and keto diets as ways to diminish the ravenous appetite for glucose (sugar) of the cancer cell.

Time-restricted eating (TRE) is another dietary approach where eating is limited to a certain number of hours each day, typically within an 8 to 12-hour window. A keto diet is a high-fat, low-carb diet that changes the body's metabolism to burn fats instead of carbs, producing ketones.

The Moss Method successfully integrates the best of complementary medicine with the cutting edge of mainstream cancer research. The Moss Method is more than a typical diet plan. It represents a lifestyle approach that joins a clean diet to nutraceuticals and supplements, offering a hopeful cancer prevention and management pathway.

The Moss Method does not replace professional cancer treatment but enhances it. Its primary objective is to empower individuals with accessible, evidence-based strategies for reducing cancer risk and enhancing overall well-being. As we explore each element of this method in the upcoming chapters, consider how these changes can positively influence your health journey and improve your quality of life.

The Moss Method is an integrated approach encompassing a clean, traditional diet, certain nutraceuticals, and carefully selected supplements as a logical method for preventing the occurrence or recurrence of cancer. As such it may involve the use of substances that are unfamiliar to your system. Under such circumstances, even if a substance is *Generally Recognized as Safe* (GRAS) it can still cause side effects.

Hopefully, you now understand the scientific and philosophical principles behind The Moss Method. I will now address the practical questions associated with this approach.

NOTE: It is essential to our method to avoid side effects as much as possible. For that reason, I encourage you to pay careful attention to your body during this period of initiating The Moss Method. If you find that a certain food or supplement upsets your stomach, for instance, stop using it. Do not proceed with the ingestion of any substance that continues to present a problem. Try to reintroduce it again at a fraction of the previous strength as before and see if that is better tolerated. Nothing that we recommend is inherently dangerous. But individual reactions differ and it is important to pay attention to this possibility.

ELEMENTS OF THE DIET

Here are some key elements of The Moss Method dietary approach:

Fruits and Vegetables: Unlimited minimally processed vegetables. This includes green above-ground vegetables, with a more limited use of starchy root vegetables. Limited use of fruits, especially in those who are overweight or have other signs of an energy-related disorder (i.e, are prediabetic).

Whole Grains: Avoid white flour. Favor ancient grains, like Kamut, emmer, einkorn, and spelt, including in their sprouted form. Limit portion sizes so as not to raise blood sugar excessively.

Fish and Seafood: Frequent consumption of essential omega-3 fatty acids. Fatty fish, like salmon, mackerel, and sardines, are crucial. These fats aren't called "essential" for no reason.

Legumes and Nuts: Beans, lentils, chickpeas, and nuts which are essential for protein and fiber. However, limit portions to half a cup at a sitting. Among nuts, one should mainly eat walnuts, almonds, and macadamia because of their low carb to fiber ratio (i.e. "net carbs"). Avoid high-carb cashews except as a treat. Pistachios are irresistible, but also relatively high in carbs.

Poultry and Eggs: Free-range chicken, other poultry, and eggs are good sources of protein. Avoid any eggs that are not "certified humane raised and handled," such as the Vital brand. Beware of eggs that are advertised as "free-range." On a personal note, when I lived in Central Pennsylvania, I visited an Amish farm where they raised "free-range" chickens. I was expecting poultry heaven, but was appalled by the overcrowded and unsanitary conditions that I found. This is not only inhumane but also not likely to be healthy for humans who eat the resulting eggs.

Almond milk: Beware of almond or nut milks that contain "mystery" ingredients. Califia Farms Organic Unsweetened Almond Milk contains only three ingredients, almonds, water and salt. In my opinion, it also has a superior taste compared to other commercial almond milk. You can also find recipes online for homemade almond milk.

Dairy Products: Considerable research now implicates an imbalance in the gut microbiome and various forms of cancer (not just of the colon). Dairy is a good source of beneficial probiotics for the gut. Kefir (a cultured liquid product) is generally superior to yogurt as a dietary source of probiotics.

(See our discussion of fermented foods and probiotics.)

Moderate intake of cheese, yogurt, and other dairy are okay, but they should be traditional, natural, and minimally processed. The commercial yogurt section of the supermarket has become yet another danger zone, especially from the point of view of added sugar, sweeteners, or fruit preserves.

Herbs and Spices: Generous use of garlic, basil, oregano, rosemary, and mint, which reduces the use of salt for flavor. In the summer you should grow your own herbs in pots and then dry or otherwise preserve your favorite herbs for use in the winter.

Red Wine: If you are not already a consumer of alcohol, do not start because of its purported health benefits. These are far outweighed by the problems it can cause. If you already drink, emphasize moderate amounts of red wine, particularly Pinot Noir, Cabernet Sauvignon, and Malbec, all of which contain some resveratrol. Women should limit themselves to one glass per day of red wine, men to two glasses.

Minimally Processed Foods: As a general rule, emphasize whole, minimally processed foods. Avoid all ultra-processed, GMO, or "Franken-foods."

(Red meat: We deal with this topic in a separate section.)

The switch from ancient dietary practices to contemporary cancer prevention strategies underscores the evolution of our understanding of health and disease management. It's remarkable how many of the tenets of the "health nuts" of yore have turned out to have a scientific foundation. The turnaround of the science about low-carb diet is one good example of this reversal of fortune. Science writer Gary Taubes' 2002 excellent article in the *New York Times* magazine launched the counter offensive (Taubes 2003).

PARADIGM SHIFT

The current mainstream cancer treatment model has been called the "one disease-one attack-one drug" approach. According to an article in the Proceedings of the National Academy of Sciences:

> *"In drug discovery, a 'one disease–one attack–one drug' approach is common practice, primarily to simplify compound screening, reduce unwanted side effects, and streamline drug registration. This approach, however, oversimplifies disease processes, which encompass complex sub-networks" (Casas 2019, edited).*

While this method has seen some successes in cancer—such as the drug imatinib (Gleevec) and other so-called targeted agents—it increasingly reveals its limitations in fully addressing the multifaceted nature of cancer, which is a disease marked by genetic diversity, metabolic problems, and a multitude of markers on the surface of the cell, which can lead to uncontrolled cell growth.

Moreover, the side effects associated not just with standard chemotherapy but with targeted drugs show the necessity for more detailed treatment strategies. Targeted drugs are designed to specifically identify and attack cancer cells by homing in on unique molecular features of those cells. The discovery and exploration of these markers set the stage for the tremendous advance in knowledge we now have about cancer cells.

The Moss Method is a wide-ranging, patient-centered approach designed to meet these challenges. This method emphasizes the importance of lifestyle modifications, including dietary changes and incorporating natural compounds like curcumin from turmeric, resveratrol from red wine, and EGCG from green tea. These changes are designed to impact various processes involved in cancer development, support cancer prevention, and offer a strategy that complements existing treatments with fewer side effects.

GROWTH OF THE HOLISTIC APPROACH

The traditional, complementary, and integrative approach to cancer is as old as humanity. For as long as we have been around as a species, our ancestors have used natural ingredients as the source of medicines. That practice continues today, where some of the most commonly used anticancer drugs are of vegetable origin. That includes taxol and Taxotere (from the Pacific yew), vincristine and vinblastine (from the Madagascar periwinkle plant), cisplatin and carboplatin (from a naturally occurring mineral), and so forth.

But I don't intend to write a history of natural medicine, much less its use in cancer. I will just note some recent history with which I was intimately involved for almost a decade. In 1993, under the direction of the U.S. Congress, the National Institutes of Health (NIH) established a modestly funded $2 million Office of Alternative Medicine (OAM) within the Office of the Director of the NIH. I am proud to have played a role in the beginning of this Center and in working as an advisor to Senator Tom Harkin of Iowa, Chair of the powerful Senate Health, Education, Labor and Pensions Committee, to increase the OAM's status and funding. Over the past 30+ years, that little office has morphed into the $183.4 million National Center for Complementary and Integrative Health (NCCIH)—an amazing amount of money being spent by top-drawer institutions on approaches that a few decades ago were almost universally derided as "quackery."

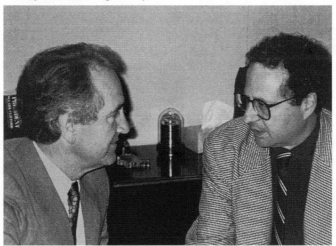

Senator Tom Harkin (D-IA) and Ralph W. Moss, Ph.D. in Washington, DC, circa 1993.
Source: Author's collection.

A 2024 report, published in the *Journal of the American Medical Association (JAMA)*, demonstrated the remarkable staying power of complementary and alternative medicine (CAM). According to the National Center for Complementary and Integrative Health, there has been a "substantial increase" in the use of non-conventional health approaches by American adults from 2002 to 2022. The seven methods they surveyed were yoga, meditation, massage therapy, chiropractic care, acupuncture, naturopathy, and guided imagery/progressive muscle relaxation.

The percentage of individuals who reported using at least one of these seven approaches increased from about 19% in 2002 to 37% in 2022. Put another way, the use of CAM practically doubled in just two decades (Nahin 2024). Little by little, CAM methods and attitudes have penetrated areas that were formerly mainstream medicine (NCCIH 2024).

When it comes to CAM, many things have changed in the last few decades. Both the conventional and the "alternative" sides continue to inch towards a common ground in integrative medicine. However, big differences remain. For a truly integrative approach, a common framework for discussion is essential. Otherwise, the two communities will continue to talk past each other. So one of the aims of The Moss Method is to show the conventional world of oncology how the practices we recommend are based on the same hard-won research findings that they also rely on.

But there are big differences between the way mainstream oncology and The Moss Method view natural products and their role in cancer. Ideally, there should be no conflict between the two, since they are not in competition. Oncology (by which we also include hematology, the study of blood diseases) is mainly concerned with the treatment of malignant disease. The Moss Method is not a treatment modality. It is concerned with preventing the occurrence and recurrence of cancer.

Put another way, oncology occupies the treatment space. It is concerned with shepherding patients through the complex maze of surgery, radiation, and chemo. In recent decades oncologists have also had to master the intricacies of so-called targeted therapies and immunotherapies as well. Considering how hard they work it is not surprising that the prevention of the disease takes a back seat to the immediate crisis of a cancer diagnosis.

EMPOWERING PATIENTS THROUGH SELF-HELP & PREVENTION

But this leaves an area that ordinary people and their families can take charge of, which is the self-help sphere focused on symptom control and prevention. That is the area that we address in *The Moss Report*. So when we contrast the two methods it is not to make a point-by-point comparison, much less to assert our superiority, but to carefully distinguish between the two.

Oncologists, in a general sense, are also sometimes concerned with lifestyle factors and there is an excellent chapter on the topic in the current edition of the DeVita textbook (Brown JC 2024). However, based on many discussions with cancer patients, I would say that it is rare for oncologists to offer more than cursory advice on this topic.

This is a result of both their training and the reality of medical practice today. Oncologists have all they can do to keep up with the demands of their busy practices. For example, according to one hospital's website "community oncologists can see up to 30 patients in a day, each with a different kind of cancer" (City of Hope 2021). **This works out to about 15 minutes on average devoted to each patient.** That kind of demanding schedule doesn't leave much time for detailed advice on lifestyle modification or prevention.

However, patients can improve that situation in two ways:

- Come prepared with questions
- Research what lifestyle changes might benefit you and write down questions for your doctor.

Express your interest: Let your oncologist know you're interested in preventive measures and how you can improve your overall health. This book could certainly be of use to you in this endeavor.

Let's now look specifically at some of the differences between The Moss Method and what oncologists do.

Almost all of the drugs used in oncology are predicated on killing cancer cells outright. They are all, to a greater or lesser degree, poisons. This fact is recognized by the inclusion of the suffix "-toxic" in their collective name of "cytotoxic chemotherapy," which means cell-killing drug treatment.

This use of toxic elements to kill off undesirable elements in the body is a very old idea in medicine. Like so many things, it dates back to Hippocrates (c. 450 BCE). "Poisons have been used for medicinal purposes for millennia. Small doses of opium, mandrake, henbane, and hemlock were all used to numb the pain of surgery for more than one thousand years" (AMNH 2013). Even one of Shakespeare's characters echoes this, saying "In poison, there is physic," meaning poisons can sometimes be used as medicine (Henry IV Part 2).

To be clear, in the context of cancer treatment, poisons are used with the utmost care under medical supervision to ensure that their benefits in fighting cancer outweigh the risks associated with their damage to healthy cells. Modern oncology also includes targeted therapies and immunotherapies that aim to further reduce side effects by focusing more precisely on cancer cells while sparing healthy ones. (That at least is the goal.)

The main difference between the natural compounds used in conventional oncology and in The Moss Method is that the former is exclusively focused on finding effective poisons for cancer cells. Our method, on the other hand, is focused on self-help and prevention, where the use of poisonous substances is always to be avoided.

Unlike chemo, the natural compounds that are a key part of The Moss Method work in a gentler way. Instead of killing cells outright, plant chemicals can alter the signals that cancer cells rely on to grow and spread. They can selectively stop cancer cells without causing much, if any, damage to healthy cells.

TARGETING OF CANCER WITH PLANT CHEMICALS

While the effectiveness of plant chemicals might initially seem too good to be true, substantial evidence supports their potential. This effectiveness manifests through several specific actions:

- *Targeted Delivery:* Cancer cells often absorb more nutrients than normal cells due to their rapid growth. Plant chemicals exploit this by getting absorbed more by cancer cells, which then become affected by the treatment while normal cells are not.

- *Cancer-Specific Actions:* These plant compounds can interfere with processes that are essential for cancer cells but not for normal cells. For example, they might block surface markers that cancer cells rely on to survive.

- *Different Processing:* Cancer cells may change and activate plant chemicals differently than normal cells. This can make these plant chemicals harmful to cancer cells while leaving normal cells unscathed.

- *Selective Harmfulness:* Some plant chemicals can cause cell damage from oxygen, specifically in cancer cells, which have less ability to handle this stress compared to normal cells.

In simple terms, plant chemicals use the unique traits of cancer cells—like their altered metabolism and specific molecular needs—to selectively attack them without damaging normal, healthy cells. This selective targeting helps in treating cancer effectively with minimal side effects.

Instead of overwhelming the body with toxins, plant chemicals can boost the immune system's natural ability to fight cancer. This is the philosophy behind immunotherapy, especially the use of immune checkpoint blocking drugs such as ipilimumab (Yervoy) and pembrolizumab (Keytruda). In their drug form, these are highly toxic for many patients. However, in The Moss Method, we suggest using natural agents to accomplish the same goal in a non-toxic way.

COMPARING THE MOSS METHOD WITH ONCOLOGY

Mainstream Oncology: The treatment of cancer involves highly specialized and complicated fields of surgery, radiation, and chemo (which come in various types— classical cytotoxic, targeted agents, and immunotherapy). These approaches have led to significant advancements in cancer survival rates and are based on rigorous scientific validation and clinical trials. For example, targeted therapies like trastuzumab (Herceptin) for HER2-positive breast cancer have shown remarkable success (Slamon 2001).

The Moss Method is focused on prevention, of both occurrences and recurrences of the disease. So they are not directly comparable. But let's explore some ways The Moss Method differs in a broad philosophical sense from the approaches that most oncologists commonly practice.

Mainstream Oncology: Mainstream cancer doctors may use natural products based on thorough scientific research, clinical trials, and studies rigorously reviewed by peers. Drugs that began as natural compounds, like paclitaxel, docetaxel, cisplatin, and vincristine, have been tested to prove their safety and effectiveness.

A so-called "active ingredient" is typically extracted, purified, and modified to develop a patented drug. But at the same time, the majority of people who take it experience side effects, such as nerve damage (peripheral neuropathy) or bone marrow suppression.

The Moss Method: Generally, our preventative approach is based on much the same scientific data as conventional oncology. However, while mainstream oncology embraces the use of cellular poisons, which may be derived from natural substances, our method is defined by its very low side effect profile. This is logically necessary by the aims and philosophy of The Moss Method. In my view, it is the only appropriate approach to preventing the occurrence and recurrence of cancer.

The U.S. Food and Drug Administration (FDA) accepts many items that we include in The Moss Method as *Generally Recognized as Safe (GRAS)*. However, the agency's GRAS list is far from comprehensive, since a substance's inclusion on the list must be initiated by a manufacturer, and not the agency itself. This greatly limits its scope.

In most cases, there is prima facie evidence of safety for the ingredients that form the core of The Moss Method. For instance, numerous studies have demonstrated the safety and efficacy of turmeric (curcumin) in reducing inflammation and supporting immune function. Similarly, green tea (EGCG) has been extensively studied for its anticancer properties.

This evidence is based on the fact that billions of people have used items such as turmeric, soy, and green tea for thousands of years without any sign of toxicity. The Moss Method aims to stay safe and to follow the teachings of Hippocrates (460-377 BCE) who wrote in his work, *On Epidemics*, that physicians had "two special objects in view with regard to disease, namely, to do good or to do no harm" (Schwartz 2004).

Mainstream Oncology: Many drugs derived from natural products are incorporated into standard cancer treatments, often used alongside surgery, radiation, or other chemo drugs. This combination is carefully planned based on solid evidence about the effectiveness and safety of these drugs when used with standard treatments.

The Moss Method: There are two basic spheres of cancer treatment: (1) The usual medical treatments of surgery, chemo, radiation, and now immunotherapy; and (2) What the World Health Organization (WHO 2023) calls the "traditional, complementary, and integrative medicine" approach. The Moss Method is grounded in science, guiding traditional therapies that doctors might not use in mainstream cancer care. These include a broader range of diet, lifestyle, and holistic methods.

For example, acupuncture, originally from Traditional Chinese Medicine, is now widely accepted in mainstream medicine for pain management and reducing side effects of cancer treatments like nausea from chemotherapy. Meditation, yoga, tai chi, and nutritional therapy have become critical to cancer care at many centers. Aromatherapy, massage, and hypnotherapy are also common.

Memorial Sloan-Kettering Cancer Center (MSKCC) is a prime example of this shift. I well remember what happened to my friend and colleague, William R. Fair, Jr., MD, chair of the Sloan-Kettering urology department, when he tried introducing a yoga course for patients there. Dr. Fair, a renowned surgeon, was himself diagnosed with

116

colon cancer in the 1990s. He underwent conventional treatments but experienced a recurrence. Seeking complementary therapies, he incorporated yoga, meditation, and dietary changes into his regimen, experiencing positive results. He then suggested introducing a yoga course for cancer patients at MSKCC. Initially, he faced fierce opposition from colleagues and administrators. (I remember his utter dismay when a pilot program was abruptly canceled just hours before it was set to begin.)

His more conventional colleagues did not view yoga (an ancient exercise and meditation practice) as a legitimate approach to healing. Despite this fierce initial resistance, Fair gathered support from other patients and clinicians who recognized the potential benefits of yoga for managing stress, anxiety, and physical side effects of cancer treatment. With persistent advocacy and growing patient interest, MSKCC finally approved a pilot yoga program in 1997. This program proved successful, demonstrating improved patient well-being and offering them a valuable coping method. Today, yoga is an accepted part of MSKCC's Integrative Medicine Service. In fact, they extol its use for nine different conditions from anxiety to generalized stress.

This service provides several treatments that were once seen as "alternative" and, therefore, unacceptable. Jun Mao, MD, head of this service at MSKCC, has noted, "Memorial Sloan Kettering has led the way in combining complementary medicine with standard care." MSKCC offers various therapies, including acupuncture, massage, meditation, and, of course, yoga. Rocco Caputo, a therapist at MSKCC, points out that "every treatment is tailored to the patient," emphasizing their approach to personalized care. This degree of integration and customization was not even dreamed of when I started as a science writer at MSKCC half a century ago, showing progress in cancer care by combining the best of mainstream and "alternative" medicine.

Mainstream Oncology: The main goal is to eliminate cancer by using treatments backed by solid evidence and medical approval. Such treatment may include surgery, radiation, chemo, hormonal agent and targeted drugs (designed to specifically identify and attack specific molecules on cancer cells), as well as immunotherapy.

The Moss Method: While valuing the importance of ridding our bodies of cancer cells, The Moss Method sees a gap in the usual approach, especially with advanced cancer or even some early-stage cancers where recurrences are common. In our opinion, this gap often involves a lack of recognition of the importance of cancer stem cells (CSCs), rare cells in a tumor that can renew themselves and drive tumor growth.

There is robust laboratory research on using natural methods to attack CSCs, which we shall deal with in this book.

Additionally, The Moss Method puts a lot of emphasis on improving life quality, managing side effects, and boosting the overall well-being of patients through a more holistic approach. This approach includes changing diet and lifestyle and using complementary therapies. Integrative Medicine Services may advise on such changes in large cancer centers or specialized holistic care clinics. *But many patients do not have access to that sort of professional advice.* Much of this approach is about self-help, enabling patients to make positive changes in their diet and lifestyle to aid treatment and recovery. This, too, is the essence of The Moss Method. While some critics may argue that integrative approaches lack the same level of scientific validation as conventional treatments, it's important to recognize that our method complements rather than replaces traditional therapies, including standard advice on cancer prevention. We advocate for a collaborative approach where patients benefit from the best of both worlds, guided by scientific evidence and clinical experience.

Mainstream Oncology: In mainstream cancer care, choices made by the patient are crucial. Patients receive options that are scientifically validated. The decision-making process often includes a detailed review of all available options. After the doctors' recommendation, a skilled medical team administers their treatment. Although patients may actively participate in choosing their treatment, the possibilities presented usually follow established medical guidelines.

The Moss Method: We emphasize ongoing, collaborative decision-making of patients and caregivers throughout the treatment process. This method strongly supports patient autonomy and informed choice, which includes exploring a broader range of treatment options, some extending beyond conventional methods. However, it is important to note that *robust scientific data support my recommended methods.*

Mainstream Oncology: This approach is widely accepted and practiced within the global medical community. Bodies like the National Comprehensive Cancer Network formalize treatments, leading to guideline-driven medicine. The Moss Method, while respecting and often aligning with guideline-driven medicine, aims to improve conventional care. My approach seeks to improve standard practices by integrating all scientifically supported methods, primarily focusing on diet and lifestyle changes.

The Moss Method: I also base my approach on an examination of Hanahan and Weinberg's ten hallmarks of cancer, showing how specific traditional foods and elements can address these hallmarks. Although it may be considered forward-thinking, often ahead of current practices by a decade or more, our approach is scientifically valid and evidence-based. *The methods I advocate, marked by low or no damage, prioritize patient safety and offer potential benefits that align with contemporary scientific understanding.*

CAVEAT: While recognizing the value of traditional, complementary, and integrative methods, it is essential to approach them with a critical eye. All cancer treatments, including complementary and alternative (CAM) methods, should be discussed with healthcare professionals to ensure they are appropriate for each individual's situation and goals. This collaborative approach between patients and healthcare providers is fundamental to ensure that all aspects of care have the best possible outcomes.

CLEAN, TRADITIONAL DIETS & LOCAL ECONOMIES

The influx of ultra-processed foods disrupts traditional diets and local food economies, usually harming ancient food cultures. The concentration of control in food production raises concerns about food security, making communities vulnerable to market changes.

In response to these challenges, a growing movement advocates for sustainable, equitable, and locally focused food systems. This movement supports practices like organic farming and community-supported agriculture. It emphasizes the importance of traditional, whole-food diets and reveals the need for sustainable and health-conscious eating practices.

The global spread of Fast Food Culture, sharply contrasting with clean, traditional diets, is a driver of the epidemic of non-communicable diseases (NCDs). This trend towards more NCDs, marked by a heavy reliance on processed foods high in sugar, salt, and flour, indicates a detachment from clean, traditional food practices.

The fast food market's growth mirrors its profound influence worldwide, with consumers often unwittingly succumbing to health risks due to corporate strategies favoring profit by selling addictive ingredients. Key concerns include the popularity of ultra-processed fast food, the decline in home cooking, and a surge in sugar and refined grain consumption. Even with some attempts by companies to offer healthier options, the trend towards processed, high-carb foods remains dominant.

Clean, traditional diets promote better health and support sustainable, culturally rich food habits by emphasizing unprocessed foods. Adopting a clean, traditional diet involves not just choosing healthy foods but also preparing them in healthful ways.

Nutritional education is critical in guiding people to use the best ingredients and cooking methods. However, ingredient availability and time constraints can block adherence to these traditional eating patterns. Research shows that older, more affluent individuals are more likely to adhere to a clean, traditional diet, possibly due to having more time for home cooking (León-Muñoz et al., 2012). Overcoming these challenges may involve using local produce and recipes that adhere to a traditional diet's principles of simplicity and seasonality (Trichopoulou 2014).

EVOLUTIONARY ADAPTATION & ANTICANCER PLANT CHEMICALS

Historically, diets consisted mainly of unprocessed or minimally processed foods. Our ancestors' diets were also rich in what we now recognize to be natural cancer-fighting ingredients. This contributed to lower cancer rates than at present.

While humans evolved in an environment that naturally reduced cancer and other diseases, the introduction of refined carbs like sugar and white flour marked the beginning of a generalized decline in health. Starting in the late 18th century, and more particularly in the last 50 years, the clean, traditional eating pattern drastically changed, first in affluent countries, and then in the rest of the world. This shift has marched hand in hand with an increase in chronic non-communicable diseases (NCDs).

The Centers for Disease Control and Prevention (CDC) notes that NCDs, such as cancer, heart disease, respiratory disease, and diabetes, are now the leading global cause of death, surpassing infectious diseases worldwide.

PLANTS' NATURAL DEFENSE METHODS

What makes a clean, traditional diet so beneficial? It is about the nutrients and how these foods interact with our bodies. Just like animals, plants have developed innate strategies against predators over centuries. These are the plant defenders. (The technical term is phytoalexins.) Plant defenders are natural compounds that plants produce to defend against threats such as germs and environmental stressors (Baur 2006b). These compounds are crucial in a plant's defense against invading microorganisms or predatory insects (Jeandet 2014).

Two German scientists introduced the concept of phytoalexins over 80 years ago. They discovered that potatoes infected by a particular microbe produced a chemical plant defender, which protected the plant from further infection (Müller 1940). Plant defenders are thus part of a plant's broad defense strategy against various germs, including bacteria, fungi, and viruses (Kuc 1984).

But it turns out that these same plant defenders can also improve human health, particularly in resisting and fighting cancer. Here are some of the methods of this surprising effect:

Antioxidant Properties: Plant defenders like resveratrol and curcumin have strong antioxidant qualities, reducing cell damage from oxygen linked to DNA damage and cancer development (Pandy 2009). Antioxidants, often found in fruits and vegetables, can prevent or slow cell damage caused by harmful free radicals.

Anti-Inflammatory Effects: Chronic inflammation contributes to cancer development. However, some plant defenders have anti-inflammatory qualities that help reduce this risk (Pan 2010).

Immune System Improvement: Compounds in garlic and green tea, such as allicin and EGCG, can enhance immune function, helping to eliminate cancerous cells (Nair 2002).

Anti-Metastatic Effects: An anti-metastatic effect is the ability of certain substances to stop the spread of cancer cells. Certain plant defenders may stop cancer cell spread, which is crucial in preventing cancer from becoming more aggressive (Roy 2002).

Cancer Stem Cell Targeting: Some plant defenders attack cancer stem cells. These CSCs, among other things, cause cancer recurrence and treatment resistance (Rayalam 2011).

Metabolic Control: Plant defenders like resveratrol are also involved in energy-related control, essential for cancer prevention as energy-related imbalances can promote tumor growth (Baur 2006a).

DNA Repair: Plant defenders support DNA repair methods, reducing changes that lead to cancer (Holloszy 2007). However, more clinical trials are needed to establish their effectiveness in humans, considering factors like dosage, availability, and individual response.

Blood Vessel Stoppage: Blood vessel blocking is the process by which certain substances prevent the formation of new blood vessels that tumors need to grow. As Judah Folkman, MD showed, blood vessel formation is crucial for tumor growth. Without it, tumors cannot grow larger than the tip of a pencil (Folkman 1992). Some studies suggest that 5-LOX inhibitors might stop blood vessel formation, as a result restricting the tumor's ability to grow and spread.

"Some plant defenders stop the formation of new blood vessels around tumors and for that reason slow cancer growth" (Nijveldt 2001, edited).

Plant defenders are crucial in the fight against cancer due to their diversity of attacks and ability to address cancer's diversity. This makes them a practical alternative to a purely drug approach, which has limitations. A modern update of a clean, traditional diet to include nutraceuticals and selected botanical substances is a practical approach to cancer prevention, a central theme of The Moss Method.

In short, plant compounds found in the nutraceuticals recommended in The Moss Method act as versatile agents for plant self-defense and also demonstrate a remarkable ability to attack abnormal cells in our bodies without harming healthy cells. The Moss Method aligns with evidence that diets evolved over centuries may inherently protect against diseases like cancer.

THE EXAMPLE OF VITAMIN C

Ascorbic acid (also known as vitamin C) is a vital nutrient known for its antioxidant qualities. It is essential for immune function and skin health. Linus Pauling suggested that humans and guinea pigs, among the few animals needing an external source of vitamin C, transferred the responsibility of making it to the abundant plant kingdom. This evolutionary adaptation saved genetic material and energy resources.

However, over time, many people lost access to fresh fruits and vegetables as they pushed on into less fertile regions, sometimes leading to the deficiency disease, scurvy. I see a similarity between this occurrence and our bodies' uses of plant defenders.

This analogy extends to cancer. The clean, traditional diets in the human race's original African homeland were rich in anticancer plant chemicals. **This provided our species with potent natural protection against cancer.**

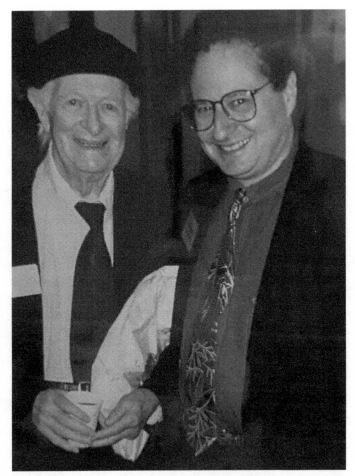

Linus Pauling and Ralph Moss, at a meeting in Tulsa, Oklahoma, November 1992.
Source: Author's collection

The gradual shift to refined white flour and sugar, which started in the late 18th century in Europe, and a gradual departure from fresh, wholesome produce, coincided with increased cancer rates. This change, along with increased exposure to cancer-causing substances (such as tobacco products), aligns with the theory that natural lifestyles of various kinds protect against cancer development.

The shift to modern diets, heavily laden as they are with refined grains and white sugar, represents a particularly dangerous departure from our ancestral dietary roots. This change, and the increased exposure to environmental cancer-causing substances closely corresponds to the rise in cancer incidence. The protective qualities of clean, traditional diets show the vital importance of returning to dietary patterns that align more closely with our physical nature. Embracing these age-old dietary practices, marked by diversity and natural ingredients, may help reduce the risk factors associated with cancer and other modern chronic diseases.

Our collective journey through the intricate relationship between diet and cancer brings us back to a fundamental truth: *Our health depends on the natural world and its bounty.* The culinary wisdom of our ancestors, often overlooked in today's fast-paced world, provides invaluable insights for achieving the best health. Reconnecting with these traditional diets offers a promising path not just in combating cancer but in fostering overall well-being.

In summarizing our exploration into the evolution of dietary patterns and their connection with health, we uncover a profound link between clean, traditional lifestyles and cancer prevention. Age-old, traditional diets exemplify the power of natural, unprocessed foods in maintaining health and preventing diseases, particularly cancer. These diets, rich in fruits, vegetables, fish, and whole grains, constituted a natural defense against cancer by our forebears. We would do well to adopt many of these "old ways" as a modern defense against chronic diseases.

FAST FOOD CULTURE

"The destiny of nations depends on how they nourish themselves."
— *Jean Brillat-Savarin,* The Physiology of Taste *(1825)*

The rise of "Fast Food Culture," as explained by Antonia Trichopolou, Ph.D., a prominent University of Athens researcher, signifies a drastic shift away from traditional (and generally clean) patterns of eating and socializing. Marked by a reliance on overprocessed foods, this trend over the past half-century has reshaped global eating habits dramatically.

Robert H. Lustig, MD, of the University of California, Los Angeles (UCLA), in his immensely popular YouTube video, "Sugar: The Bitter Truth," has defined fast food as without exception *fiber-less* food:

"I dare you to go to any fast food restaurant and find anything on their menu that they actually have to cook that has more than one gram of fiber in it. There isn't any. And that's on purpose, because they take the fiber out. That way they can freeze it, ship it around the world, cook it up fast, and not only is it fast-cooking, but it's fast-eating" (Lustig 2009).

This is a formula for economic success–and nutritional disaster. The fast food industry has a current valuation of nearly $700 billion, which is predicted to increase to $931.7 billion by 2027 (Anonymous 2020). To put this in perspective, this single industry is now worth more than the gross domestic product (GDP) of *all but the top 20 countries* in the United Nations (World Bank 2022).

In the U.S., the cradle of Fast Food Culture, an alarming 36.6% of adults consume fast food daily—a figure echoed globally, with notable increases in countries as far-flung as South Africa and China (Fryar 2018, Popkin 2022). The rapidity of this change is breathtaking. This is perhaps the greatest shift in eating patterns since Neolithic times.

On a personal note, when my wife and I first crossed the U.S. by car in 1966, to take up our residence at Stanford University's married student housing, we encountered our first fast food outlet in Salt Lake City, 2,000 miles from our starting point. This was of course a McDonald's, when the number of burgers sold was still listed beneath the double arches in front of the restaurant.

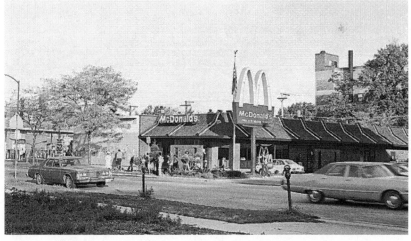

McDonalds used to list how many burgers had been sold. But when it passed a billion they stopped counting.
Source: *Wikimedia Commons*

We ate some hamburgers, remarkable for their saltiness, and then continued to the Bay Area without encountering another fast food restaurant along the way. Of course, not every roadside diner we ate at was a culinary delight, but generally, the food was cooked from scratch with local ingredients. Just as importantly, local diners were not only places to eat but social hubs for many communities across the country.

However, by the 1970s, Fast Food Culture was well on its way to conquering America and then the rest of the world. According to *Time* magazine:

> *"McDonald's managers have taken a familiar American institution, the greasy-spoon hamburger joint, and transforming it into a different though no less quintessentially American operation: A computerized, standardized, premeasured, super clean production machine efficient enough to give even the chiefs of General Motors food for thought" (Anonymous 1973, edited).*

Three decades later, when my son Ben and I drove across the country on a book tour, there were *almost nothing but* fast food restaurants from which to choose. McDonald's still ruled the roost. But Starbucks, Chick-fil-A, Taco Bell, and Dunkin' Donuts were not far behind. The roadside diner had become a "retro" curiosity. Traveling the interstate system in the 1990s, our idea of a "health food restaurant" was Wendy's, because it alone had a salad bar, although it featured iceberg lettuce and pallid tomato slices.

You too may have observed how families, once the cornerstone of culinary traditions and shared meals, have been engulfed in this pervasive corporate culture. The dining room table, once emblematic of a family's solidarity, is now more often than not a platform for computers and bills. The car's interior has become the "dining room" of today, with the drive-thru emerging as our contemporary kitchen. This shift has not only undermined the essence of family meals but also mirrored behaviors disturbingly similar to drug addiction, fueled by the convenience and allure of what the industry calls "quick service" or "pay-before-you-eat" restaurants (Jiao 2015).

But the phenomenon of "fast food" is not just something people get from a drive-thru off the freeway. It also includes things to eat at home, including chips, soda, cookies, candy, breakfast cereals, "protein" bars (loaded with sugar and other carbohydrates), French fries, burgers, pizza, white flour baked goods, and other high-calorie, low-nutrient foods. You can eat them rapidly and they are absorbed very quickly into the bloodstream (Fuhrman 2018).

The fast food business is not only gigantic but it continues to grow. One company, Yum Brands Inc, boasts that it has over 55,000 restaurants in 155 countries and territories, including three of the leading brands in the world, Taco Bell, Pizza Hut, and KFC. Its revenue in 2023 was U.S. $7 billion. In other words, this one company's revenue was greater than the gross domestic product (GDP) of more than 30 entire countries. And there are more than a dozen such fast food conglomerates now straddling the globe. Geographically, they range from a Subway sandwich shop in Alaska, 330 miles north of the Arctic Circle, to a Pizza Hut in southern New Zealand, 8,300 miles away.

The domination of fast food, propelled by this dirty dozen of expanding multinational corporations, has far-reaching consequences—eroding biodiversity, spreading plant monoculture (the cultivation of a single crop in a given area), and presenting huge challenges to small-scale farmers. Furthermore, the environmental effects of long-distance food transport, coupled with aggressive marketing, have set in motion a litany of health issues, including the twin epidemics of obesity and diabetes.

I do not think that we as "political animals" (as Aristotle called us) can do much to influence this trend, at least in the short run. Fast food has been woven into the American way of life. It is almost synonymous with America. I will never forget the look of confusion on our companions' faces on a ride from Guangzhou to Xi'an, China, when we refused their generous offer of KFC and Coca-Cola and asked for Chinese food instead. However, we, as individuals, can at least save ourselves from the ravages of Fast Food Culture by making consistently better food and lifestyle choices. This is a part of The Moss Method. Avoid all fast food outlets and over-processed foods. Instead, adopt a clean diet that is most appropriate to your circumstances. Then augment that wholesome diet with carefully selected nutrients from around the world.

The Moss Method is of course focused on the risk of cancer and its recurrences. However, it is noteworthy that **the same program that prevents the occurrence of cancer also prevents numerous other serious conditions**, such as heart disease and diabetes. It also has a positive effect on longevity. You could therefore also call it a "Save Yourself Diet" as much as an anticancer program.

RISE OF COUNTER MOVEMENTS

I am not alone in rejecting Fast Food Culture. As a reaction to the subjugation of our best food traditions, there has been a rise of various counter-movements. These take many forms, such as the farm-to-table movement, slow food, and an ever-increasing interest in organic and locally sourced foods. By choosing to resist the convenience of fast food and embracing the principles of The Moss Method, we can each make a powerful statement for our health and the health of our families.

A CLEAN, TRADITIONAL DIET

> *"Diet is among the most important influences on health in modern societies. An injudicious diet is among the leading causes of premature death and chronic disease. The best eating practices are associated with **increased life expectancy** and the dramatic **reduction in one's lifetime risk of all chronic disease**."*
> —*David L. Katz, MD, MPH, Yale University (2014 edited)*

The foundation of The Moss Method is adherence to a "clean, traditional diet." This refers to a way of eating that emphasizes whole, unprocessed foods similar to those consumed by previous generations before the advent of modern food processing and industrial agriculture. The term "traditional" reflects a return to the eating habits of earlier times when diets were naturally rich in nutrients, varied, and closely tied to seasonal and local food sources. This type of diet focuses on natural foods, organically grown (wherever possible), and minimally processed, with an emphasis on preserving nutritional value and avoiding additives, pesticides, and genetically modified organisms (GMOs).

The key traits of a clean, traditional diet include:

- *Whole Foods:* Favoring foods in their natural state or with minimal processing. This includes whole grains, legumes, nuts, seeds, fruits, and vegetables.

- *Organic and Locally Sourced:* Whenever possible, choose organic foods to reduce exposure to pesticides and support local farms to ensure freshness and minimize the environmental impact of transportation.

- *Sustainable Seafood and Grass-fed Meats:* Opting for wild-caught, sustainable seafood and meats from animals that have been pasture-raised or grass-fed, which are often higher in helpful nutrients like omega-3 fatty acids and lower in contaminants.

- *Healthy Fats:* Incorporating sources of healthy fats such as olive oil, avocados, and nuts, while avoiding trans fats and limiting saturated fats.

- *Limited Added Sugars and Refined Carbs:* Reducing intake of added sugars and refined grains, such as white bread and pasta, in favor of whole, complex carbs.

- *Fermented and Traditional Foods:* Including fermented foods like yogurt, kefir, sauerkraut, and kimchi, which support gut health, alongside traditional staples of various cultures that have been shown to offer health benefits.

- *Herbs and Spices:* Use herbs and spices not only for flavor but also for their health-promoting qualities, as many contain antioxidants and anti-inflammatory compounds.

- *High fiber content:* Favor foods rich in fiber to support digestive health and promote a feeling of fullness, which can aid in weight management. Dietary fiber, found in roasted chicory root (inulin), fruits, vegetables, whole grains, and legumes, plays a crucial role in maintaining heart health and adjusting blood sugar levels.

A clean, traditional diet is also not just about what is eaten, but also how it is prepared and consumed. It encourages cooking from scratch, mindful eating, and enjoying meals with others as part of a healthy lifestyle. This approach to eating is aligned with many principles of sustainable living, emphasizing the environmental and social impacts of food choices.

In essence, this type of diet seeks to reconnect individuals with the origins of food and its preparation, promoting a healthier relationship with food that is both nourishing and sustainable. This way of eating is flexible and can be adapted to fit various cultural traditions and personal preferences, making it a potentially enriching approach to nutrition and overall well-being.

One question I grappled with as I began this project was why not center it around the Mediterranean Diet? After all, *U.S. News & World Report* has ranked it the "best diet overall" in the world for the year 2024. But even they caution about the misinterpretation of this diet:

"It's also a top-rated diet for those looking for a heart-healthy diet, a diabetes-friendly diet or to promote bone and joint health. But don't confuse Americanized Mediterranean menus – which often feature too much refined pasta, beef and cheese – with healthy eating."

So the "Mediterranean Diet" that they advocate is actually an idealization of what certain public health experts think the American or European public should be eating, rather than a strict set of rules based on actual current practices. As U.S. News correctly states, there isn't actually a single Mediterranean Diet.

"Greeks eat differently than Italians, and Turks eat differently from the French and Spanish. There's even a Costa Rican version of the Mediterranean diet."

While the general contours of the Med Diet are reasonable, I find the whole concept to be disturbingly Eurocentric. After all, every culture on earth has something to recommend it, and the point of The Moss Method is to discover and share those elements that have been shown to have the greatest positive impact on cancer. But how can you do that if you limit yourself to just one traditional dietary pattern? Yes, we want the benefit of extra virgin olive oil (EVOO), which is a prominent part of the cuisine and the economy of countries bordering that vast inland sea. But we also need contributions from other regions and climes. We must also have yogurt and kefir from the Caucasian mountains, turmeric/curcumin from India, tofu and soy products from China, Gyokuro tea from Japan, to name just a few.

I believe that any traditional diet, once cleaned up, can serve as a framework for a program aimed at cancer prevention. To this foundational diet, however, I add selected nutraceuticals and plant chemicals, each backed by substantial scientific research for their potential to address cancer's underlying methods. It is crucial to recognize the role of diet in cancer therapy.

(See our discussion, A Global Approach that follows.)

The research into plant chemicals that attack CSCs underscores the potential of natural compounds found in traditional diets, like the Mediterranean diet, in supporting cancer treatment. These diets, rich in plant-based foods, offer a wealth of bioactive compounds that may aid conventional therapies by attacking the very methods that allow CSCs to drive disease growth and resistance. As we shift focus from the specific actions of plant chemicals in a clinical context to the general principles of traditional diets, it becomes apparent that these eating patterns embody more than just nutritional guidelines; they represent a holistic approach to health that has been sustained across cultures and generations.

This perspective not only enriches our understanding of diet's role in cancer prevention but also reveals the importance of integrating traditional dietary wisdom into contemporary cancer care strategies.

A traditional diet is more than a health-focused eating plan. It is an embattled way of life in many countries around the globe. We can take, as an example, the famous Mediterranean diet, which is a heavily curated version of a traditional dietary pattern.

One very important takeaway from the Mediterranean diet is that it favors extra virgin olive oil (EVOO), as well as fruits, vegetables, whole grains, legumes, fish, and nuts. It involves a relatively low use of red meat, dairy, sweets, and moderate red wine intake with meals (Bloomfield 2015). This, at least, was the case in Italy, Spain, Greece, and a dozen other countries before the invasion of what is called the "quick service restaurant industry." But according to a report on the website Statista.com:

> *"The revenue of the quick-service restaurant industry in Spain continued to increase in 2022, surpassing by nearly 16% the 2019 figure. In total, this restaurant segment generated around 4.7 billion euros of revenue in the European country" (Lopéz 2023).*

When I speak about the "Mediterranean Diet" I am speaking about a historical phenomenon that has to be reinterpreted to conform with the beliefs of contemporary health authorities and experts.

As a result, Antonia Trichopoulou, Ph.D., has described the Mediterranean Diet as the dietary pattern prevalent in **olive-growing regions during the late 1950s and early 1960s.** This time was before American-style Fast Food Culture took hold in many places. Trichopoulou (2001) makes the point that the diet in the Mediterranean region *today* bears little resemblance to the diets of yesteryear.

When I speak of the diet of a particular region I am talking about a *traditional* diet, part of the so-called "old ways," which contrasts with modern Fast Food Culture. As a side note, my wife and I experienced this cuisine on our first trip to Europe (which included several months in Greece) in 1966. We have since returned to the

Mediterranean area several times. The diet and lifestyles we encountered on that first trip bore little resemblance to the Fast Food Culture that increasingly encroaches on that way of life, which Trichopoulou deplores.

The Moss Method generally avoids all ultra-processed foods, trans fats, refined grains, and sugar in many forms. This method is international, cosmopolitan, and highly adaptable since it encompasses many different culinary practices from not just southern Europe, northern Africa, and western Asia but from the rest of the world. My approach includes essential contributions from China, India, and Japan (for example).

But The Moss Method is more than a diet. It is a summation of our global cultural heritage with scientifically supported food and supplement recommendations. It embodies the ancient Greek concept of "diaita" (δίαιτα), integrating food, physical activity, and overall lifestyle for balance and harmony.

Central to The Moss Method are fresh, seasonal foods. Unlike the typical Western diet's emphasis on heavily processed and adulterated foods, The Moss Method necessarily includes a healthy portion of extra virgin olive oil (EVOO) and fish rich in omega-3 fatty acids. I do not suggest taking up the alcohol habit for health reasons. But if you already consume alcohol without experiencing any negative effects, I suggest a moderate intake of red wine with your meals. Resveratrol is the leading healthy compound in red wine (as well as in grape juice and peanuts).

Admittedly, the amount of resveratrol in wine is rather small. But if you are going to drink alcoholic beverages, you should concentrate on American Pinot Noir, or its French equivalent, Burgundy.

WHOLE FOODS FOCUS

Clean diets all have a whole foods focus, emphasizing unprocessed foods, which are rich in nutrients and low in artificial additives and preservatives. They limit refined sugars and grains. This minimizes the intake of refined carbs and sweeteners, which are linked to various health issues, such as type 2 diabetes (T2D). Very importantly, they incorporate traditional sources of natural fats.

Natural fats are typically extra virgin olive oil from the Mediterranean region, but also fatty fish and other sources of omega-3 fatty acids (as in the Nordic diet), avocados (a Mexican discovery), and butter from grass-fed cows. Animal fats such as butter and lard were usually stored and cherished. They emphatically did not know such modern innovations as ultra-refined vegetable cooking oils, partially hydrogenated vegetable oils, or rancid fats of any kind.

The re-use of vegetable oils by fast food restaurants is a particular health concern. Fast food chains, by the nature of their high-volume frying operations, often reuse oils multiple times. This practice is driven by economic considerations but can lead to the accumulation of harmful byproducts. But when oils are repeatedly heated, they undergo chemical changes that produce harmful compounds, such as trans fats and polycyclic aromatic hydrocarbons (PAHs). These compounds have been linked to various health issues, including increased risks of cardiovascular diseases and cancer. Studies have found that oils used in fast food restaurants often exceed safe limits for these harmful compounds, posing health risks to consumers. Therefore, it's important for fast food establishments to manage oil use carefully to minimize these risks.

Clean diets incorporate fermented foods, which we now know support gut health by enhancing the microbiome. By necessity, they focused on foods that were in season and locally sourced, supporting both nutritional content and environmental sustainability. They intuitively grasped the importance of eating in moderation to maintain a healthy body weight and prevent overuse. In many cultures, gluttony was a sin.

Above all, they championed the role of meals in fostering community connections and cultural traditions, which contribute to overall well-being. Communal meals have been an essential part of human culture, serving as a means to strengthen community bonds, celebrate important events, and express cultural and religious identities.

These principles support physical health and align with sustainable and environmentally conscious food practices, showcasing the wisdom embedded in clean diets for our contemporary health challenges. We cannot of course time-travel our way to before the introduction of Fast Food Culture. Nor do I forget all the negative elements in our culture at that time–when, for example, 42% of the U.S. adult population smoked tobacco (U.S. Department of Health 1964). In the U.S. at least, the variety and often the quality of produce is much better than it was 50 or so years ago.

But we can–and should–reintroduce some of the helpful aspects of food culture from that period because it aligned better with our physiology and human health in general. The general idea is to *clean up* traditional diets to benefit from the health-promoting qualities and minimize harm.

A GLOBAL APPROACH

The concept of a "clean, traditional diet" is applicable to different regions and populations, reflecting local agriculture, cultural practices, and historical influences. While modern globalization and urbanization have introduced processed foods into almost every corner of the world, including the Mediterranean, there remain areas where traditional dietary practices are still closely followed.

Innumerable sources are urging us to adopt a Mediterranean diet. These include the World Health Organization (WHO), the American Heart Association (AHA), and the National Cancer Institute (NCI). Here is how the NCI describes the Mediterranean Diet:

"The diet plan includes olive oil, fish, legumes, whole grains, and fruits and vegetables. It is low in n-6 polyunsaturated fats (PUFA) and high in plant-based foods and monounsaturated fats (MUFA) [such as extra virgin olive oil, ed.].

"Specifically, the daily dietary goals are to consume seven to 10 high-MUFA foods, one to two servings of dark green vegetables, one to two servings of orange and yellow vegetables, one to two servings of red vegetables, one to two servings of other vegetables, one serving of dark green culinary herbs, a liberal portion of allium vegetables, two servings of fruit (one serving of vitamin C fruit and one serving of other fruit), and three or more servings of whole grains. In addition, foods high in omega-3 [such as fatty fish, ed.] should be consumed at least twice per week" (NCI 2023a).

Studies have shown that strict adherence to the Mediterranean diet can indeed reduce the risk of cancer death by up to 23% in women and 24% in men (Liese 2015). Cancer survivors following healthy diets also had up to an 18% lower death risk from all causes (Morze 2020, Morze 2021).

According to several studies, people who strictly follow the Italian version of the Mediterranean Diet have a 50% reduction in overall cancer risk, a 56% reduction in the risk of colon cancer, and a 59% reduction in rectal cancer (Agnoli 2013.) We ignore such astounding results at our peril.

Scientists from the University of Navarra, Spain, have written:

> *"The Mediterranean Diet is defined as a traditional eating pattern found among populations living in the Mediterranean Basin during the 50s and 60s of the 20th century,* **but, unfortunately, not today"** *(Martínez-González 2019).*

But, as good as the Mediterranean diet may be, the fight against cancer transcends any specific country or regional tradition. So pomegranate, chia, quinoa, turmeric, spirulina, and many other nutraceuticals bring unique anticancer qualities from around the world. Their inclusion in The Moss Method represents our globally inclusive approach to nutrition, where many different foods contribute to cancer prevention and health improvement. This broad perspective shows the importance of exploring and integrating global nutritional wisdom in our collective battle against cancer, embracing various natural, health-promoting foods worldwide.

The Moss Method is meant to help people all over the world who are trying to prevent an occurrence or recurrence of their cancer. We live in the age of social media, where information flows at lightning speed around the globe.

Our company, *The Moss Report*, has had an internet presence since 1995, and has colleagues and connections all over the globe. So although based in the U.S., we are international in our outlook. This doesn't mean that we favor the homogenization of cultures that is characteristic of globalization. *We believe that people should cherish what is helpful in their cultural traditions relating to food. This is not a negation of the Mediterranean diet, but advocates its inclusion as a well-researched form of a clean, traditional diet.*

This doesn't make any one diet a panacea for people all over the globe. It is ludicrous to tell natives of, for example, Japan, South Korea, East Africa, or South America that they should abandon their own traditions and adopt the diet of the Mediterranean instead. There is simply no good reason for them to do so.

Most of the time people are most comfortable with their native cuisine. And since there are good features to be had in all traditional food cultures and traditions, it is better to build on those traditions than to dogmatically adhere to a different tradition.

People can also construct perfectly good health-promoting diets based on their own national or regional dietary regimens. We agree with the members of the Danish Cancer Society who wrote:

> *"Attempts should be made to* **promote a healthy regional diet, instead of promoting a Mediterranean diet worldwide;** *this might ensure the compliance of people of lower socio-economic status and also ensure cultural diversity, respect for heritage, and protection of the environment" (Kyrø 2013).*

All traditional cultures around the world have much to offer. As David L. Katz, MD, of Yale University, has put it:

> *"***The established superiority of any one specific diet over others is exaggerated.*** The weight of evidence strongly supports a theme of healthful eating while **allowing for variations** on that theme. A diet of minimally processed foods close to nature, mainly plants, is associated with health promotion and disease prevention" (Katz 2014, edited).*

The UNESCO Chair at the University of Naples also has recognized the impracticality of exporting the diet of one particular region to fundamentally different cultures. They advocate a Mediterranean-type diet that is appropriate to different cultures, "by using the food products available in the different areas of the world." They called this new model the 'Planeterranean' diet, a word that combines the words "Planet" and "Mediterranean" (Colao 2022). This is fully in line with The Moss Method.

THE BLUE ZONES

A useful way of understanding the international dimensions of health is to study the so-called Blue Zones; these are regions identified by longevity researchers where people live longer lives, often with less chronic disease. The diets in these areas, such as Okinawa (Japan), Sardinia (Italy), Nicoya (Costa Rica), Icaria (Greece), and Loma Linda (California), emphasize fresh produce, whole grains, and healthy fats, with a focus on plant-based foods and small amounts of red meat.

- *Okinawa, Japan:* The traditional Okinawan diet is low in calories yet nutrient-rich, including a variety of vegetables (notably sweet potatoes), legumes (especially soy in the form of tofu), and fish, with minimal meat and dairy intake. Okinawans also practice "Hara Hachi Bu"" eating until they're 80% full.

- *Sardinia, Italy:* Particularly in the mountainous Barbagia region, in the heart of Sardinia, the diet leans heavily on whole-grain bread, beans, garden vegetables, fruits, and in particular, a type of Locatelli Pecorino Romano cheese made from grass-fed sheep's milk. There is also a moderate intake of wine.

- *Nicoya, Costa Rica:* The diet, from Costa Rica's Pacific coast, is based on staples like corn, beans, rice, squash, and tropical fruits. The inhabitants consume legumes and whole grains, with a focus on fresh, local products.

- *Icaria, Greece:* Icaria is a small island in the Aegean Sea, near Samos. The inhabitants consume a Mediterranean diet that includes a lot of wild greens, legumes, potatoes, goat milk, and honey. They also use a lot of olive oil and some wine.

- *Loma Linda, California:* This community in San Bernardino County consists largely of Seventh-day Adventists, many of whom follow a vegetarian diet rich in fruits, vegetables, nuts, and whole grains, adhering closely to their religious beliefs about health and diet.

GLOBAL SOLUTIONS TO PREVENT CANCER & IMPROVE HEALTH

Each traditional diet is "clean," in that it emphasizes whole and minimally processed foods, and healthy fats, alongside moderate use of animal products.

(See my discussion of the Question of Red Meat.)

The health benefits of all of these diets are supported by a variety of research studies, mainly population-based in nature, showing their potential to reduce the risk of chronic diseases, improve lifespan, and promote overall health. Avoiding a strict adherence to any one diet, The Moss Method takes a mixed or eclectic approach, leveraging key elements from traditional cultures across the globe. This powerfully bolsters the diet's role in sustaining and restoring health for cancer prevention. My approach is underpinned by the incorporation of hundreds of medical research papers, which demonstrate how dietary ingredients can combat ten hallmarks of cancer.

Starting with lifestyle modifications, I advocate the avoidance of fast food and a shift back toward the diets that people ate for thousands of years—a regimen abundant in minimally processed whole foods.

Historically, the act of sharing meals with friends and family was and is important. This sharing not only strengthened family bonds but also nurtured well-being. It was epitomized by the "Roseto Effect," a long-forgotten concept that is discussed later in this work.

NUTRACEUTICALS OF THE MOSS METHOD

The Moss Method is a dietary and lifestyle program that has been carefully designed to not only be effective at preventing cancer but to cause the least possible damage to the individual and to society. In my view, that is the only sort of prevention program that is sustainable over a person's lifetime. In fact, it should not just be sustainable, but enjoyable, because the more pleasant a regimen, the more likely it is to be maintained.

As we explore the details of this method, let's start by emphasizing the nutraceuticals on which it is based. We have divided these into two categories. The first ten primary substances are things **we try to get every day.** The secondary ones are elements we try to get a few times per week. These foods and food groups come from different parts of the globe, but all are crucial to the various clean, traditional diets that contribute to *The Moss Method*. They are essential for anyone using a dietary approach to cancer prevention, regardless of which traditional diet serves as their starting point.

This chapter includes information on the rationale, modes of action, and specific clinical trials in support of these measures. This will provide a look at how these chemicals function at the molecular level, their impact on cancer markers, as well as information on enhancing their availability. This section also discusses the synergy of substances to increase their effectiveness, grounded in research studies and clinical trials. It also contains practical info on availability and challenges.

HOW DOES IT WORK?

We could in fact write a separate book on the intricate dance of chemicals involved in our program. But in a work intended for a broad non-specialized audience, such a level of detail would be unnecessary and counterproductive.

There are at last count about 1,400 natural medicines and supportive therapies available in the U.S. (NatMed 2024). One can't discuss all of them, of course, nor are they of equal importance. So I lay particular emphasis on those easily available *plant chemicals that attack cancer stem cells* (CSC). This narrows the field considerably.

It is important to note that research in this area is ongoing, and scientists around the globe are still exploring the effectiveness and methods of these and other agents. Before launching into our discussion of the elements, I want to address a common criticism of our approach. Some people believe that we should hold off before implementing any program that has not gained FDA approval and other signs of wide-scale acceptance.

THE PRECAUTIONARY PRINCIPLE

This is where I apply the Precautionary Principle. In the late 20th century, environmentalists suggested the Precautionary Principle. According to a classic declaration:

> *"Where there are threats of serious or irreversible damage, lack of full scientific certainty shall not be used as a reason for postponing cost-effective measures to prevent environmental degradation" (Gollier 2011).*

Or, according to another classic definition:

> *"A lack of full scientific certainty should not be used as a reason for postponing measures to avoid or minimize such a threat," in the case of threats to the environment (NOAA 2024, edited).*

I would argue that the same logic applies to many time-honored diets, such as the Mediterranean Diet, and to most *Generally Recognized as Safe* (GRAS) dietary substances. The Precautionary Principle impels us not only to avoid harm–its usual interpretation–but also to **embrace harmless things that could be of great benefit.**

The preponderance of evidence proves that the approaches suggested in this book are harmless and are associated with a reduced risk of cancer and other diseases. It is therefore justifiable to embrace this approach in advance of conclusive proof of its effectiveness through randomized clinical trials. There is little to lose and potentially much to gain by doing so.

A NOTE ON ORGANIZATION

In this section of The Moss Method, I have sorted 20 plant chemicals into two groups: Primary and Secondary Elements. I have sorted them, roughly speaking, in order of importance. I have made these determinations by looking at how much published research there is, how consistent the results have been, and how much they help in preventing and managing cancer.

I will be the first to admit there is an element of subjectivity in this selection. Also, these lists are dynamic, in the sense that new research is constantly emerging. For example, while I was writing this book, over 1,800 PubMed articles have appeared in PubMed that at least mention the topic of curcumin, or about six every calendar day. So inevitably even the most conscientious researcher will have to impose order on this mass of data, and that involves some subjectivity.

For that reason, this list reflects my own understanding of the strength, importance, and promise of the various elements. For example, I put sulforaphane and olive oil into the first rank, reflecting what I take to be the high quality of the data on each of these, such as the outstanding work at Johns Hopkins University on broccoli sprouts or the PREDIMED clinical trial of olive oil in Spain (Toledo 2015). It also reflects on my intuitive sense of what is most likely to be effective based on 50 years of research into the world literature and conversations with thousands of cancer patients.

THE 10 PRIMARY ELEMENTS

The 10 Primary Elements are plant chemicals that have shown consistent, robust, and promising results across a variety of study types. These compounds not only have a higher volume of supportive research but also have effectiveness in cancer risk reduction according to current scientific understanding, such as an understanding of the molecular targets involved in their action. This robust data and the substantial anti-cancer potential they present make them foundational to The Moss Method. They are emphasized for their critical roles and are essential for anyone looking to incorporate anticancer strategies into their daily regimen. **I consider this section the core of this book and of The Moss Method, more generally.** On a personal note, on most days I prepare and eat food and drink for my wife and myself that includes most of the primary elements mentioned in this book.

In considering these elements, I have used a combined reductionist and organicist approach. For example, we note that curcumin, derived from turmeric, specifically inhibits the NF-κB pathway, which is crucial for cancer cell survival and proliferation (Singh & Tuli 2022). This sort of insight is typical of a reductionist approach, reducing a substance's effects to the smallest element. And we rely on many such studies to build a picture of curcumin's beneficial effects.

However, within The Moss Method, we also realize that curcumin is also part of a broader organicist strategy. Organicism means, essentially, that wholes are greater than the sum of their parts. Organicists believe that the whole system has properties that cannot be explained by simply studying its individual components. Furthermore, the parts of a system are interconnected and interdependent and a change in one part affects all the other parts. Thus, we believe that all the elements in turmeric are greater than the effects of isolated chemicals. We also believe that the ingredients in a well-prepared meal, or for that matter, an entire cuisine, are more powerful than any particular ingredient.

In our method we are seeking to maximize synergy, and therefore include compounds from various cultures, such as EGCG from green tea and resveratrol from grapes, to create a comprehensive defense against cancer. We respect the granular details that reductionism provides, but we harness that to a higher purpose—which is to create an entire program that will seriously impact one's chances of avoiding the occurrence or recurrence of "the dread disease" (Patterson 1987).

1. EXTRA VIRGIN OLIVE OIL (EVOO)

The Mediterranean diet is celebrated for its health benefits, particularly in preventing chronic diseases. There are sixteen countries and one overseas territory (Gibraltar) that border the Mediterranean Sea. But, reduced to its simplest form, one thing they all have in common is the liberal use of olive oil. And not just olive oil, but its highest grade, which is called Extra Virgin Olive Oil (EVOO). EVOO is not only a fundamental culinary ingredient but also a source of crucial plant chemicals, which have been recognized all over the world for their cancer-fighting qualities and many other health benefits (Marshall 2024).

THE HEALTH BENEFITS OF EVOO

EVOO's class of antioxidants (called polyphenols) play a crucial role in reducing cell damage from oxygen and inflammation, two processes in the development of diseases such as cancer and heart disease. The PREDIMED trial shows that a Mediterranean diet enriched with four or more tablespoons of EVOO per day reduces the risk of breast cancer among women. Specifically, incorporating this much EVOO daily led to an astonishing **68% reduction in breast cancer risk** (Toledo 2015).

To underscore these results, this randomized controlled trial (RCT) paper was published in the prestigious *JAMA Internal Medicine* and had 21 authors affiliated with 19 separate institutions, including Harvard School of Public Health, Brigham and Women's Hospital, and Harvard Medical School, all of Boston, Massachusetts. The paper in question has been viewed over 84,000 times and has been cited over 300 times by other authors.

The antioxidant qualities of EVOO are pivotal in protecting cells from damage that could lead to cancer and other diseases. These benefits are primarily ascribed to several antioxidants in EVOO, which improve heart health and improve overall well-being by combating inflammation. (As we have explained, chronic inflammation, as part of the tumor microenvironment, is considered the "seedbed of cancer.")

Extracting oil from the fruit of the olive tree (*Olea europaea*) was among the first signs of civilization and one of the main items of trade in the ancient world; it is still a huge part of the economy of many of the Mediterranean-area countries. Even today, thousands of years later, it is a major item of trade. The global EVOO market is substantial and experiencing steady growth. In 2023, the market was valued at approximately US $9.5 billion and is projected to grow to around US $10.08 billion in

2024. By 2032, it is expected to reach US $14.41 billion, exhibiting a compound annual growth rate of about 5.30% (Fortune 2024).

Naturally, there is also a chance for organized crime to take advantage of the worldwide demand for good quality oil from the leading producers. According to 60 Minutes, there is a criminal enterprise involved in the production and distribution of counterfeit or adulterated food products, particularly olive oil. Because many consumers are willing to pay a premium for good quality oil, a lot of the EVOO that winds up in restaurants and kitchens has been secretly diluted with cheap vegetable oils. This makes the consumer's task difficult, but not impossible. Finding genuine EVOO involves a combination of sensory, chemical, and regulatory considerations.

Taste: From a sensory point of view, genuine EVOO should have a fruity taste characteristic of fresh olives. There is a particular sensation that is associated with EVOO that is high in healthy chemicals, which is a tickling, peppery or even a pungent or bitter sensation in the back of the throat. EVOO should never taste rancid, musty, or sour, as these are signs of oxidation, fermentation, or poor-quality olives.

Seals of approval: Look for quality seals or certifications from reputable organizations such as the North American Olive Oil Association's (NAOOA) *Certified Quality Seal* in the U.S., PDO and PGI labels the European Union, or the DOP seal in Italy. I generally avoid blends of oils from different countries, such as you commonly find in supermarket brands.

Harvest date: Check for the harvest date on the label. Unlike wine, olive oil does not improve with age, and only a harvest date from the previous fall's harvest indicates the product's freshness and therefore its relatively high polyphenol content. Avoid oil that only has a "best-by date," as this tells you nothing about when and how the olives were harvested or the oil was produced. (The oil should be extracted without heating within hours of the harvest.)

In the Northern hemisphere, including the three main European producers (Spain, Greece, and Italy), the olive harvest begins in the Fall and new products begin to appear on shelves in Europe and America in January. So come the New Year, you should ask for a product that has a harvest date of the previous year, and not a year or so earlier. The exception to this rule is for oils that originate in South America. Their harvest begins in April and stretches into July. Their products start showing up in the market in the Fall.

Shopping tips for olive oil: Securing a fresh product can be challenging. For example, in the spring of 2024, I visited a market chain that boasts a wide selection of EVOOs from renowned olive-growing regions. It looks like a gourmet selection on the shelf. But *all* the bottles and tins that I checked had a harvest date from the fall of 2022, not the expected 2023.

Also, because of EVOO's relatively high prices, it is tempting to look for bargains. But be aware that grocers often discount their older stock to clear shelf space for fresher products. These older oils have lost some of their beneficial polyphenols (Mancebo-Campos 2023). So steer clear of them.

A good strategy is to purchase directly from producers online. Engage with the manufacturers to confirm the harvest and pressing dates, and inquire about the total polyphenol content and specific amounts of hydroxytyrosol and its derivatives in 20 grams of olive oil. They know this, but they are not always willing to share it with the consumer.

The EU permits health claims for olive oil only if it contains at least 5 milligrams (mg) **of hydroxytyrosol** and its derivatives per 20 grams of oil.

To expect health benefits, consumers should get a minimum of 20 grams of EVOO daily, which equals about one and a half tablespoons (Mancebo-Campos 2023). Ideally, consume this quantity **raw** to maximize health benefits, as cooking can destroy about half of the beneficial compounds. But remember that the breast cancer preventive quality of Spanish EVOO in the PREDIMED trial was correlated with a consumption of **four or more tablespoons** per day.

Robust-flavored oils typically have higher polyphenol content; some we've found online contain over 600 milligrams per kilogram (mg/kg), with a **hydroxytyrosol content of 9.0 mg per 20 grams**—double the amount required by European law to make health claims. For cooking, less concentrated and less expensive EVOOs are typically used.

Single source: You want, if possible, to know the specific source of the olive oil. The more generic the oil, the greater the chance that it has been mishandled. The best oil comes from single estates, but that is rare. Next in quality is EVOO from a particular designated region. Then come oils from a particular state or country. Finally there are blends from various regions or even continents.

You must be cautious, because fakes abound. One common trick is to stamp "product of Country X" on the label. But this doesn't necessarily mean that the olives in question actually *grew* in Country X. They might have been imported from anywhere around the world and then bottled in a country known for its excellent EVOO. Sometimes there are little two letter abbreviations of the country of origin on the bottle (good luck in interpreting these cryptic signs). According to news reports, some oils can sit in the hull of a ship for years, before being foisted off as "fresh EVOO" on unsuspecting customers abroad.

WHAT ARE POLYPHENOLS?

Most of the antioxidants in EVOO are classified as polyphenols. These are natural pigments that give some flowers, fruits, and vegetables, including olives, a great variety of colors. They have a basic chemical structure that includes rings—think of them as little circles made up of carbon atoms. Attached to these rings are other molecular parts made of oxygen and hydrogen. These structures help polyphenols act as antioxidants, where they protect our cells and keep us healthy.

There are at least 16 polyphenols in EVOO. **The overall polyphenol content is the single most important thing to know about the healthfulness of any particular olive oil product.** Unfortunately, very few EVOO labels state their polyphenol content. This in part because that number fluctuates depending on the condition of the olives at the time of the pressing of the olives. The temperature used in the pressing and other factors involved in the conversion of the fruit into "juice" can also affect the polyphenol content. But manufacturers or importers could more generally give the latest "certificate of analysis" (COA) results of the oil. This provides a great deal of information, not just on polyphenols but on acidity, peroxides (a measure of harmful oxidation), pesticide residues, contaminants, and the like.

Companies do not generally release this information, even if you ask for it. They (and, sadly, many consumers) seem more focused on the creative label designs than the scientifically verified analysis of the container's content.

But we are not completely in the dark. An independent testing lab has analyzed the polyphenol content of a dozen EVOOs typically available to American or European consumers. Leaving aside a single oil that enhanced its product with powdered olive leaves (a cheap source of some antioxidants), the polyphenol content ranged from as little as 149 milligrams per kilogram (mg/kg) for an North Africa EVOO to an impressive 441 mg/kg for an American brand, _Life Extension California Estate Extra Virgin Olive Oil_.

I have used this Life Extension Foundation oil and in general have been very pleased with it. (By way of transparency, I am on the LEF's scientific advisory board.)

146

(The independent testing lab analysis is available to consumers, but is part of a paid subscription. See Cooperman, 2024, in our Bibliography.)

You should be able to call or email the various manufacturers and ask their customer representative for the polyphenol content of their products. This should be contained in the certificate of analysis. California Olive Ranch (which also owns the Italian-origin brand, Lucini Extra Virgin Olive Oil) was particularly forthcoming with results when I did so. Any company's inability or refusal to provide such information may be indicative of problems with the product, which I would therefore avoid.

DAILY INTAKE RECOMMENDATIONS

Integrating EVOO into your diet isn't just about using it in your cooking; it is about making it a staple of your entire dietary regime. You should strive to *have some raw olive oil on a daily basis*–**between one and four tablespoons** per day. I not only cook with olive oil, but add it raw to many dishes, such as tabbouleh, to vinegar-and-oil salad dressings, or add it at the last minute to many cooked dishes.

There is no FDA or USDA established recommended daily requirement for EVOO or polyphenols. We have mentioned the PREDIMED clinical trial in Spain (Toledo 2015, Estruch 2018). Participants in the EVOO arm of that study were recommended by the scientists to take *four tablespoons per day* or more of the high quality Spanish EVOO supplied as part of the study.

In another study, in *JAMA Internal Medicine,* the dose was almost the same four tablespoons per day for men and three for women (Ferrara 2000). This study was highly positive for lowering blood pressure compared to people getting equivalent amounts of sunflower oil.

NUANCES OF FLAVOR

Different EVOO brands have nuances of flavor that I find fascinating to explore. At the moment, I am using EVOO from Spain, Greece, Italy, Palestine, and California, which I choose based on the taste enhancement I am looking for. I am presently using a Spanish oil that I purchased at a small food market in my town; some *California Olive Ranch* propellant-free spray; a Spartan oil that comes from a farm owned by the proprietors of a local Greek restaurant; some California oil from Life Extension EVOO (mentioned above); an Italian oil that I bought online; and another Greek oil that I also bought online because of its freshness and proven polyphenol content; and both *Graza* oils— Drizzle" for dressing, and "Sizzle" for cooking, which won the *New*

York Times product review website's recognition as "the best all-around olive oil you can buy at the store." (They did not consider the polyphenol content.)

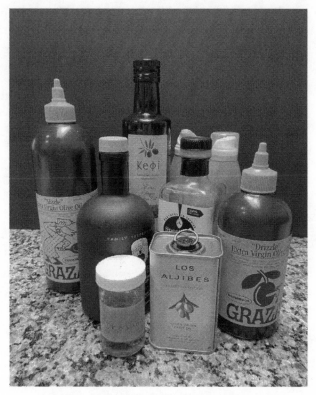

Some of the olive oils in the Moss household pantry.

It is a common misunderstanding that EVOO cannot be used in cooking because of a low smoke point. Actually, EVOO works fine for sautéing foods. But you should use it at low to medium heat to maintain its polyphenol content, about half of which on average is lost in the heating process.

The widespread acclaim of EVOO is well-deserved. Its benefits extend beyond just enhancing food flavor—it is a powerful health ally against chronic diseases, particularly heart disease and cancer. The PREDIMED trial and other studies provide compelling evidence of its protective effects, particularly through its rich polyphenol content. As part of a balanced diet, EVOO can offer health benefits, making it a central part of health-conscious dietary practices worldwide. It is also the key ingredient that binds the various national variations together to make up the Mediterranean Diet.

Guasch-Ferré Study (2022)

A study from the famed Department of Nutrition, Harvard T.H. Chan School of Public Health, Boston, found that higher consumption of extra virgin olive oil (EVOO) is associated with a significantly lower risk of total and cause-specific mortality among U.S. adults. Involving over 60,000 women and 30,000 men, the study revealed that those who consumed **more than half a tablespoon of olive oil per day** had a 19% lower risk of cardiovascular disease mortality, 17% lower risk of cancer mortality, 29% lower risk of neurodegenerative disease mortality, and 18% lower risk of respiratory disease mortality compared to those who rarely or never consumed olive oil. Additionally, substituting 10 grams per day of margarine, butter, mayonnaise, or dairy fat with olive oil was linked to an 8%-34% lower risk of total and cause-specific mortality, underscoring the potential health benefits of replacing less healthy fats with olive oil in the diet. (Guasch-Ferré 2022)

2. GREEN TEA (EGCG)

Green tea is globally recognized not only for its cultural and historical significance but for its health-promoting qualities. It contains several powerful chemicals, a type of polyphenols called **catechins,** the most abundant of which is epigallocatechin gallate (EGCG). This potent ingredient plays a pivotal role in cancer prevention, particularly through its ability to target and disrupt cancer stem cells (CSCs).

(Catechins are natural antioxidants of the flavonoid family found in various plants, which help protect cells from damage and may provide health benefits such as reduced inflammation and lowered risk of certain diseases. Some other dietary sources are berries, pomegranate seeds, apples, grapes, pecans, and hazelnuts.)

A great deal of research shows EGCG's ability to block many of the cell signals that help cancer cells grow and spread (Kciuk 2023). It can thereby help prevent various types of cancer, including breast, prostate, and colorectal cancers.

Between 8 and 12 ounces of high quality green tea taken every day is an essential part of The Moss Method. We suggest taking this first thing in the morning, before breakfast.

The Bettuzzi Clinical Trial (2006)

An important clinical trial from Parma, Italy, in the flagship journal of the American Association for Cancer Research, explored the effects of green tea catechins on prostate cancer. Researchers found that these compounds were highly effective in preventing cancer in men at high risk. Specifically, men with a precancerous condition of the prostate gland called PIN showed a dramatic decrease in cancer development when treated with GTCs.

In this double-blind study, 60 men with PIN were divided into two groups: one group received daily GTC capsules (600 milligrams total), while the other received an inactive placebo. After one year, scientists looked at the incidence of prostate cancers in the two groups. According to their article in *Cancer Research:*

> *"After one year, only one tumor was diagnosed among the 30 green tea extract-treated men (the incidence was approximately 3%), whereas nine cancer cases were found among the 30 placebo-treated men (for an incidence of 30%)"* *(Bettuzzi 2006, edited).*

This first-of-its-kind study not only confirmed the safety and effectiveness of green tea in preventing a prostate cancer-related condition but also noted improvements in symptoms of benign prostate hyperplasia (BPH), which is a non-cancerous but often troublesome enlargement of the prostate gland that commonly affects men as they age. No significant side effects of the green tea extract were reported (Bettuzzi 2006). Although cited in over 260 other scientific publications, according to clinicaltrials.gov, there has been no follow-up with larger Phase III clinical trials of this concept.

Henning Study (2015)

In a study at the University of California, Los Angeles (UCLA) exploring the potential of green tea and black tea in preventing prostate cancer, 113 men with the disease were divided into three groups. Each group consumed either six cups of brewed green tea, black tea, or water daily before undergoing surgery for prostate cancer. The main goal was to observe changes in cancer markers in the tissue of the participants when they subsequently underwent surgery for prostate cancer (Henning 2015).

The findings showed that drinking green tea significantly reduced inflammation markers (specifically nuclear factor kappa B or NFκB) in the prostate tissue compared to the group that drank water. Green tea also reduced oxidative stress in the body, as indicated by lower levels of markers of oxidation in the urine.

Additionally, 32 out of 34 participants who drank green tea had detectable levels of tea polyphenols in their prostate tissue and experienced a small but significant *decrease* in the levels of prostate-specific antigen (PSA), a marker often used to diagnose and monitor prostate cancer.

Black tea did not show the same beneficial effects as green tea (ibid.)

The article was published in the journal *Prostate* in 2015, but has not been further pursued at UCLA or elsewhere to our knowledge. To paraphrase a comprehensive review article from 2024:

> *"Drinking green tea may lower the risk of developing prostate cancer, including its more aggressive forms. Lab studies show that components of green tea can inhibit tumor growth, trigger cancer cell death, and affect key biological pathways involved in prostate cancer development and progression. Clinical trials and human studies also support these findings, showing that green tea consumption is linked to lower levels of prostate-specific antigen (a marker for prostate cancer) and other tumor markers, suggesting that green tea might help slow the progression of the disease" (Liu GH 2024).*

A COMPARISON OF GREEN TEAS

Choosing a high-quality bulk green tea is based on a combination of its EGCG (and overall polyphenol) content, as well as its flavor profile. Since this is something we recommend taking every day, it is important that you enjoy it. Here is a breakdown of the main varieties of bulk green teas on the market:

Matcha

- *Polyphenol Content:* Very High

- *Characteristics:* Bright green, powdered tea with a rich, creamy texture and a slightly sweet, grassy flavor. It involves consuming the whole tea leaf in powdered form, which provides a concentrated source of nutrients and antioxidants. (A great source of polyphenols, but *definitely an acquired taste. We do not recommend starting your acquaintance with green tea with home-brewed Matcha tea.*)

Gyokuro

- *Polyphenol Content:* High
- *Characteristics:* Deep green, needle-shaped leaves with a smooth, umami-rich (savory) flavor. It is shaded for about three weeks before harvest which increases its amino acids and reduces bitterness, enhancing its sweet notes. *(Author's note: this is our household's regular early morning tea.)*

Kabusecha

- *Polyphenol Content:* Moderately High
- *Characteristics:* Similar to Gyokuro but with a shorter shading period (about one week), leading to a slightly lighter flavor that balances sweetness with a touch of astringency, and a fresh vegetal quality. (*Less expensive than gyokuro.*)

Sencha and Shincha

- *Polyphenol Content:* Moderate

Characteristics: The most popular tea in Japan, Sencha, has a refreshing, grassy, and slightly sweet flavor. It is grown in full sun, resulting in a bright green color and a well-rounded flavor profile that includes a pleasant vegetal bitterness.

(In the Spring, we drink Shincha, which is the first tea harvest of the year in Japan. These are extra-high-quality leaves, which are tender and rich in nutrients. But the taste is more mild and subtle than Gyokuro. Unless you live in Japan you will probably have to buy this online.)

Bancha

- *Polyphenol Content:* Low
- *Characteristics:* Harvested later than Sencha, Bancha leaves are larger and have a coarser feel. The flavor is milder and somewhat grassier compared to Sencha, with a light astringency and a woody, slightly nutty undertone.

Hojicha

152

- *Polyphenol Content:* Low
- *Characteristics:* Roasted green tea with a reddish-brown color and a toasty, caramel-like flavor. The roasting process reduces caffeine content and bitterness, making it mild and smooth with a comforting warmth. A nice drink, but too low in polyphenols to be your daily drink.

Genmaicha

- *Polyphenol Content:* Low
- *Characteristics:* A blend of green tea, usually Bancha or Sencha, and roasted brown rice. It has a light-yellow hue and a distinctive nutty flavor. The rice adds a rich and popcorn-like taste, which complements the astringency of the green tea. People who do not generally like green tea sometimes find this variety desirable. *(We like this as well and since its caffeine content is low, we can drink this later in the day without upsetting our sleep cycle. But not a sufficient source of polyphenols for daily consumption.)*

Chinese Green Teas (e.g., Longjing, Bi Luo Chun)

- *Polyphenol Content:* Variable (Moderate to High)
- *Characteristics:*
  - *Longjing (Dragon Well):* Known for its flat, spear-shaped leaves and a gentle, sweet flavor that sometimes exhibits a slight bitterness. It has a soft, orchid-like aroma with a clean finish. *(Note: We were first introduced to high-quality green tea at the Kempinski Hotel in Beijing. But in general, we find Chinese green teas to be far less subtle or enjoyable than the Japanese.)*
  - *Bi Luo Chun:* Spirally shaped leaves that unfurl when brewed, known for its delicate floral aroma and a crisp, vegetal flavor with a lingering sweet aftertaste.

Brewing Tips

- As with olive oil, you should attempt to get the latest season's crop. In Japan, the green tea harvest typically starts in mid-May and lasts for a few weeks. This period is known for the picking of the freshest tea leaves, often called Shincha, which is prized for its superior flavor and nutrient content. Shincha starts to become available online in the first few weeks of June. In the premier Kyoto region, the harvesting season includes several rounds throughout the year, with additional harvests in summer and fall for other types of green tea.

153

- Leaf teas like Gyokuro, Kabusecha, and Sencha are best brewed at lower temperatures (60-70° Celsius) for 1 to 3 minutes depending on personal taste preferences, which allows their delicate flavors and antioxidants to infuse the water without releasing too many tannins.

- Obtain the freshest green tea you can afford. If you are used to the price of supermarket tea bags you may experience "sticker shock" when you see how much you have to pay for high quality bulk teas. But green tea is one area where, if possible, you do not want to economize. If you must, the latest tests of which we are aware ranks Trader Joe's Organic Green as tops for polyphenol content. But in our opinion the taste profile is

A Dollop of Pepper Sauce

According to the research of Professors James and Dorothy Morré of Purdue University, the anticancer effect of green tea is greatly increased by taking it with a little of the plant chemical capsaicin from red peppers. Their pepper of choice was guajillo, which they chose because it was the mildest red-pepper they could find. I had no trouble finding guajillo chili powder over the Internet, and use it regularly. As the Morrés wrote in 2006:

> "*EGCG and red pepper chemicals together are* **10 to 100 times more effective** *than either is alone" (Morré 2006, Hanau 2014, edited).*

Other research shows that in a study of micronutrients, the most potent two item combination was EGCG and vitamin C. They were particularly effective at inhibiting chemicals that promote the "invasion and metastasis of malignant tumors" (Roomi 2010).

I have only found one product on the market that contains both guajillo pepper extract and vitamin C. It is **Cholula Hot Sauce Chili Lime®.** I routinely take a dollop of this on a postage stamp-size bit of cracker just before drinking a pint or so of green tea in the morning.

THE "BROWNING" OF GREEN TEA

The "browning" of green tea after it stands for a while is a phenomenon related to the tea's chemical composition and the brewing process. This change in color is primarily due to the oxidation of healthful compounds (polyphenols) found in the tea leaves.

But the change is more than cosmetic; it reveals important insights into the tea's quality, flavor profile, and potential health benefits.

According to Chinese researchers:

"Light, temperature, and acidity affect the color of green tea infusions by shifting its color from bright green to yellowish/brown, which lowers its quality" (Dai 2017, edited).

Some teas (especially from cheap tea bags for sale in supermarkets) are not green at all but emerge a murky yellow/brown color. Others start out green but turn yellow/brown within a few minutes. This color change indicates the rapid oxidation ("rusting") of chlorophyll and other compounds. One of these is EGCG, which is a powerful antioxidant.

The browning of green tea is usually a sign of oxidation that can lead to the degradation of desirable compounds, including both chlorophyll and EGCG. Exposure to air, light, or prolonged heat during storage can also trigger oxidation reactions, leading to changes in the chemical composition of the tea. To maximize the amount of EGCG and other antioxidants, green tea should be stored in a cool, dark place, in an airtight container to minimize exposure to air. While the browning of green tea may indicate a loss of some antioxidants, it does not necessarily mean that all health benefits are lost. However, for the greatest benefits, fresher, properly stored green tea is preferable.

High temperature water also changes the color of tea from green to yellowish/brown. It is, therefore, essential to keep the temperature of the tea water below 70° Celsius 158° Fahrenheit), and to avoid all old or stale products. When you brew tea, you should not subject the tea to boiling water. This is not good for either the tea or your esophagus since esophageal cancer has been linked to the habitual drinking of very hot tea.

The International Agency for Research on Cancer (IARC) has classified all hot drinks at temperatures above 65° Celsius (149°F) as possibly cancer-causing in humans. This classification is based on studies that have found a higher risk of esophageal cancer associated with the drinking of very hot beverages (Loomis 2016). This is indeed why I aim for a brewing temperature of 64º Celsius (147°F) for my Gyokuro each morning, which is warm enough to be pleasant but not so hot that it could cause heat damage–to me or to the tea itself.

Thermal injury to the esophagus can cause chronic inflammation and increased cell turnover, which may therefore increase the risk of cancer (Islami 2009). It is important to note that it is the temperature of the beverage *at the time of ingestion* (i.e., drinking), rather than the specific type of beverage, that is the key factor in this increased risk.

In short, when it comes to green tea, do not settle for inferior products, when really high-quality ones are available over the internet for most consumers. And brew it with the utmost care, for the sake of both the tea and your anatomy. It will take a little effort to get really excellent green tea, but it will certainly be worth it.

THE ISSUE OF LIVER TOXICITY

According to a scientific panel of the European Food Safety Authority (EFSA), an intake of 300 milligrams of EGCG per day (which they defined as a moderate intake) was *Generally Recognized as Safe* (GRAS). Since eight fluid ounces of green tea provides an average of 168 milligrams of EGCG, one should be able to safely consume slightly more than *12 fluid ounces per* day without risk. This is enough to reap its health benefits without risking the potential side effects that are associated with higher doses (EFSA 2018). However, EGCG supplements may contain more than this, and such products should be approached with caution.

It may surprise people that there have been cases of elevated liver enzymes in people taking excessive amounts of green tea extract, which is defined as over 800 mg of EGCG per day. To be sure, the literature on green tea consumption and its effects on the liver is mainly positive in nature. But high-doses of chemically extracted EGCG and other catechins can be a problem.

A 2018 review of 159 studies concluded that some concentrated, catechin-rich green tea preparations resulted in liver problems when ingested in large single doses. But this did not occur when EGCG was obtained through brewed tea or as part of food. The authors suggested that a safe level of EGCG is approximately 700 milligrams per day (Hu 2018). Others state that problems could start at 800 mg of EGCG (the pure chemical, mind you, not the amount of liquid tea) per day.

So what about my recommendations of a daily intake of green tea? Is this risky? The amount of EGCG in various green teas varies. But a reasonable estimate is that 12 fluid ounces of Gyokuro tea from Japan contains between 120 and 240 milligrams of EGCG. The exact amount will vary depending on the specific variety of tea and how it is brewed. But even at the high end for Gyokuro, this is well within the upper end of the safe limit. Genmaicha has less EGCG (since it contains toasted rice kernels) and

Matcha has more (because it is made from powdered leaves). But most people only consume about two to four ounces of Matcha. As a general rule you will be within the safety zone if you limit your intake to **no more than 12 ounces per day.**

Given the widespread occurrence of non-alcoholic fatty liver disease (NAFLD), which now affects about one-third of the world population, it is a good idea not to put any additional stress on your liver by taking more than the safe amount (Wong V 2023). Plus, despite what some people may tell you, a purified chemical EGCG is not the same as a finely brewed cup or two of green tea. It certainly isn't as pleasurable.

If you want to make sure, you should pay attention to your liver enzyme scores on your next annual physical. You should ask your primary care physician (PCP) with help in interpreting these results. They are generally designated as ALT, AST, ALP, and GCT. These can be elevated for a variety of reasons, but you should definitely discuss your green tea consumption with your PCP if they are.

On a personal note, I have never heard of anyone having elevated liver enzymes just from drinking high quality green tea. However, cheap supermarket green tea bags can have numerous problems, including pesticide residues and micro plastics. So pay close attention to what you are putting in your body, and always emphasize quality.

DIETARY SYNERGIES

Research continues to explore the ways through which EGCG interacts with cancer and other health challenges. Innovations in how EGCG can be formulated to improve its absorption are also ongoing, which may eventually lead to more effective methods of cancer prevention and health maintenance.

EGCG stands out as the principal ingredient in green tea with profound health benefits, especially in cancer prevention. Don't take it alone, but remember that green tea also contains other potentially beneficial compounds abbreviated EC, ECG, and EGC.

Green tea's integration into your daily routine will not only add to your enjoyment but also contribute to health improvement. By maintaining a reasonable intake of up to 12 fluid ounces per day and staying informed about the latest developments, you can maximize green tea's anticancer potential while enjoying the cultural and culinary delights that it has to offer. This approach ensures that it can be a safe and effective addition to one's regimen, with many health benefits, particularly for those trying to prevent cancer.

3. CURCUMIN/TURMERIC

Turmeric has been used for its medicinal and culinary properties since ancient times, with evidence of its use dating back to at least 2,500 BCE in regions near modern-day New Delhi. This long-standing incorporation into Ayurvedic (traditional Indian) medicine shows its importance in ancient health practices and their enduring relevance in modern times.

The World Health Organization's Regional Director for Europe, Hans Kluge, recently supported the integration of traditional practices into modern medical models; he recognized the potential benefits that natural products hold for contemporary health issues (Kluge 2023). The use of turmeric certainly fits into that picture.

Research into the topic of curcumin, the main ingredient in turmeric, is certainly robust. There are almost 25,000 articles that at least mention the topic of curcumin in PubMed, about one-third of which concern cancer. For the half century between 1949 to 1999, articles on curcumin appeared at a rate averaging ten per year. Now they appear at a rate of over six per calendar day.

Curcumin has a remarkably broad range of beneficial effects. These are too extensive to review here. However, according to the MSKCC "About Herbs" website (where it is discussed under the heading of "Turmeric"), research suggests that turmeric may help with depression, improve cognitive performance in elderly Asians, and alleviate symptoms of gastrointestinal issues, irritable bowel syndrome, and ulcerative colitis. It can reduce arterial stiffness in type 2 diabetes patients and benefit children and adolescents with asthma. Turmeric is also safe and effective for treating knee osteoarthritis but does not affect knee effusion or cartilage. Topical turmeric can also reduce vitiligo lesions.

Combined with aerobic exercise, it improves vascular function in postmenopausal women. However, its effects on cholesterol are inconsistent. Both turmeric and curcumin may help with non-alcoholic fatty liver disease. Curcumin combined with antipsychotics can aid in managing chronic schizophrenia and reduce inflammation markers and triglyceride levels in hemodialysis patients.

TURMERIC & CANCER

Turmeric and its curcumin-like compounds (called curcuminoids) have been shown to kill cancer cells in more than half a dozen ways. These include:

- Cell cycle control
- Triggering programmed cell death
- Reducing cell growth
- Enhancing cell survival
- Preventing invasion
- Blocking blood vessel formation
- Halting cancer spread
- Reducing inflammation (PDQ 2024)

Preliminary research suggests that turmeric supplements can improve quality of life and blood parameters in breast cancer patients (Kalluru 2020), and reduce hand-foot syndrome rates following the standard drug capecitabine (Scontre 2018).

In a small clinical study from the M.D. Anderson Cancer Center on advanced pancreatic cancer, a very difficult situation, curcumin was well--tolerated and showed promising results. One patient experienced stable disease for over 18 months, and another saw a significant 73% reduction in tumor size. Additionally, curcumin was found to reduce levels of harmful proteins associated with cancer progression. These findings suggest that curcumin could offer potential benefits for pancreatic cancer patients, providing hope for improved outcomes with this natural supplement (Dhillon 2008).

In a study on post-menopausal breast cancer patients taking hormonal therapy, a combination of hydroxytyrosol (from olives), omega-3 fatty acids, and curcumin was tested for its effects on inflammation and pain. After one month, patients saw a significant drop in C-reactive protein (CRP) levels, a marker of inflammation, from an average of 8.2 mg/L to 5.3 mg/L. Pain scores also improved, showing less discomfort. The treatment was well-tolerated with no major side effects, and those with the highest baseline CRP levels experienced the most significant reductions (Kanai 2010).

(We discuss the 2019 Leicester, UK, clinical trial of curcumin with standard FOLFOX chemotherapy, elsewhere.)

Despite its proven benefits, curcumin, an active ingredient in turmeric, suffers from poor availability. This means that when consumed in traditional forms, curcumin's absorption into the bloodstream is minimal, which could seemingly contradict the claims of its health benefits.

To overcome this challenge, research has focused on improving how well curcumin can be absorbed when ingested. One effective strategy is the addition of piperine, an active ingredient of black pepper, which has been shown to increase curcumin's availability **20-fold,** at least compared to when curcumin is consumed on an empty stomach (Shoba 1998).

Consistent with practices from the Leicester clinical trial, consuming curcumin with a fat-rich meal, such as those containing extra virgin olive oil (EVOO), also enhances its absorption due to curcumin's fat-soluble nature (Howells 2019).

To further address the availability issue, several specialized formulations have been developed:

- *C3 Complex:* This formulation includes three different curcumin-like substances and piperine to improve absorption and effectiveness.

- A specially formulated type of curcumin mixed with lecithin improves how it is absorbed by the digestive system (Matthewman 2023).

The typical dosages for curcumin supplements range from 500 to 2000 milligrams (mg) per day. These dosages typically include substances like piperine that help the body absorb the drug, which is crucial for its effectiveness. In fact, it is rare these days to find a curcumin supplement that has not been chemically modified to enhance absorption.

Curcumin is generally safe; however, it can improve the effects of blood thinners and antidiabetic drugs, and may interact with drugs that deliberately suppress the immune system (such as those used by transplant recipients). Therefore, talking to healthcare providers before beginning any new supplement regimen is crucial (Howells 2019).

Adding turmeric to foods not only enhances their flavor but also contributes health benefits, particularly when included in golden milk or savory dishes. These uses allow for the integration of curcumin into daily diets and reflect its role in both traditional and modern healing practices (Matthewman 2023, Kroon 2023).

Case Study from the University of Newcastle (2019)

A pivotal clinical trial at the University of Newcastle, NSW, Australia, tested curcumin's availability in three different forms—fresh grated turmeric root, turmeric powder, and pure curcumin powder. The study found that:

- Turmeric powder increased blood curcumin levels compared to other forms.

- The matrix effects of the various plant chemicals in turmeric improved curcumin's usability in the body (Nasef 2019).

Turmeric and its most active ingredient curcumin have evolved from ancient remedies to staples in modern supplement arsenals, demonstrating the potential of traditional practices to improve contemporary medical treatments. Through advanced formulations and proper dietary practices, the benefits of curcumin can be maximized, making it a valuable part of preventive health strategies and adjunctive therapies for various conditions.

A NOTE ON PIPERINE

Piperine, a substance found in black pepper, significantly increases how well our bodies can absorb nutrients, especially curcumin from turmeric, making it up to 20 times more effective (Shoba 1998). It works by slowing down the breakdown of curcumin in the body, allowing more of it to enter the bloodstream and be more effective. Typically, supplements suggest taking 5 to 20 milligrams of piperine, usually together with curcumin, to get the most health benefits.

Piperine's effectiveness stems from its ability to:

- Stop certain liver processes that break down drugs.
- Block mechanisms that eject drugs and other substances from cells.
- Help the body absorb nutrients better.
- Increase blood flow to the digestive system and make it easier for the intestines to absorb what we eat and drink.

These methods ensure that substances like curcumin are less broken down in the body and are more available for absorption.

Incorporating black pepper in recipes not only adds flavor but also contributes to improved nutrient uptake. Creative uses include seasoning for eggs, avocado toast, and additions to beverages like Golden Milk.

(See our discussion and recipe for The Moss Method Golden Milk.)

High-quality supplements verified for purity and potency are recommended, and users should be aware of potential interactions with drugs due to piperine's effect on nutrient absorption.

Historically, black pepper has been highly valued not only for its flavor but also for its preservative qualities and health benefits. Ancient texts such as India's *Charaka Samhita* (an ancient Sanskrit text of Ayurvedic medicine) and traditional Chinese medicine have documented black pepper's health-enhancing qualities, including its anti-inflammatory and digestive stimulant effects (Norouzkhani 2022).

In ancient Europe, pepper was a culinary luxury as well as a healing item, used for its health-enhancing qualities, even before its biochemical nature was understood. This deep-rooted historical value reflects not only trade but also in its enduring application in health and cuisine.

Piperine's role in enhancing the effectiveness of anticancer agents and other nutrients by facilitating their absorption makes it a critical ingredient in dietary supplements. Its combined culinary, preservative, and drug qualities have made it a substance of immense value across different cultures and eras, underscoring the "coincidence" of its prized status and profound health impacts. This aligns with the historical appreciation of its benefits, which were empirically observed long before the advent of modern scientific research.

---

4. VITAMIN D: THE SUNSHINE VITAMIN

Vitamin D, commonly known as the "sunshine vitamin," is pivotal in the realm of oncology for its potential roles in bone health, immune function, and particularly, cancer prevention. This vitamin, which the body chiefly obtains through sunlight exposure, diet, and supplements, is crucial not just for calcium metabolism but also for its possible anticancer qualities.

Vitamin D exists in two primary forms: Vitamin D2 (Ergocalciferol) and Vitamin D3 (Cholecalciferol). Vitamin D2 is sourced from plants and certain fungi and is not naturally synthesized by humans. It is converted in the liver to 25-hydroxyvitamin D2, an active form used by the body. Found in fortified foods and UV-exposed mushrooms, D2 is less potent compared to D3 but still effective in raising vitamin D levels. On the other hand, Vitamin D3 is the more active form of vitamin D, produced in the skin through exposure to UVB radiation from sunlight. It can also be derived from animal-based foods like fatty fish and egg yolks. Vitamin D3 is converted in the liver to 25-hydroxyvitamin D3, the primary circulating form of vitamin D, and is more effective than D2 in maintaining sufficient levels in the blood.

Research indicates that vitamin D can influence various processes that may prevent cancer development. It promotes the differentiation of cells, reducing the risk of cells becoming cancerous. Vitamin D also exhibits anti-proliferative effects, stopping the growth of cancer cells and reducing their metastatic potential. Additionally, it can initiate programmed cell death, helping to eliminate cancerous cells. Moreover, vitamin D enhances the immune system's ability to detect and destroy cancer cells. Higher levels of vitamin D3 are associated with a reduced risk of breast cancer, with studies suggesting that sufficient vitamin D3 levels can lead to smaller, less aggressive tumors, particularly in premenopausal women (Manocha 2023). Women with higher vitamin D levels at diagnosis have been shown to experience less advanced disease stages and lower recurrence rates (De Sousa 2017).

Early research indicated that higher vitamin D levels might reduce the risk of prostate cancer, although recent studies provide more nuanced results where higher levels may increase the risk of non-aggressive prostate cancer due to detection biases (Travis 2019). Adequate levels of vitamin D are also linked with a decreased risk of colorectal cancer. High serum levels of 25(OH)D, are correlated with better outcomes in colorectal cancer patients, suggesting that vitamin D sufficiency should be maintained to improve prognosis (Chandler 2015).

Vitamin D's role extends to influencing the microenvironment around tumors, particularly affecting cancer stem cells (CSCs), which are crucial for cancer's growth. It may impact CSCs by promoting their differentiation into non-cancerous cells, halting CSCs at specific cell cycle phases to prevent their growth, triggering programmed cell death in CSCs, preventing new blood vessel formation necessary for tumor growth, and improving the immune system's ability to attack cancer cells, including CSCs (So 2015).

For general health, a supplemental dose of 1,000 IU of vitamin D is commonly recommended, though individual requirements, especially in winter months or higher latitudes, might be higher. Routine blood tests to monitor vitamin D levels can help tailor the dosage to achieve the best levels, potentially enhancing cancer preventive effects. Vitamin D3, particularly in its role against CSCs, presents a promising avenue for cancer prevention and treatment. Ongoing research continues to unravel the complex interactions of vitamin D with the cell methods of cancer, showing its potential as a part of integrative cancer therapy strategies. Larger clinical trials and research are needed to establish effective guidelines and harness the full potential of vitamin D in oncology.

BEST USE & DOSAGE

For general health, a supplemental dose of 1,000 IU of vitamin D is commonly recommended, though individual requirements, especially in winter months or higher latitudes, might be higher. Routine blood tests to monitor vitamin D levels can help tailor the dosage to achieve the best levels, potentially enhancing cancer preventive effects.

Vitamin D3, particularly in its role against CSCs, presents a promising avenue for cancer prevention and treatment. The ongoing research continues to unravel the complex interactions of vitamin D with the cell methods of cancer, showing its potential as a part of integrative cancer therapy strategies. Larger clinical trials and research are needed to establish effective guidelines and harness the full potential of vitamin D in oncology.

---

5. CRUCIFEROUS VEGETABLE SPROUTS

"Sprouts are in essence a microcosm of the larger plants which they will grow up to become, but they are fresh, extremely inexpensive, and incredibly fast to grow. Anybody can grow them indoors, anywhere there's a square foot or so of free space, and commercially grown sprouts are widely available."
–Jed Fahey, Sc.D. and Thomas Kensler, Ph.D., Johns Hopkins University, Baltimore (2021)

Sprouts are essentially young plants that quickly grow from seeds and are extremely cost-effective. They require very little space, and with a little practice, are easy to make at home and much more delicious and nutritious. Scientists from Johns Hopkins University, including my summertime neighbor, Paul Talalay, have shown sprouts to be compact powerhouses of nutrients, readily available both home-grown and in stores (Fahey 2021)

There's a strong link between cancer prevention and the *Brassica* family of vegetables, which includes broccoli, cauliflower, kale, Brussels sprouts, and radishes. These vegetables are grouped together as **cruciferous** because their flowers form the shape of a cross ('crux' in Latin). Among them, broccoli sprouts are particularly notable for their health benefits, packed with up to a hundred times more glucosinolate—a key nutrient—than mature broccoli plants (Fahey 1997, Lee 2006).

Though I have aimed to keep technical terms to a minimum in this book, understanding a few key concepts is essential to grasp this important topic:

- *Glucosinolates:* These sulfur-containing compounds are found in cruciferous vegetables like radishes, broccoli, kale, and cabbage, and are of great interest for their potential health benefits, particularly their role in cancer prevention.

- *Isothiocyanates:* These compounds are produced when glucosinolates break down, facilitated by the enzyme myrosinase.

- *Sulforaphane (SF):* This is the most notable isothiocyanate, especially when considering anticancer activity. It's produced in high amounts in broccoli sprouts and plays a key role in fighting cancer. In radishes, a similar but slightly different compound called sulforaphene is produced—importantly, not a typo (Fahey 1997).

SULFORAPHANE: A CRUCIAL CHEMICAL

SF serves as a form of chemical defense for the plant against predators like caterpillars. When these pests chew on the plant, they cause the plant to release SF, effectively acting as a natural pesticide. For humans, SF helps detoxify the body and is safe in consumed amounts. Research by Paul Talalay, MD, of Johns Hopkins Hospital, Baltimore, found that these sprouts activate an enzyme that protects against carcinogens, highlighting the protective effects of SF (Fahey 1997).

(Carcinogens are substances or agents capable of causing or promoting cancer development in living tissue.)

While laboratory tests show that adding an enzyme to broccoli sprouts converts nearly all their glucosinolates into SF, this conversion is more efficient when sprouts are eaten either raw (as in a salad) or warmed (as in the last moments in an omelet). Cooking can destroy myrosinase, thus stalling this conversion, and the presence of epithiospecifier protein (ESP) might convert chemicals called glucosinolates into a less beneficial compound, called SF nitrile, rather than SF (Fahey 1997).

ESP is found in certain vegetables like broccoli, cabbage, and Brussels sprouts. It affects how these vegetables produce certain chemicals when they are broken down. Normally, these vegetables can produce compounds that may help fight cancer. However, when ESP is present, it can change these beneficial compounds into different forms that might not have the same health benefits. So ESP can influence how much of the good, cancer-fighting chemicals we get from eating these vegetables (Matusheski 2001, Matusheski 2004).

While broccoli sprouts are rich in **sulforaphane,** radish sprouts contain **sulforaphene,** a similar compound. Both chemicals are formed when the plant's

165

glucosinolates break down through damage, reacting with the enzyme myrosinase. These compounds are effective in stimulating enzymes that stimulate the removal of toxic compounds, contributing significantly to their anticancer effects (Zhang Y 1992, Posner 1994). Though studies on broccoli sprouts are more frequent, research by Tim J. O'Hare, Ph.D., from the Queensland Alliance for Agriculture and Food Innovation, has demonstrated that *radish sprouts have even greater anticancer potential* (O'Hare 2008, O'Hare 2009, O'Hare 2024).

THE HUMBLE RADISH SPROUT

Radish sprouts, members of the same *Brassica f*amily as the other cruciferous vegetables, come without the complications of making broccoli sprouts as they don't require soaking, a necessary step to remove the ESP. The lack of epithiospecifier protein (ESP), allows them to produce **sulforaphene (SFE)** efficiently without the unwanted conversions to less useful compounds (Fahey 1997).

Moreover, for under $20, you can purchase a pound of radish seeds, about 50,000 to 70,000 seeds, which offers great value and a long-lasting supply. Their sprouts also have a peppery flavor, which many find more appealing than the somewhat bitter taste of broccoli sprouts.

The optimal daily intake of sulforaphane/sulforaphene is estimated between 30 to 60 milligrams. Achieving this requires about three tablespoons of radish sprouts daily, depending on the variety. The more pungent the sprout, the higher its sulforaphene content, thus enhancing its anticancer efficacy. It's crucial to consume these sprouts raw or minimally heated to preserve the sulforaphene content; for instance, if adding them to an omelet, fold them in at the final stage to avoid overheating (O'Hare 2008, O'Hare 2009).

I currently use a mix of three radish seed types: Red Arrow, Purple Triton, and White Daikon. These varieties are chosen for their high levels of glucosinolates, enhancing their health impacts:

- *Red Arrow:* Known for its high glucosinolate levels similar to other red radish varieties.

- *Purple Triton:* Features striking purple stems and a milder flavor, but like Red Arrow, it is high in glucosinolates.

- *White Daikon:* These sprouts from Daikon radish seeds are used widely in Asian cuisine for their flavor and health benefits, particularly their glucosinolates that convert to sulforaphane, noted for its anti-cancer properties.

Radish sprouts offer a nutritious, flavorful, and easy-to-prepare option for enhancing your diet with superfoods. They overcome some biochemical challenges posed by broccoli sprouts, provide substantial nutritional value, and are a delightful addition to meals with their zesty flavor. Whether grown at home or purchased, when incorporated into your diet, radish sprouts are a straightforward and potent health food choice, robust in growth and flavor, alongside their significant health benefits. These qualities make them a superior choice for those seeking practical and effective nutraceutical options.

To maximize the cancer-fighting benefits of cruciferous vegetables:

- Eat broccoli sprouts and radish sprouts fresh, whenever possible.
- Lightly steam rather than boil or fry to minimize the loss of beneficial enzymes.
- Include a variety of these vegetables in your diet to take advantage of their diverse protective compounds.

This approach not only enhances your overall health but also supports a natural and potent defense against cancer development. Understanding these key components and their interactions helps us appreciate the profound benefits cruciferous vegetables offer in cancer prevention and overall well-being.

SAFE HANDLING & USE

Following food safety guidelines when preparing and consuming sprouts is crucial to avoid potential foodborne illnesses. Ensure they are stored properly and washed thoroughly before eating. Dispose of any sprouts older than a week to prevent the risk of contamination.

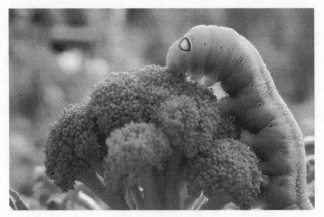

A caterpillar attacking a cruciferous vegetable. Sulforaphane may give it the equivalent of indigestion.
Source: OpenAI

6. PROBIOTICS & FERMENTED FOODS

There is, arguably, no topic more important to natural medicine than that of probiotics and fermented foods. To a surprising degree, the state of one's microbial "hitchhikers" determine your underlying health as well as your response to mainstream treatments. The existence and importance of the microbiome (more technically, the microbiota) came to light in the late 19th century.

The greatest food source of probiotics is a drink known as kefir (pronounced kuh-**feer**). This is similar to a thin yogurt. The "grains" that serve as a starter for milk kefir are made of various microorganisms including lactic acid bacteria, acetic acid bacteria, and yeasts, which are naturally present in kefir starter (Culpepper 2022). You can buy these grains, use them in making a batch of kefir, and then laboriously reclaim them from the liquid with a strainer. Or you can do as I do, and buy a powdered starter, whose end product can be used repeatedly as a starter (up to seven times).

In the West, interest in kefir began with an enthusiastic report by a German doctor, Edward Kern, in 1881. An English medical journal article from 1884 then noted that kefir was the chief article of diet among a long-lived population: the mountaineers of the Caucasus mountains on the border between Russia and Georgia (Anonymous 1884). The word kefir seems to be of Turkic origin, but its original meaning is unknown.

168

Kefir had a vogue of interest in the West in the 1880s. At the time there were literally dozens of books and articles touting it as a kind of medical miracle. As early as 1885, the *American Medical Digest* reacted by stating that "although the most extravagant praise has been bestowed upon this new remedy, more careful observations are still necessary" in order to define its precise therapeutic value.

The pioneering zoologist and immunologist, Elie Metchnikoff (1845-1910), became internationally known for his work on probiotics. Ukrainian by birth, he became deputy director of the Pasteur Institute of Paris and shared the 1908 Nobel Prize in Physiology or Medicine with Paul Ehrlich for their work on immunity. He was also the author of a popular book, *The Prolongation of Life: Optimistic Studies*, in which he established the relationship between the gut microbiome and good health (Metchnikoff 1908).

Metchnikoff's interest in probiotics stemmed from his observation of rural populations in Bulgaria who consumed large amounts of fermented milk products and generally lived longer, healthier lives. He theorized that the lactic acid bacteria in fermented products, particularly *Lactobacillus bulgaricus*, could improve consumers' health by inhibiting the growth of harmful bacteria in the gut. This idea laid the groundwork for the modern field of probiotics, which studies how beneficial microorganisms can enhance gut health and overall well-being.

Probiotics are living microbes that, when consumed in adequate variety and amounts, confer important health benefits. They are commonly found in fermented foods such as kefir, yogurt, sauerkraut, tempeh, kimchi, and miso paste. These foods help restore the natural balance of gut bacteria, crucial not just for effective digestion (they aid in regularizing bowel movements) but also in robust immune functions, and overall health. **Prebiotics,** in contrast, are compounds typically found in fibrous foods like roasted chicory root (a core ingredient in New Orleans style coffee), as well as garlic, onions, asparagus, bananas, and oats. They nourish these beneficial bacteria, thereby enhancing gut health.

From this reference to Metchnikoff, and the current intense interest, you may have the impression that there has been a steady development of the topic for 100 or more years. But this is emphatically not the case. Metchnikoff himself was mocked by most of his colleagues for implying a link between the state of the bowels and health. After his death, the topic went "underground" as it were and became a favorite theme of non-scientific "health enthusiasts."

When I entered the cancer field in 1974, there were almost no modern scientific studies on the topic. According to PubMed, the first article on the microbiome and cancer appeared in 1979. In the latter part of the 20th century such articles appeared at a rate of one per year. By 2010, however, they began appearing once per week. Now they appear at a rate of almost 10 per calendar day. There are few topics in medicine that have seen such an extraordinary rise. Scientists now routinely talk of the "cancer-microbe-immune axis" (Vadhwana 2023).

There is considerable clinical data on the health benefits of kefir, although very little of this directly concerns cancer patients:

Colitis and Crohn's Disease: In a study, kefir was found to contain a high count of beneficial bacteria. When people with ulcerative colitis and Crohn's disease drank kefir, their gut bacteria levels significantly improved. For Crohn's disease patients, inflammation markers decreased, hemoglobin levels increased, bloating reduced, and their overall well-being improved. This suggests that kefir can positively impact gut health and reduce symptoms in these conditions (Yilmaz 2019).

Metabolic syndrome: In a clinical study, 62 participants with metabolic syndrome were given either 180 milliliters (mL) [6 ounces or ¾ of a cup] of probiotic kefir or unfermented milk daily for 12 weeks. Results showed that kefir consumption improved cholesterol levels and reduced inflammation. Specifically, those drinking kefir had increased levels of a beneficial protein (apolipoprotein A1) and decreased bad cholesterol (LDL-C) and inflammatory markers. Both kefir and milk helped lower blood pressure. This suggests that kefir, as part of a balanced diet, may be particularly beneficial for managing metabolic syndrome.

THE COMBINED ROLE OF PREBIOTICS & PROBIOTICS

In 2019, a disturbing report from the Parker Institute for Cancer Immunotherapy (PICI) and M.D. Anderson Cancer Center suggested that taking over-the-counter probiotic supplements could actually *reduce* the effectiveness of cancer immunotherapy, specifically with anti-PD-1 checkpoint inhibitors like pembrolizumab (Keytruda) (Spencer 2019). In fact, according to a Parker Institute press release,

> *"In melanoma patients, taking over-the-counter probiotic supplements was associated with a **70 percent lower chance of response** to cancer immunotherapy treatment" (Dang 2019, edited).*

This abstract, presented at the American Association for Cancer Research (AACR), received significant attention due to its alarming implications (Dang 2019). However, the full paper published in 2021 in *Science* provided a surprising update: there were that

> *"...no statistically significant differences in progression-free survival or odds of response in patients who reported taking probiotics compared to those who did not" (Spencer 2021, edited).*

That alarming 70 percent lower chance evaporated into non-significance, not the first time that a headline-generating finding disappeared upon further consideration. However, what did remain was a strong recommendation to eat more fiber, especially one particular kind, called inulin, which is abundantly present in the root of the chicory plant. This revelation points to the complexity of gut microbiota's role in therapy and underscores the importance of dietary fiber, which feeds these microorganisms.

There remains a lingering suspicion that the microbiome's *diversity*, rather than merely supplementing with probiotics, plays a critical role in treatment outcomes. One top-selling probiotic contains 12 billion CFUs, which stands for "colony forming units." However, all 12 billion are of a single bacteria strain, highlighting a lack of microbial diversity in this and many other commercial products (Spencer 2021).

DIVERSE MICROBIAL DIET OVER SUPPLEMENTS

The most effective sources of probiotics are **living foods**, which typically are found along the perimeter of the supermarket's floor space, such as in the refrigerator cases. In general, we avoid the portions of the supermarket that contain an endless array of canned or packaged goods. These are "dead" foods from the point of view of the microbiome.

Here's a list of living foods and their benefits:

- *Kefir:* Our preferred sources are made from 100% grass fed milk, containing many different species of healthy bacteria. Maple Hill is made from grass fed milk. Lifeway Organic has the widest variety of probiotics. *I do not buy commercial kefir, except for research purposes, since making my own is so simple and successful.* But you will need a starter to begin the process.

171

- Making your own kefir is a simple process that only requires a source of whole milk and a kefir starter. I use a dehydrated and freeze-dried packet of kefir starter powder, such as from *Cultures for Health* (available online). It contains the following probiotic strains: *Lactobacillus acidophilus, Lactobacillus delbrueckii subsp. bulgaricus, Lactobacillus helveticus, Lactococcus lactis subsp. lactis, Lactococcus lactis subsp. cremoris, Leuconostoc mesenteroides,* and *Streptococcus thermophilus.*

- Another good brand of Kefir starter is Yogourmet (imported from France). It takes about one day at room temperature to turn plain milk into delicious kefir, packed with probiotics. You can then use that kefir several times to start new batches. It contains *Lactococcus lactis, Lactococcus cremoris, Lactococcus diacetylactis, Lactobacillus acidophilus, Saccharomyces cerevisiae,* and *Kluyveromyces lactis.* I sometimes mix these two starters to get the maximum variety of probiotics from my kefir.

- *Yogurt:* I recommend whole milk, unsweetened, whole-milk yogurt that has at least six strains of bacteria. It is similar to kefir, but does not generally contain as many bacterial strains. *Stonyfield Organic Whole Milk Probiotic Yogurt* stands out for containing a wide variety of probiotic strains. It includes live and active cultures such as *Streptococcus thermophilus, Lactobacillus bulgaricus, Bifidobacterium BB-12, Lactobacillus acidophilus, Lactobacillus paracasei, and Lactobacillus rhamnosus.*

- *Pickles:* Bubbies Kosher Dill Pickles, Baby Kosher Dill Pickles, and Kosher Dill Relish, all contain the probiotic strains *Lactobacillus plantarum* and *Lactobacillus brevis.* NOTE: Check the labels, though, as *Bubbie's Bread & Butter* snacking pickle chips contain both sugar and vinegar, the latter of which kills probiotic bacteria.)

- *Sauerkraut:* Only consider varieties sold in the refrigerator section of the supermarket, made without vinegar or preservatives. The best ones we have found are *Bubbies* and *Cleveland Kitchen.* Bubbies sauerkraut contains *Lactobacillus plantarum, Lactobacillus brevis, Leuconostoc mesenteroides,* and *Pediococcus pentosaceus.*

- *Miso paste:* Miso is a traditional Japanese seasoning made by fermenting soybeans with salt and kōji (a type of fungus). Choose unpasteurized (raw), organic, non-GMO miso. Many varieties are available, but we favor aged soybean miso. The brand I favor is *Miso Master Traditional Red* (soybean-

172

based) miso paste, which is aged for one year. This contains *Lactobacillus spp., Pediococcus spp., Leuconostoc spp.,* and the fungus *Aspergillus oryzae.*

Avoid any miso product that you find on the dry good shelf and ONLY use the kind found in the refrigerator section. That is because only the refrigerated type of miso contains live bacteria, especially Lactobacilli. Also, look for the "red miso" type for its health benefits. The white varieties are tasty but do not have the same amount of healthy bacteria.

- *Cottage Cheese and Sour Cream:* Look for organic products that contain strains of live cultures and states so on the label. I favor the Good Culture brand, which contains *Lactobacillus acidophilus, Bifidobacterium lactis,* and *Streptococcus thermophilus (in the cottage cheese).*

- *Kimchi:* A fermented cabbage condiment. Look for kimchi that contains at least three strains of good bacteria and has only minimal amounts of added sugar. I like the Cleveland Kitchen brand, which contains *Lactobacillus plantarum, Lactobacillus brevis,* and *Leuconostoc mesenteroides.*

- *Natto:* A traditional Japanese food made from fermented soybeans. It is known for its strong smell, distinctive flavor, and sticky, slimy texture. The fermentation process is carried out by the bacterium Bacillus subtilis, which gives natto its unique characteristics. It's definitely an acquired taste.

Here is a list of several dozen probiotic strains you can get from foods available in most supermarkets:

- *Bacillus coagulans GBI-306086* (GT's Pure Kombucha)
- *Bacillus subtilis* (natto, tempeh)
- *Bifidobacterium BB-12* (Stonyfield Organic Yogurt)
- *Bifidobacterium bre*ve (Lifeway Organic Yogurt)
- *Bifidobacterium lactis* (Lifeway Organic Yogurt, Good Culture Cottage Cheese)
- *Bifidobacterium longum* (Lifeway Organic Yogurt)
- *Kluyveromyces lactis* (Yogourmet Kefir Starter)
- *Lactobacillus acidophilus* (Cultures for Health Kefir Starter, Yogourmet Kefir Starter, Stonyfield Organic Yogurt, Good Culture Cottage Cheese, Lifeway Organic Yogurt, Miso Master Traditional Red Miso)

- *Lactobacillus brevis* (Bubbies Sauerkraut, Cleveland Kitchen Sauerkraut, Cleveland Kitchen Kimchi, Bubbies Kosher Dill Pickles)

- *Lactobacillus casei* (Lifeway Organic Yogurt)

- *Lactobacillus casei Shirota* (Yakult)

- *Lactobacillus delbrueckii subsp. bulgaricus* (Cultures for Health Kefir Starter, Stonyfield Organic Yogurt)

- *Lactobacillus helveticus* (Cultures for Health Kefir Starter)

- *Lactobacillus paracasei* (Stonyfield Organic Yogurt)

- *Lactobacillus plantarum* (Bubbies Sauerkraut, Cleveland Kitchen Sauerkraut, Cleveland Kitchen Kimchi, Bubbies Kosher Dill Pickles, Lifeway Organic Yogurt)

- *Lactobacillus reuteri* (Lifeway Organic Yogurt)

- *Lactobacillus rhamnosus* (Stonyfield Organic Yogurt, Lifeway Organic Yogurt)

- *Lactococcus cremoris* (Cultures for Health Kefir Starter, Yogourmet Kefir Starter, Lifeway Organic Yogurt)

- *Lactococcus diacetylactis* (Yogourmet Kefir Starter, Lifeway Organic Yogurt)

- *Lactococcus lactis* (Cultures for Health Kefir Starter, Yogourmet Kefir Starter, Lifeway Organic Yogurt)

- *Leuconostoc mesenteroides* (Cultures for Health Kefir Starter, Bubbies Sauerkraut, Cleveland Kitchen Sauerkraut, Cleveland Kitchen Kimchi, Miso Master Traditional Red Miso, Lifeway Organic Yogurt)

- *Pediococcus pentosaceus* (Bubbies Sauerkraut)

- *Pediococcus spp.* (Miso Master Traditional Red Miso)

- *Saccharomyces boulardii* (GT's Pure Kombucha) [See note below.]

- *Saccharomyces cerevisiae* (Yogourmet Kefir Starter)

- *Saccharomyces florentinus* (Lifeway Organic Yogurt)

- *Streptococcus thermophilus* (Cultures for Health Kefir Starter, Stonyfield Organic Yogurt, Good Culture Cottage Cheese)

Most shoppers will only encounter these beneficial bacteria in the form of heavily sweetened yogurt. And this only affects a minority of the population. In fact, according to the authoritative National Health and Nutrition Examination Survey

174

(NHANES), "The data show that approximately 6.4% children and 5.5% adults consume yogurt" (Cifelli 2020). Yet there is an abundance of data to show that numerous aspects of health are linked to the intake of prebiotics and probiotics such as are mentioned in this list.

NOTE: According to MSKCC's "About Herbs" website, patients who are immunocompromised, or have a central venous catheter or critically ill should not take probiotics containing *S. boulardii* (Cohen 2010)

It is important to never heat fermented foods like miso over 115° F (46° C). (Use your food thermometer to make sure you don't exceed this temperature.) That is the point at which the *Lactobacilli* in miso experience a rapid die-off. When heating miso, it is advisable to avoid boiling it or subjecting it to high heat to preserve these beneficial microorganisms. For culinary uses, such as in soups, it's best to add miso at the end of cooking and allow it to dissolve in warm, but not boiling, water. This approach helps maintain the probiotic benefits of miso. This is a good general rule when dealing with live foods.

Living foods not only improve gut microbial balance but also support overall health and could influence cancer prevention and treatment.

PREBIOTICS

We have mentioned that our approach also emphasizes the daily consumption of roasted chicory root, a rich source of inulin—favored food for the microbiome—combined with ground coffee to create a "synbiotic," a combination of pre- and probiotic elements (Pandey 2015), a mixture promoting a healthy gut. Getting a wide variety of probiotics is fine, but these are living organisms, which need regular care and feeding.

The main food for healthy gut bacteria is fiber. Inulin and oligofructose are both types of fructans, which are carbohydrates composed of fructose molecules. They are classified as prebiotics, which means they promote the growth of beneficial bacteria in the gut. Oligofructose is often derived from the enzymatic breakdown of inulin and is found in similar plants. It is more rapidly fermented in the gut compared to inulin due to its shorter molecular chain length.

Inulin is contained in over 3,000 plants, including asparagus, leek, onion, banana, wheat and garlic. So if you eat vegetables you probably get a trace amount. But the most abundant sources are Jerusalem artichokes, dandelion greens and especially **roasted chicory root.**

This is readily available online and in some specialty food stores. Chicory root also contains various antioxidants, including polyphenols. This helps combat oxidative stress and reduce inflammation in the body. The brand I favor is Micro Ingredients™ Organic French Chicory Root, which comes in two-pound sealed packages.

Roasted chicory root is often used as a caffeine-free coffee substitute or blended with coffee to reduce its caffeine content. The root is roasted and ground, just like coffee beans. A common ratio in NOLA-style coffee is approximately 2/3 coffee to 1/3 chicory. This ratio can be adjusted to taste, with some blends containing up to 50% chicory. Chicory adds a slightly bitter, earthy flavor and can reduce the caffeine content of the coffee. It is an ingredient in several brands of New Orleans-style ground coffee, such as "Café du Monde" and "French Market."

Chicory contains 15-20% inulin by weight and a cup of New Orleans-style coffee made with a typical 1/3 chicory blend may provide approximately 0.5 to 0.66 grams of inulin. So if you drink two cups of New Orleans-style coffee you would get about one gram of inulin.

You should try to include this in your morning coffee (my formula for pour-over coffee is equal amounts of roasted chicory root, caffeinated, and decaffeinated grounds). That way, you can create your own "synbiotic," which is defined as a combination of pre- and probiotic elements (Pandey 2015).

A more concentrated source of inulin is to brew an ersatz coffee with just roasted chicory root. This will probably provide you with 1.5 to 2.0 grams of inulin per cup. There is no recommended daily allowance of inulin. But in 2019, the FDA accepted chicory root powder as a *Generally Recognized as Safe* (GRAS) ingredient in foods (Carlson 2019). That does not mean that chicory root powder cannot, in all circumstances, cause any side effects. The most likely of these is gastric distress. So, as with any new item, it is best to start with a small dose, and only work up to larger amounts if you do not experience any negative consequences.

(See our recipe for Roasted Chicory Root Coffee.)

It is essential to balance a diversity of bacteria from your diet with adequate fiber intake. In *The Moss Method*, we stress the importance of integrating living foods with prebiotics for a holistic approach to gut health and overall well-being.

FERMENTED WHEAT GERM EXTRACT SUPER CONCENTRATE

While on the subject of fermentation, we will mention a product that originated as a fermented food but has now transitioned to a very refined and specialized food supplement. Fermented Wheat Germ Extract (FWGE). Formerly known by various brand names, such as Ave Ultra and Avemar, in the United States it is now called Metatrol. It plays an important role in supporting immune function and regulating cell metabolism. This extract is particularly effective in repairing defective mitochondria in cancer cells, potentially changing them back to normal at the molecular level (Matson 2018, Vetizou 2018).

This product was based on the thinking of the Nobel laureate Albert Szent-Györgyi, MD, Ph.D. The isolation of the most bioactive fraction was achieved under the direction of another Nobel laureate, James D. Watson, Ph.D., Chancellor Emeritus of Cold Spring Harbor Laboratory, New York. According to the manufacturer, American Biosciences, Inc., 41 mg of Metatrol has the same health effect as 5,500 mg of whole FWGE and 17,000 mg of spray-dried FWGE. The label dose is two capsules per day.

Uzsoki Hospital Study (2005)

The Uzsoki Hospital, a teaching hospital of Semmelweis University, in Budapest demonstrated that FWGE could prevent the spread of tumors in colorectal cancer patients post-surgery when used alone or with chemo, showcasing its potential as a supplementary cancer treatment (Jakab 2000, Farkas 2005).

The integration of probiotics and prebiotics, particularly through the eating of varied fermented foods and specific supplements like FWGE (Bencze 2020), plays a crucial role in The Moss Method. These elements help maintain a healthy gut microbiome, which is essential for effective immune function and cancer prevention. Adopting a diet rich in these nutrients can offer health benefits and improve the quality of life for cancer patients and survivors.

7. SOY/GENISTEIN

The history of soybean use dates back to at least the 11th century BCE in North China, showing its longstanding cultural and nutritional importance. Introduced to the United States by 1765, soy has become a staple in various products including soy sauce and miso (soybean paste), reflecting its global culinary versatility (Hymowitz 1970).

177

Isoflavones, especially genistein, found in soy, act like the human hormone estrogen and can block estrogen receptors in the body. Soy helps keep hormones balanced and can ease menopausal symptoms, offering a natural option instead of hormone replacement therapies (Setchell 1984).

A NOTE ON PLANT ESTROGENS

The term "plant estrogens" may sound scary to some people who know about the breast cancer-promoting effects of human estrogen. However, the opinion of most scientists is that estradiol, the main human form of estrogen, is around *1,000 times stronger* than the plant estrogens in soy (Autrup 2020). So rather than stimulating tumor growth, plant estrogens take up the estrogen receptors on breast cells, thereby preventing the human estrogen from stimulating growth (Bilal 2014). So its mode of action is similar to the widely used drug tamoxifen, but without tamoxifen's many potential side effects.

In studies, taking 50 milligrams (mg) of genistein daily for two months increases the variety and amount of good gut bacteria, particularly the elusive but important *Akkermansia muciniphila*. This microbe, which thrives on the mucinous lining of the gut, could potentially improve the effectiveness of cancer treatments, such as modern immunotherapy (Hilakivi-Clarke 2022). We don't have space here to go into the fascinating *Akkermansia* story in detail. But it is a microbe that has an intimate relationship to good health. Consider this statement from Belgian researchers:

> *"A lower amount of Akkermansia muciniphila has been associated with many diseases in both lab rodents and in humans. Akkermansia muciniphila has proven effectiveness to improve obesity, type 2 and type 1 diabetes mellitus, fatty liver, intestinal inflammation and different cancers in mice" (Cani 2022, edited).*

That's a tall order for such a tiny organism that is so elusive that it was only discovered 20 years ago (Derrien 2004).

Soy isoflavones can be found in various foods. According to soy expert Mark Messina, one serving of soymilk typically provides about 25 mg of isoflavones (Messina 2016). However, the Edensoy brand of organic unsweetened soy milk offers 75 mg of isoflavones per 8-ounce (250 mL) serving, three times the average amount. Other rich sources include tofu and tempeh, which are versatile and can be used in numerous dishes. Soybeans and miso, being less processed, offer wholesome isoflavones, while edamame, young soybeans usually steamed and consumed as a snack, also provide beneficial compounds. Opting for whole, minimally processed forms like organic, non-GMO soy products can enhance the absorption of isoflavones and maximize their health benefits.

Incorporating soy into your diet is straightforward and does not require major dietary changes. You can add tofu or tempeh to salads or stir-fries, use soy milk in smoothies or baked goods, or snack on edamame. These methods offer simple ways to enjoy the health benefits of soy. While isoflavone supplements can provide concentrated doses (30-100 mg daily), incorporating natural food sources like soy into your diet can offer these plant chemicals along with other essential nutrients. The appropriate intake levels should be tailored to individual health needs and goals (Kurzer 2002).

Soy isoflavones have shown promise in supporting prostate health. A notable study from the Netherlands demonstrated that a dietary supplement containing soy isoflavones slowed the growth of prostate cancer by prolonging the PSA doubling time from 445 days to 1150 days, indicating a slower rate of disease progression (Schröder 2005). Soy and its isoflavones have been studied for safety and effectiveness. A study from Vanderbilt University involving over 9,500 breast cancer survivors indicated a 25% reduction in tumor recurrence with higher soy intake, affirming its safety and beneficial impacts on health (Nechuta 2012).

Although soy is not officially designated as *Generally Recognized as Safe* (GRAS) by the FDA, the agency recognizes the safety of soy for consumption, especially noting that soy protein is considered GRAS. This underscores its health benefits and long history of safe use (FDA 1999).

Historical and scientific insights into soy and isoflavones, particularly genistein, highlight their potential to enhance health, especially through hormonal balance and cancer prevention. Soy's versatile use in culinary practices worldwide further supports its incorporation into diets for its functional benefits. Embracing soy in its various forms—whether through traditional soy foods or modern dietary integrations—can contribute to a balanced diet and overall well-being.

---

8. QUERCETIN

Quercetin is a powerful pigment found in a variety of fruits, vegetables, and grains, notably in onions, apples, berries, and kale. Quercetin was first discovered and named by the Hungarian scientist Albert Szent-Györgyi, MD, Ph.D., in 1936. His pioneering work in isolating and identifying various plant chemicals, including the bioflavonoid quercetin, significantly contributed to our understanding of their biological activities and potential health benefits.

(See Free Radical, my biography of Albert Szent-Gyorgyi, MD, Ph.D., who also discovered the chemical nature of vitamin C.)

Renowned for its antioxidant qualities, quercetin combats dangerous free radicals, supports heart health, and provides anti-inflammatory benefits. In the context of cancer, quercetin has attracted attention for its ability to stop the growth and spread of cancer stem cells (CSCs), particularly in breast, colon, and prostate cancers.

Henning Study of Green Tea & Quercetin (2020)

A 2020 study from Suzanne M. Henning, Ph.D., and colleagues at the University of California, Los Angeles (UCLA) suggested that green tea might play a significant role in enhancing the absorption of quercetin. When consumed together with green tea, the levels of quercetin in the body increased dramatically.

This effect is thought to be due to the interaction between quercetin and the active compounds in green tea, such as the antioxidant EGCG, which may facilitate better uptake and retention of quercetin in the blood and tissues (Henning 2020).

In a controlled study, participants were given either a pill with **800 milligrams** (mg) of quercetin or a placebo. This amount of quercetin would be hard to achieve with food alone, and would require supplementation. There are numerous formulations where two capsules of quercetin add up to 800 mg or slightly more.

Those who consumed a green tea extract alongside this amount of quercetin showed a *14-fold increase* in the blood plasma levels of quercetin compared to those who consumed quercetin with the placebo (ibid.)

This suggests that the natural chemicals in green tea, such as EGCC, enhance the availability of quercetin, potentially by affecting the way it is broken down and absorbed. By my calculation, the amount of liquid green tea necessary to achieve this effect would be 12 ounces of brewed Gyokuro tea from Japan (or a smaller amount of Matcha tea). Ordinary commercial tea bags are unlikely to have this effect, since they vary greatly in their antioxidant content, but are almost always less. In fact, some of them contain virtually no EGCG at all.

AVAILABILITY & DIETARY SOURCES

Quercetin's effectiveness is influenced by its availability, which can vary depending on the food source and preparation methods. It is most bioavailable in its natural form when consumed in foods that are minimally processed. For instance:

- Onions provide a relatively high amount of quercetin, especially red onions, which contain up to 415 mg/kg of this plant pigment.

- Apples are another prime source, with the skin or peel of the apple containing the majority of its quercetin. Apple peel powder is available online. It contains most of the benefits of apples, without almost all the carbs.

- Berries like blueberries and blackberries also offer meaningful amounts.

- Kale and other leafy greens provide quercetin along with a host of other good nutrients.

Integrating these foods into your diet not only enhances quercetin intake but also benefits overall health due to their rich nutrient profiles.

While dietary quercetin provides health benefits, supplements can offer more concentrated doses, which are often used in clinical studies investigating healing effects. Standard dosages for quercetin supplements typically range from 500 to 1,000 mg per day. The European Food Safety Authority considers up to 1,000 mg daily safe for adults, aligning with dosages used in various studies. However, doses exceeding 1,000 mg daily may pose some risks, such as potential kidney damage and interactions with drugs, particularly blood thinners and certain types of antibiotics. (See "Possible Interactions," below.)

Quercetin's health benefits are numerous, attributed to its role in adjusting several processes. It has notable antioxidant and anti-inflammatory effects, reducing inflammation and cell damage from oxygen, which are linked to various chronic diseases, including cancer. In terms of cancer prevention, quercetin promotes normal cell death in cancer stem cells (CSCs) and interferes with their ability to multiply, helping to prevent tumor growth and spread. Additionally, quercetin supports heart health by reducing inflammation and protecting against lipid peroxidation, thereby lowering the risk of heart diseases. Furthermore, quercetin enhances immune function with its antiviral qualities and ability to modulate immune responses, making it a supportive nutrient for overall immune health.

POSSIBLE INTERACTIONS

The combination of polyphenols, such as quercetin, and cancer chemotherapy is complicated. A 2023 review concluded:

> *"Some polyphenols work in synergy with chemotherapeutic drugs, but some polyphenols can act antagonistically, so caution is always required" (Jakobušić Brala 2023).*

Quercetin's interaction with drugs is a concern, especially for individuals on drugs such as blood thinners or undergoing chemo. It can affect the body's ability to process drugs due to its influence on enzymes involved in drug metabolism.

That is why, in this book, we have avoided the question of the interaction of plant chemicals with chemotherapy, except for our one chapter on *Cancer Treatment & The Moss Method*. If you are under medical treatment of any sort, especially cancer chemotherapy, you should only introduce supplements such as quercetin with the active participation of your treating physician. In fact, under such circumstances, please have your oncologist review the recommendations of The Moss Method before implementing them.

To maximize the absorption and effectiveness of quercetin in foods, it is advisable to pair quercetin-rich foods with healthy fats. Consuming these foods with fats such as olive oil can improve quercetin's bioavailability. Additionally, applying gentle cooking methods, such as steaming or sautéing vegetables lightly, helps retain their quercetin content compared to boiling.

Quercetin is a versatile plant pigment that offers a range of health benefits, from reducing inflammation and supporting heart health to providing a potential defense against cancer. Whether through dietary sources or supplements, it is important to consider individual health needs and potential interactions with drugs. Talking with a healthcare provider can help tailor the use of quercetin to maximize its benefits while ensuring safety, especially for those with underlying health conditions or those on medications. But as part of a balanced diet, quercetin can contribute to overall health and well-being, showing its importance within The Moss Method.

In summary, incorporating quercetin into your daily diet or as a supplement should be done with an understanding of its benefits and risks. The optimal dosing, attention to food sources and preparation, and a look at individual health conditions are key to utilizing quercetin effectively to improve your health and potentially reduce the risk of various chronic diseases.

9. OMEGA-3 FATTY ACIDS

Omega-3s are essential polyunsaturated fatty acids (PUFAs) crucial for maintaining heart health, reducing inflammation, and supporting brain functions. These nutrients are primarily found in fatty fish, such as salmon and mackerel, and plant sources like flaxseeds and walnuts. Supplements are also widely available as fish oil, krill oil, and algae-based options, catering to different dietary preferences, including veganism.

Fatty fish are an excellent source of essential fatty acids (EFAs), particularly omega-3 fatty acids like EPA (eicosapentaenoic acid) and DHA (docosahexaenoic acid). Some of the fatty fish that are high in EFAs include:

- *Salmon:* One of the best sources of omega-3 fatty acids, especially wild-caught salmon.

- *Mackerel:* A rich source of omega-3s, often consumed smoked or canned.

- *Sardines:* These small fish are packed with omega-3s and are usually available canned.

- *Herring:* Another fatty fish high in omega-3s, often eaten pickled or smoked.

- *Anchovies:* Small and oily, anchovies are rich in omega-3s and often used in salads and as a pizza topping.

- *Tuna:* Especially the albacore variety, which contains higher levels of omega-3s.

- *Trout:* Particularly lake trout, which is high in omega-3 fatty acids.

Other natural dietary sources include plant-based options like flaxseeds, chia seeds, and walnuts. Supplements are available in the form of fish oil, krill oil, and algae oil, providing flexibility in meeting omega-3 needs.

For general health, the daily recommended intake of EPA and DHA (the primary forms of omega-3s) is between **250 to 500 mg per day.** However, for specific conditions, supplements of higher doses of up to 4,000 mg may be used under medical supervision. The effectiveness of omega-3 supplements can vary based on the product's purity and the body's ability to absorb these fats. It is crucial to choose supplements certified for purity to ensure they are free from contaminants like mercury and are sourced sustainably.

Omega-3 fatty acids offer numerous health benefits. They play a pivotal role in lowering triglyceride levels, thereby helping to prevent heart disease. These fatty acids also support brain health functions, potentially reducing the risks of dementia and mental decline. Additionally, their anti-inflammatory effects can help manage arthritis and other inflammatory conditions.

OMEGA-3s & CANCER

Research has explored the relationship between omega-3 fatty acid intake and cancer risk. For example, in an analysis of 26 studies involving almost 900,000 total participants and over 20,000 breast cancer cases, higher intake of marine-derived omega-3 fatty acids (PUFAs) was linked to a *14% reduction* in breast cancer risk. In other words, those with the highest omega-3 intake had a relative risk of 0.86 compared to the lowest intake group. Each 0.1 gram per day increase was associated with a 5% decrease in breast cancer risk. These results suggest that it is the marine omega-3s in fatty fish that helps in breast cancer prevention through dietary changes (Zheng 2013).

Omega-3s' anti-inflammatory qualities may also reduce the risk of colorectal cancer by reducing chronic inflammation, a known risk factor.

OMEGA-3 & CVD RISK

There is similar data on the benefit of fish and omega-3 consumption and the heart. In a huge meta-analysis involving over 2 million participants, researchers found that eating fish is linked to a lower risk of dying from cardiovascular disease (CVD). Specifically, those who ate more fish had a 9% lower risk of CVD death. Additionally, higher intake of marine omega-3 fatty acids further reduced this risk by 13%. For every 20 grams of fish or 80 milligrams of omega-3s consumed daily, the risk decreased by 4%. This study suggests that incorporating fish and marine omega-3s into your diet can help reduce the risk of fatal heart disease (Jiang L 2023).

An international study that reviewed 18 papers, covering over 1.4 million people, found that eating more fish can reduce the risk of cardiovascular disease (CVD). People who ate more fish had an 8% lower risk of CVD. Eating 50 grams of fish per day was linked to a 9% reduction in both fatal and non-fatal CVD events. Consuming two to three portions of fish per week (each portion being 150 grams) resulted in an 8% reduction in CVD risk. The recommended two portions of fish per week can lower the risk of CVD by about 10%, and eating a full portion of fish daily can reduce the risk by up to 30% (Ricci 2023).

Incorporating omega-3s into your diet can be straightforward. It is recommended to **eat omega-3-rich fish two to three times a week**, alongside plant-based sources. For those who find it difficult to source fatty fish, options such as canned mercury-free and pole-caught albacore tuna (however, not skipjack tuna), sardines, and mackerel are viable alternatives. For individuals unable to meet their omega-3 needs through diet alone, high-quality supplements are advised. Consulting with a healthcare provider before starting supplements, especially at high dosages, is essential.

Practical tips for maximizing the benefits of omega-3s include not overcooking fish to preserve its benefits and storing omega-3-rich oils in the refrigerator to maintain their effectiveness. Additionally, it is crucial to balance omega-3 and omega-6 fatty acid intake to avoid promoting an inflammatory diet.

SAFETY & SIDE EFFECTS

While helpful, omega-3 supplements can cause side effects such as a fishy aftertaste, digestive discomfort, and interactions with drugs like blood thinners. Awareness and management of mercury exposure from certain fish is also necessary.

Omega-3 fatty acids are a vital part of a healthy diet, contributing to heart, brain, and overall health while also offering potential cancer-fighting benefits. Whether through diet or supplements, it is important to ensure a balanced intake of these essential nutrients for the best health outcomes. Consultation with a healthcare provider is crucial to tailor omega-3 intake appropriately based on individual health needs and conditions.

---

10. VITAMIN C

Vitamin C, known for its multifaceted health benefits, holds a prominent place within *The Moss Method*. Its role encompasses supporting the immune system, serving as a potent antioxidant, and even showing potential in attacking cancer stem cells (CSCs). As we delve into the details of incorporating vitamin C into your health regimen, it becomes evident that its benefits extend beyond the familiar immune support that it provides (Dresen 2023)

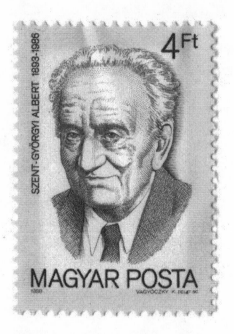

A Hungarian postage stamp paid homage to the discoverer of vitamin C and quercetin, Albert Szent-Györgyi, MD, Ph.D. Source: National Library of Medicine

HISTORY OF VITAMIN C'S DISCOVERY

Scurvy, a severe deficiency disease, caused the sickness and agonizing death of thousands of early explorers and seamen. Some Native American tribes used pine needle tea as a traditional remedy for scurvy long before its vitamin C content was scientifically understood. This remedy provided essential nutrients during winter months when fresh fruits and vegetables were scarce (Schick 1943).

In the 1530s, the French explorer Jacques Cartier witnessed the effectiveness of this remedy firsthand. During his second voyage in 1535-1536, most of Cartier's crew became sick and were dying of scurvy in the harsh Québec winter. Cartier observed an interpreter, previously stricken with scurvy, who had recovered remarkably. The interpreter revealed he had been healed by a beverage made from the leaves and bark of a tree.

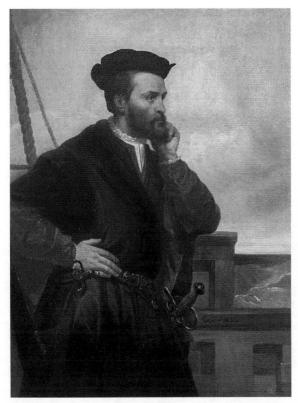

Explorer Jacques, by painter Theophile Hamel (1844). Source: Wikimedia Commons

In a memorable passage in an account of the voyages of the French explorer Jacques Cartier (1491-1557), the Canadian author, Stephen Leacock, wrote of this landmark discovery. On their second voyage in 1535-1536, most of Cartier's crew became sick in the winter and were dying of scurvy, in the harsh Québec winter. What happened next was truly remarkable:

> *"One day Cartier saw a band of Indians coming over to him from Stadacona [now Québec City, ed.]. Among them was an interpreter, whom Cartier had known to be stricken by scurvy only ten days before, but who now appeared in abundant health. On being asked the manner of his cure, the interpreter told Cartier that he had been healed by a beverage made from the leaves and bark of a tree.*

"The bark and needles were to be boiled, and the drink thus made was to be taken twice a day. The potion was duly administered, and the cure that it caused was so rapid and so complete that the pious Cartier declared it a real and evident miracle. An entire tree—probably a white spruce—was used up in less than eight days. The scourge passed and the sailors, now restored to health, eagerly awaited the coming of the spring" (Leacock 1915, edited).

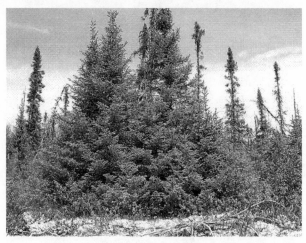

The black spruce, or Picea Mariana, *whose bark, needles, and cones were the most likely source of Cartier's anti-scurvy medication. Source: Wikimedia Commons*

Two centuries later, the Scottish physician James Lind, MD (1716-1794) featured the pine needle cure for scurvy in his historic work, *A Treatise of the Scurvy*. Lind noted Cartier's remedy, referring to it as the "tree of life," and identified the tree as the black spruce (*Picea mariana*), which thrives in cold, moist environments and is common in Canadian forests:

"But the last and most sovereign remedy was the ameda, mentioned by Cartier, which he called the 'tree of life.' Monsieur Champlain, who was then up country, [i.e., further inland] had orders to search for ameda among the Indians, and to lay up a store of it for the preservation of their colony." (Lind 1772, edited).

Lind stated that "a simple decoction of the tops, cones, leaves [needles], or even green bark and wood of these trees is an excellent antiscorbutic [anti-scurvy] medicine," and even more so when fermented with molasses into "spruce beer." However, black spruce was not readily available to British sailors, leading Lind to conduct one of the world's first clinical trials. He demonstrated that lime juice could significantly improve naval health by administering citrus to sailors on long voyages, giving the British navy a distinct advantage and coining the term "limey."

However, he remarks that the spruce cure was "known only to a few physicians."

Lind quotes at length from the harrowing account of the surgeon of the British sailing ship, *America*, which lost a third of its crew to scurvy. In November 1762, this doctor wrote from Manila:

> *"Every captain, and surgeon, who had any lime juice, experienced great benefit from it in this disease" (Ibid.)*

At the time that Lind wrote, scurvy was considered an incurable disease, as incurable as most late-stage cancers are considered today. In his 1772 book, Lind wrote:

> *"The world has almost despaired of finding out a method of preventing this dreadful calamity at sea; and it is the received opinion that it is altogether impossible in long voyages, either to prevent or cure it" (p. 145, edited).*

To overcome this negativism, Lind performed one of the world's first clinical trials, to show that what he called "lime juice" could significantly improve naval health by administering it to sailors on long voyages. In discussing the prevention of scurvy, however, it is important to clarify the terminology used in historical contexts. Lind, in his great medical classic, referred to both lemons and limes. However, historical records indicate that he was actually using what today we know as lemons. During that time, the terms 'lime' and 'lemon' were often used interchangeably, particularly within the British navy.

The long search for a chemically defined anti-scurvy element—later identified as vitamin C—culminated in 1931 when the Hungarian-American biochemist Albert

Szent-Györgyi, MD, Ph.D., succeeded in isolating and naming ascorbic acid from Hungarian paprika (red pepper). Szent-Györgyi's work, along with that of pioneering vitamin researcher Sir Frederick Gowland Hopkins, led to both scientists receiving Nobel Prizes.

(I tell the full story of this discovery in my authorized biography of Szent-Györgyi, Free Radical.)

LINUS PAULING & VITAMIN C

Linus Pauling, Ph.D. (1901-1994), a renowned American chemist and himself a two-time Nobel laureate, was a prominent advocate for the health benefits of vitamin C. In 1970, he published *Vitamin C and the Common Cold,* promoting the idea that high doses of vitamin C could effectively prevent and alleviate that all too frequent condition. Pauling's recommendations sparked widespread interest and led to significant public and scientific discussion regarding the potential health benefits of higher than typical doses of vitamin C, extending beyond just cold prevention to include potential effects on cancer and other diseases.

Despite his lack of medical qualifications–he was a chemist–Pauling's assertions had a profound impact on the public's perception of dietary supplements. He continued to champion the use of high-dose vitamin C throughout his life, proposing that it could extend the average human lifespan and improve overall health. His views were controversial and met with skepticism in the medical community, which often criticized the lack of randomized trial evidence to support his claims. Nevertheless, Pauling's enthusiasm contributed significantly to the popularity of vitamin C as a dietary supplement and sparked further research into its potential health benefits. Some of this research is now confirmatory of the positive role of vitamin C in cancer.

(See my discussion of Pauling and the vitamin C controversy in my book, The Cancer Industry.)

THE IV-C CONTROVERSY

I have no intention of entering into a prolonged discussion of cancer *treatment,* which (with the exception of one specialized chapter), is beyond the scope of this book on prevention. However, I do have to clarify that there is a big difference between vitamin C taken as a food ingredient or oral supplement and "IV-C," which is vitamin C administered, usually in large doses, intravenously (IV).

The method by which ascorbic acid is administered has a big impact on the amount that becomes available in the body. A 2004 study by Mark Levine, MD, Sebastian J.

Padayatty, and others at the National Institutes of Health (NIH) showed that much more vitamin C gets taken up when it is given via the intravenous (IV) route than when the vitamin is taken orally (Padayatty 2004).

In this study, 17 healthy volunteers were hospitalized and given either oral or intravenous doses of vitamin C, and blood plasma levels were calculated for a dose range of 1 to 100 grams. The authors reported that peak plasma vitamin C concentrations were:

> *"...higher after administration of intravenous doses than after administration of oral doses...and the difference increased according to dose" (ibid.)*

In fact, the blood concentration of vitamin C when given intravenously was *6.6 times greater* than when the same amount was given orally. This finding was of great importance in explaining the difference between the results reported by Linus Pauling, Ph.D., and Ewan Cameron, M.D., using a combination of oral and IV vitamin C (Cameron 1978) and those of the Mayo Clinic, which only used the oral form (Creagan 1979).

BREAST CANCER & VITAMIN C

In a meta-analysis from the famed Karolinska Institute in Sweden and Brigham and Women's Hospital, Boston, researchers found a positive relationship between vitamin C consumption and the prevention of breast cancer. This comprehensive review looked at how both vitamin C supplements and dietary intake of vitamin C relate to the risk of death from breast cancer and from all causes (Harris 2014).

- *Supplement Use:* Women who took vitamin C supplements after their diagnosis had a 19% lower risk of dying from any cause and a 15% lower risk of dying from breast cancer specifically.

- *Dietary Intake:* Increasing vitamin C intake by 100 mg per day from food was linked with a 27% lower risk of dying from any cause and a 22% lower risk of dying from breast cancer.

Vitamin C, whether through supplements after diagnosis or as part of a daily diet, appears to be beneficial in reducing mortality for breast cancer patients. This finding supports the inclusion of vitamin C-rich foods and possibly supplements in the diets of those diagnosed with breast cancer (Ibid.)

STOMACH CANCER & VITAMIN C

A massive 2024 meta-analysis from the *Stomach Cancer Pooling (StoP) Project* has shown that a diet high in vitamin C may reduce the risk of stomach cancer. This study was thorough, taking into account how much fruit and vegetables people ate, which has often been overlooked in the past. It had three dozen authors who spanned the globe from Italy to China (Sassano 2024).

For this meta-analysis, researchers looked at 14 different studies involving over 5,000 people with stomach cancer and over 11,000 people without it. They compared those who consumed a lot of vitamin C in their diets to those who didn't, while also considering their intake of fruits and vegetables. Here is what they found:

- People who had the highest amount of vitamin C in their diet were 36% less likely to have stomach cancer compared to those who had the least.

- Even after adjusting for how many fruits and vegetables people ate, those with the highest vitamin C intake still had a 15% lower risk of developing the disease.

- The most significant drop in risk (46% lower) was seen at vitamin C intakes of **150-200 milligrams (mg) per day.** Higher intakes did not show additional benefits.

This study suggests that vitamin C could be a powerful factor in protecting against cancer, particularly if you consume **about twice the daily recommended amount (which is just 90 mg for men and 75 mg for women).** It shows the importance of considering vitamin C as part of a cancer-preventive diet, especially given the complexities of dietary factors and cancer risks. By demonstrating a clear link between vitamin C intake and a lower risk of stomach cancer, this research adds another piece to the puzzle of how diet can influence cancer development.

This goal of 150-200 mg per day of vitamin C is quite doable. Here are some possible food choices:

- One medium red bell pepper provides about 152 mg of vitamin C.

- One cup of cooked Brussels sprouts provides about 97 mg of vitamin C.

- One large orange provides about 98 mg of vitamin C.

- Try our High Vitamin C, Low-Carb Fruit Salad Recipe (which can also be made into a Smoothie).

UNDERSTANDING DOSAGE & FORMS OF VITAMIN C

When considering vitamin C supplements, understanding the recommended dosage is a fundamental step. Typically falling within the range of 500 to 1000 mg daily, the specific amount may vary depending on your health objectives. Beyond dosage, the form in which vitamin C is consumed can influence its absorption. Different formulations are available, and some include plant pigments. These are complex compounds found in many fruits and vegetables, including citrus fruits. Some authors believe that they aid in the absorption of vitamin C, which has the potential to improve the body's uptake of this essential nutrient. However, there is a great deal of controversy over the proper form and dosage. What is more certain is that eating foods containing between 150 and 200 mg per day (as in our High Vitamin C, Low-Carb Fruit Salad) is more likely to yield the maximum benefit.

WIDE-RANGING HEALTH BENEFITS

The health benefits associated with vitamin C are many and far-reaching. It plays a pivotal role in bolstering the immune system, a function that is crucial for overall well-being. Additionally, vitamin C is recognized for its contribution to collagen creation, an essential part of skin health. Its antioxidant qualities offer protection against cell damage from oxygen, while ongoing research explores its potential impact on heart health and mental well-being.

To incorporate vitamin C naturally into your diet, you can turn to a variety of sources. Citrus fruits, berries, bell peppers, and leafy greens are rich in this vital nutrient. Furthermore, culinary creativity allows you to infuse your meals with vitamin C, whether it is through salads, smoothies, or snacks. The culinary landscape provides ample opportunities to harness the nutritional benefits of this essential vitamin.

When opting for vitamin C supplements, quality and safety are most important. Favoring high-quality products that undergo third-party testing ensures that you receive the intended benefits. It is advisable to begin supplements with lower doses to judge tolerance, as high doses may lead to potential GI discomfort.

In specific contexts, such as high-dose therapy for cancer care, collaboration with a healthcare provider, particularly an oncologist, is recommended. The choice of oral supplements matters, with options including ascorbic acid or stomach-friendly formulations. Pairing vitamin C with plant pigments and iron-rich foods can improve its absorption, and distributing high oral doses throughout the day can contribute to your overall health.

While the benefits of vitamin C are substantial, it is essential to be aware of potential side effects. These may include GI discomfort, headaches, and, in some cases, a risk of kidney stones when consumed at high doses. Additionally, understanding potential interactions with drugs, such as blood thinners and certain drugs, as well as its impact on iron absorption, is crucial.

SECONDARY ELEMENTS

The secondary elements of The Moss Method are also helpful and backed up by scientific research. However, while important, they have either less data, show variability in results, or are emerging in their scientific evidence with promising but yet fully confirmed outcomes.

This category includes ten plant chemicals that are supportive in nature and improve the impact of ten primary elements. They contribute to broadening the anticancer potential of an individual's diet but are generally introduced after the primary elements to optimize well-being without overwhelming those new to The Moss Method.

---

11. POMEGRANATES & OTHER FRUITS

"An overwhelming body of research has now firmly established that the dietary intake of berry fruits has a positive and profound impact on human health, performance, and disease."
— Navindra P. Seeram, Ph.D., UCLA Center for Human Nutrition (2008)

When we in the West think of berries we normally think of blackberries, black and red raspberries, blueberries, cranberries, and strawberries. However, in recent years we have also been introduced to several "exotic" species, including acai, goji, and maqui, which are celebrated for their high antioxidant content, particularly their water-soluble pigments called anthocyanins.

(Anthocyanins are natural pigments found in fruits and vegetables that give them red, purple, or blue colors and have antioxidant properties that may offer health benefits.)

But berries contain an amazing array of nutrients, many of them of importance in the prevention of cancer:

"Some of the known preventive agents in berries include vitamins A, C, and E and folic acid; calcium and selenium; beta-carotene, alpha-carotene, and lutein;

polyphenols such as ellagic acid, quercetin, and several anthocyanins; and three different forms of phytosterols" (Stoner 2016 edited).

BLACK RASPBERRIES

Berries such as black raspberries, raspberries, cranberries, blueberries, blackberries, strawberries, and Indian gooseberries are rich in bioactive components that offer significant health benefits. Black raspberries (*Rubus occidentalis*) are particularly notable due to their high content of beneficial compounds like various polyphenols (such as ellagic acid and quercetin). These compounds contribute to the positive health effects of black raspberries.

Recent studies have focused on how black raspberries and their plant chemicals can help prevent various cancers. For example, research has shown that black raspberries can inhibit the growth of cancer cells, reduce inflammation, and trigger pathways that lead to cancer cell death. They also change the immune system, positively affect the gut microbiome, and decrease oxidative stress.

In studies involving head and neck cancers, dietary black raspberries significantly reduced tumor incidence in animal models exposed to carcinogens. For instance, a study found that mice fed a diet with 5% black raspberries had a reduced tumor incidence from 70% to 46.7%, along with a decrease in harmful DNA adducts in the oral cavity (Chen KM 2020).

Another study using hamsters demonstrated that black raspberries could reduce tumor numbers and incidence when applied topically or consumed in the diet (Casto 2002).

In a human trial at the Ohio State University involving a black raspberry gel applied to oral premalignant lesions showed a regression in some patients, along with significant reductions in certain cancer-related markers. These findings highlight the potential of black raspberries in cancer prevention and suggest further research to explore their effectiveness when combined with other cancer treatments (Shumway 2008).

Other fruits are also important to The Moss Method due to their high antioxidants, vitamin, and fiber content, and we try to eat some every day. They contain ingredients that are crucial in combating cell damage from oxygen, and reducing inflammation, which can lower cancer risk.

Incorporating fruits like berries and citrus into the diet is a culinary pleasure and a strategic health choice. The antioxidants and anti-inflammatory compounds in these fruits underscore the importance of The Moss Method in reducing the risk of chronic diseases, including cancer. Routine eating of citrus fruits, rich in vitamin C, may contribute to a broader strategy against cancer, emphasizing the potential of natural, non-toxic approaches in oncology.

POMEGRANATE EXTRACT

Pomegranate (*Punica granatum L.*) has a special place in The Moss Method. It contains many plant chemicals (Olvera-Sandoval 2022). Pomegranate has been used as a fruit for thousands of years. It is a nutritional powerhouse, whether eaten fresh, frozen, or concentrated into no-sugar-added molasses. One difficulty with pomegranate is how to get its considerable benefits, without adding to one's carbohydrate load.

One medium-sized pomegranate contains 52 grams of carbs and 11 grams of fiber. The glycemic index of pomegranate is 60 to 70, and the glycemic load of half a cup of arils is 10 to 11, both of which are considered moderate.

(The glycemic index (GI) measures how quickly a food raises blood sugar levels, while the glycemic load (GL) judges the actual impact on blood sugar, taking into account the amount of carbs in a serving of the food.)

Opinion is divided on whether pomegranate juice will raise or lower fasting blood glucose and other markers of type 2 diabetes (T2D). According to a meta-analysis (study of studies) of the question, 32 randomized controlled trials (RCTs) with pooled results revealed that eating pomegranate had a positive impact on metabolism-related health markers. Specifically, pomegranate intake lowers fasting blood glucose, fasting insulin levels, and the A1c level. These findings support the potential benefits of pomegranates in managing important key indicators related to blood sugar and insulin resistance (Bahari 2024a, Bahari 2024b).

In our household, we use pomegranate in several different forms:

- *Raw pomegranate arils:* These fleshy seeds can be obtained fresh in season or, more conveniently, frozen. Since many markets only carry fresh pomegranates during part of the year, you can buy them then and carefully open them with a knife, separating out the "arils" or seeds. I then place them on a tray and put them in the freezer for an hour or more, later moving them to a plastic freezer bag for storage. You can then have them as a snack or put them into your unsweetened kefir, as I do. Three tablespoons equal six grams of carbs and one gram of fiber, for a "net carb" load of five grams. Taken in moderation they allow one to enjoy a delicious fruit at a small cost in terms of net carbs. I also keep a bag of commercial frozen pomegranate seeds in the freezer for when I do not have access to fresh sources. The product I favor at such times is Woodstock Organic Pomegranate Kernels.

- *Organic pomegranate juice:* One ounce contains 19 calories and 4.7 grams of net carbs. Because of its intense flavor, you will not want to drink this in abundance as you might with, for example, orange or apple juice.

- *Unsweetened pomegranate molasses:* This is a little-known product from the Middle East. Some products contain added sugar, but this is not necessary or desirable. One teaspoon of unsweetened pomegranate molasses contains approximately 16 to 20 calories and 5 grams of net carbs. It can be used to flavor unsweetened yogurts. But a little goes a long way.

RESEARCH BASE ON POMEGRANATE

There are now over 3,500 articles concerning pomegranate in PubMed. The first appeared in the early 19th century. That concerned the case of tapeworm (*taenia*) cured by a decoction of pomegranate, prepared by boiling the fresh bark of the root of the plant in water (Pollock 1814). This was a traditional East Indian remedy, perhaps of Arabic origin. According to a contemporary catalog of Indian healing plants and drugs, both the rind and the root of the plant yielded useful drugs, the latter mainly used for the expulsion of tapeworms (Fleming 1810, p. 33). After this, the topic of pomegranate's health benefits disappeared from the Western medical record for two centuries! When interest revived, it was mainly to "suspect the sharp crushed pomegranate seeds" of irritating the esophagus and possibly causing esophageal cancer (Ghadirian 1987, Ghadirian 1992).

However, it wasn't until the 21st century that modern research into pomegranate's health benefits really got underway (Kim 2002). A study from South Korea studied pomegranate parts, such as fermented juice, skin extract, and seed oil, for their potential to help prevent or treat breast cancer. Pomegranates contain natural compounds that can significantly reduce the activity of aromatase, an enzyme that converts androgens into estrogens, by 60-80%. This is beneficial because reducing aromatase activity can lower estrogen levels in the body, which may help prevent the growth of estrogen-sensitive cancers, such as certain types of breast cancer (Kim 2002).

The Pantuck Trial (2006)

Between 2006 and 2017 pomegranate products were tested in several clinical trials. All of these concerned prostate cancer (Freedland 2013, Paller 2013, Stenner-Liewen 2013, Paller 2017).

The most positive result was a non-randomized clinical trial for men who had increasing prostate-specific antigen (PSA) levels following surgery or radiotherapy. It slowed the growth of the cancer, based on the PSA score. Participants were given 8 ounces of pomegranate juice daily of the so-called "Wonderful" variety. Each portion contained 570 mg of polyphenols (antioxidants). Furthermore, lab tests on prostate cancer cells before and after treatment showed a 12% decrease in cell growth and a 17% increase in programmed cell death. There were also reductions in cell damage from excess oxygen. No serious side effects were reported (Pantuck 2006).

The POMx Trial (2013)

In a 2013 study from the Prostate Cancer Research Program, Sidney Kimmel Comprehensive Cancer Center at Johns Hopkins, Baltimore, a commercial pomegranate extract called POMx was tried as a treatment for men with recurrent prostate cancer. The extract extended their PSA doubling time (PSADT) from an average of **11.9 months to 18.5 months,** indicating a significant slowdown in their cancer's growth (Paller 2013).

The POMI-T Trial (2014)

In 2014 a double-blind, placebo-controlled, randomized trial examined a whole food supplement called POMI-T in men under active surveillance for prostate cancer. The study was done at the Primrose Research Unit of Bedford Hospital, Bedford, UK,

POMI-T contained four minimally processed food extracts. The intervention consisted of one capsule taken three times per day, for six months. Each capsule contained:

- Broccoli powder (*Brassica oleracea*) 100 mg (milligrams)
- Turmeric powder (*Curcuma longa*) 100 mg
- Pomegranate whole fruit powder (*Punica granatum*) 100 mg
- Green tea (*Camellia sinensis*) in a 5:1 extract. As a result, 20 mg of the powder was equivalent to 100 mg of green tea.

The median increase in the Prostate Specific Antigen (PSA) score in those taking the supplement was a slower rise of **14.7% in their PSA scores versus a rapid rise of 78.5%** in those getting the placebo pill. This notable difference (of 63.8%) suggested real benefit (Thomas 2014).

What made this trial unusual was that it involved four natural food factors taken at the same time. Plus, unlike most such studies, the investigators administered concentrated food powders instead of refined chemicals—for example, turmeric root powder instead of purified curcumin. As the authors stated:

> *"Up to now, research has focused on supplements containing specific, extracted chemicals believed to be the anti-cancer candidates" (ibid.)*

While using food powders does not allow for the same degree of standardization as ultra-refined plant chemicals, it captures more of the complexity of actual foodstuffs.

University of Wisconsin Study (2021)

Scientists at the University of Wisconsin, writing in the journal *Prostate*, reported on 30 men who had early-stage prostate cancer. They found that taking 1,000 milligrams (mg) of a pomegranate extract daily for a year was well-tolerated, with no significant side effects. Out of the initial participants, almost all (29) completed the study. The men taking pomegranate extract showed highly significant increases in beneficial metabolites, urolithin A and urolithin A-gluc, in their urine and blood plasma (Jarrard 2021).

Additionally, tissue analysis revealed notable reductions in markers of DNA damage (8-OhdG levels decreased) and androgen receptor expression in prostate tumors. These changes suggested that pomegranate extract can positively affect biomarkers associated with prostate cancer progression, supporting further investigation into its use as a preventive treatment for men on active surveillance.

MAQUI BERRY POWDER

Maqui (*Aristotelia chilensis)* is a perennial evergreen shrub that produces a profusion of deep purple berries. It is native to the Patagonia district of Chile and parts of Argentina. It came to my attention because it is among the lowest in carbs of all the berries. Each teaspoon of the dehydrated berries has just 2 grams of carbs, one of which is fiber. So it is an excellent food for people concerned with borderline diabetes or T2D.

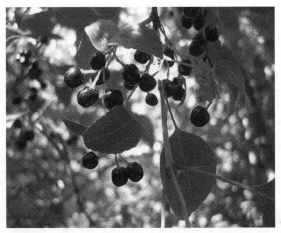

Maqui berries, native to Patagonia in southern Chile. Source: Wikimedia Commons

(Maqui is a key ingredient in our Purple Smoothies.)

But maqui is also a powerhouse of desirable chemicals. These include plant pigments, ellagic acid, resveratrol, and quercetin. Native people in South America are said to use the leaves as an infusion, and for the treatment of diarrhea, sore throats, and mouth sores (Muñoz 2001). According to a dozen authors:

> *"For the local Mapuche people, maqui is one of the sacred plants, a symbol of peaceful intention and goodwill. The Spanish conquerors described maqui as a healing plant to treat sore throats, intestinal tumors, diarrhea, fever, or wounds"* *(Otero 2023, edited).*

Of course, the fact that native inhabitants used a plant for millennia doesn't prove that it is effective, but neither does it rule out the possibility that it has a scientific basis, as UNESCO recognizes.

Most of the health impacts of maqui are related to the high content of antioxidants in their fruits. It is particularly rich in plant pigments called anthocyanins, which gives the berry its dark purple color. As a result, maqui fruit has up to four times the amount of antioxidants as blueberries, red raspberries, blackberries, strawberries, and pomegranate (Fredes 2014). It has almost ten times as much of this plant pigment than the nearest contender, which was the blackberry. That is reason enough to make it part of your smoothie recipes.

ACEROLA CHERRIES

Acerola cherries (*Malpighia emarginata*), also known as Barbados cherries or West Indian cherries, are small, bright red fruits native to the tropical regions of the Western Hemisphere, particularly found in the Caribbean, Central America, and northern South America. They grow on a small shrub-like tree that produces gorgeous pink blossoms. These fruits are not only notable for their vibrant color and tart flavor but also for their exceptionally high vitamin C content and various health benefits. They figure prominently in our recipe for <u>High Vitamin C, Low-Carb Fruit Salad.</u>

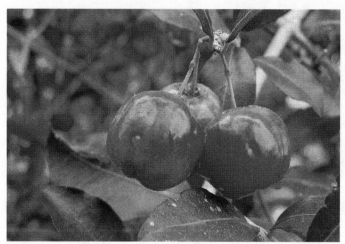

Acerola cherries, one of the world's best sources of vitamin C. Source: Wikimedia Commons

There is not a lot to say about the health effects of Acerola, other than the fact that it is an outstanding source of vitamin C. This could change, as scientists in Brazil and elsewhere begin to explore the beneficial effects of this native plant. One interesting study showed that Acerola acts synergistically with green tea to combat inflammation (Souza 2020).

Acerola figures in The Moss Method as a valuable contributor of natural vitamin C to our fruit mixture. They are rather tart, with about half as sweet as apples and one-third as sweet as bananas and so do not raise one's blood sugar excessively.

12. RESVERATROL

Resveratrol, a plant chemical found in grapes, berries, peanuts, and notably in red wine, is widely recognized for its health-enhancing qualities. This compound serves as a potent antioxidant and exerts anti-inflammatory, cardio-protective, and anticancer effects, making it a valuable component of The Moss Method for holistic cancer prevention.

Resveratrol's ability to inhibit cancer is rooted in its interaction with cancer stem cell (CSC) growth pathways. Key research findings highlight its potential in disrupting growth signaling, which is crucial for the self-renewal and survival of breast cancer stem cells. By interfering with these growth signals, resveratrol helps prevent the spread of cancer cells (Fu Y 2014). Additionally, resveratrol blocks CSCs' ability to migrate and invade healthy tissues, further illustrating its role as a deterrent to cancer metastasis (Shankar 2011). These mechanisms underscore resveratrol's dual role in both preventing cancer development and curtailing the growth and spread of existing cancer cells.

While dietary sources of resveratrol provide some benefits, the concentrations in these foods are generally low. Thus, it is assumed that supplements are often necessary to achieve levels needed for clinical benefits. There is no established upper limit for dietary resveratrol, indicating its safety when consumed as part of food. Clinical trials frequently use doses of 250-500 mg daily, which have been well-tolerated and considered safe for short-term use.

While moderate doses of resveratrol are generally safe, high doses can lead to gastrointestinal discomfort and potential interactions with medications. Symptoms such as diarrhea and nausea are common at higher doses. Additionally, due to its anticoagulant properties, high-dose resveratrol should be used cautiously in individuals taking blood thinners or those with bleeding disorders.

RESVERATROL & METABOLIC SYNDROME

Resveratrol supplements have been extensively studied for their health impact. For instance, a study involving patients with metabolic syndrome (pre-diabetes) found that taking 500 mg of resveratrol three times daily significantly improved energy-related markers, including reductions in weight, BMI, and insulin levels (Méndez-del Villar 2014). Another study on type 2 diabetes patients demonstrated that a daily intake of 1,000 mg of resveratrol supplements enhanced cellular defenses against damage and inflammation (García-Martinez 2023). This can indirectly contribute to cancer prevention by improving overall health and resistance to disease.

Integrating resveratrol into the diet involves more than just supplements. Red wines such as Burgundy, Pinot Noir, and Malbec are the greatest natural source of resveratrol. However, alcohol presents so many other health challenges that we do not generally advocate its use. Incorporating resveratrol-rich foods like grapes and berries into meals can enhance daily intake naturally. For those looking to harness these benefits within The Moss Method, a balanced approach combining dietary sources and supplements, mindful of dosage and potential interactions, is recommended. This comprehensive strategy ensures the maximization of resveratrol's potential while maintaining safety and effectiveness in cancer prevention and overall health improvement.

Scientific interest in resveratrol peaked in the pre-pandemic years (2020-2021), although there are still groups researching its effect on cancer. The scientific consensus is still up in the air. To quote scientists at Leicester, UK:

> *"There is currently no conclusive clinical evidence to advocate its recommendation in any healthcare setting....Over the last 20 years, there have been almost 200 studies evaluating resveratrol across at least 24 indications, including cancer, menopause symptoms, diabetes, metabolic syndrome, and cardiovascular disease. There are currently no consensus treatment regimens for any given condition or endpoint, beyond the fact that resveratrol is generally well-tolerated at a dose of up to 1 g/day" (Brown K 2024).*

13. GARLIC/ALLICIN

Garlic, renowned for its pungent aroma and rich flavor, boasts a treasure trove of health benefits, including its potential as a potent weapon against cancer stem cells (CSCs) through its most active ingredient, allicin. Garlic can be enjoyed in various forms. Eating raw garlic, especially when chopped or crushed to activate the release of allicin, provides the greatest health benefits. Consuming one to two cloves of fresh garlic daily in this way is recommended. In culinary use, incorporating garlic into dishes like sauces, soups, stews, and dressings not only enhances flavor but also boosts its health-promoting qualities.

For those opting for supplements, it is advisable to aim for 600-1200 mg of garlic extract daily, divided into doses to ensure consistent allicin intake. Selecting high-quality supplements with standardized contents is crucial to guarantee effectiveness and minimize variability. Garlic offers many health benefits. It aids in reducing blood pressure and cholesterol levels, promoting heart health. Its robust antimicrobial and antioxidant properties bolster overall health and fortify the immune system. Extensive research supports garlic's role in reducing the risk of cancers, particularly prostate and breast cancer.

When utilizing garlic, it is beneficial to add it towards the end of cooking or consume it raw to preserve its helpful compounds. However, be mindful of potential side effects like gastrointestinal discomfort and headaches, especially with high doses. Garlic may interact with drugs, so it is essential to consult healthcare providers, particularly regarding interactions with blood thinners, diabetes drugs, and immunosuppressants used for organ transplants. Gradually introducing garlic into your diet allows for a review of tolerance to it, while selecting firm, fresh bulbs and proper storage ensures the best quality.

Pairing garlic with onions and other anticancer foods like turmeric enhances their collective benefits. Combining garlic with other healthy ingredients amplifies their cancer-fighting potential. Garlic, with its multifaceted health advantages and cancer-fighting prowess, stands as a stalwart ally in the quest for holistic well-being. By thoughtfully incorporating garlic into your diet and supplement regimen, you unlock its full potential in cancer prevention and overall health improvement.

GARLIC & CANCER

In one large trial, published in the *BMJ* (*British Medical Journal*) long-term garlic supplementation was linked to a lower risk of dying from gastric cancer, although it did not reduce the incidence of the cancer itself. There were over 2,000 participants, all of whom were at high risk of stomach cancer. In this long-term study spanning over 22 years, garlic supplementation was associated with a significant **34% reduction in deaths from gastric cancer**. While garlic did not significantly reduce the *incidence* of gastric cancer, its role in lowering mortality is a positive finding (Li WQ 2019).

Moreover, the study found that the beneficial effects of garlic on reducing gastric cancer mortality became evident around 12 years after starting supplementation. These results suggest that garlic may have long-term protective effects, making it a valuable component in dietary strategies for cancer prevention. However, it is important to consult with healthcare professionals before starting any supplementation, especially for individuals on anticoagulants or those with platelet dysfunction (Ibid.)

The Colorectal Cancer Meta-Analysis (2020)

A meta-analysis of 11 studies involving over 12,000 cases found that high garlic consumption was associated with a 20% reduction in the risk of colorectal cancer (CRC). The analysis showed significant variability among the studies but tests confirmed the stability of the results. No significant publication bias was detected. This evidence supports the potential role of garlic in reducing the risk of colorectal cancer. This study added to a growing body of evidence suggesting that including garlic in your diet could be a simple and natural way to help reduce the risk of colorectal cancer (Zhou 2020).

National Cancer Institute Study (2002)

Both population-based and laboratory studies suggest that garlic and other allium vegetables like onions, scallions, and leeks have anti-cancer properties, according to the NCI. A population-based study found that men who consumed more than 10 grams (a third of an ounce) of allium vegetables per day had about half the risk of developing prostate cancer compared to those who ate less than 2.2 grams per day.

Specifically, high garlic intake was linked to a 53% lower risk and high scallion intake was linked to a 70% lower risk of prostate cancer. These findings were consistent regardless of body size, intake of other foods, and total calorie intake, and the protective effect was even stronger for localized prostate cancer. This study highlights the potential benefits of incorporating garlic and other allium vegetables into your diet to help reduce the risk of prostate cancer (Hsing 2002).

---

14. NUTS, SEEDS & LEGUMES

Nuts, seeds and legumes are essential to most traditional diets. They offer a treasure trove of nutrients that contribute to one's health and lifespan. They are particularly renowned for their roles in reducing cancer risk when incorporated with balance and mindfulness into one's daily diet. Nuts and seeds, including almonds, walnuts, and flaxseeds, are powerhouses of nutrients good for cancer prevention. They contain various vitamins, minerals, and antioxidants, each bringing its unique blend of healthy qualities. For example, almonds and walnuts are rich in vitamin E, known for its antioxidant qualities. These may help interrupt processes that lead to cancer development.

These small yet powerful dietary staples contain bioactive compounds such as antioxidants and omega-3 fatty acids. These compounds are celebrated for their anti-inflammatory and antioxidant effects, offering a protective shield against various health issues, including cancer. Studies have shown that these nutrients can control cell growth and survival, adding another layer of defense in our fight against cancer.

IMPACTING LIFESPAN & HEALTH

The use of nuts and seeds goes beyond enjoying their rich flavors; it taps into their profound health benefits. Research, including large-scale studies like the Nurses' Health Study, has revealed that frequent use of nuts and seeds is linked with a reduced death rate. The Nurses' Health Study (NHS) was part of a massive population-based study headquartered at the Harvard T.H. Chan School of Public Health, Boston. It ran from 1986 to 2014 and included over 67,000 women. A companion study called the Health Professionals Follow-Up Study contains data on over 45,000 men. The NHS was augmented by another study of over 93,000 younger women. So obviously, this study was extremely strong in terms of the number of participants and the prestige of its researchers. In these studies, nut and seed intake was associated with a notable increase in health, including factors related to cancer prevention.

Su Study (2010)

Scientists at Brigham and Women's Hospital and Harvard Medical School, Boston, found that higher consumption of nuts during adolescence was associated with a reduced risk of benign breast disease, a condition considered a marker for increased breast cancer risk. In a study of almost 30,000 women who completed a high school diet questionnaire in 1998, those who consumed two or more servings of nuts per week during their teenage years had **a 36% lower risk** of developing this precancerous condition compared to those who consumed less than one serving per month (Su X 2010).

Aune Meta-Analysis of Nut Consumption (2016)

Dagfinn Aune, Ph.D., of Imperial College London, London, UK, is a copious researcher in the field of cancer and diet in this comprehensive meta-analysis in *BMC Medicine,* which included 20 studies and 29 publications, he found that increasing nut intake by one ounce per day was associated with a notable reduction in several health risks. The results were similar for tree nuts and peanuts. The total cancer risk was reduced by 15% and the risk of all-cause mortality by 22%. Even more noteworthy was the **reduction of diabetes risk by 39%, respiratory disease deaths by 52%, and infectious diseases by a staggering 75%**. The authors, from nine different institutions including the School of Public Health, Imperial College London, make an extraordinary statement:

"If the associations are causal, an estimated 4.4 million premature deaths in the America, Europe, Southeast Asia, and Western Pacific would be attributable to a nut intake below 20 grams per day in 2013" (Aune 2016).

J. Long Meta-Analysis (2020)

A 2020 meta-analysis from China confirmed the previous results. The authors looked at 33 separate studies that included more than 50,000 cancer cases. When comparing the highest with the lowest category of nut intake, high consumption was associated with a 10% decreased overall risk of cancer. The protective effect of nuts was especially apparent against cancers from the digestive system, with a 17% decrease. Among different nut classes, significant associations were only obtained for intake of **tree nuts (not peanuts).** There was a clear dose-response relationship between nut consumption and cancer: That is, every 20 grams (less than an ounce) increase in nut consumption was associated with a 10% decrease in overall cancer risk (Long J 2020).

The PREDIMED Findings (2013)

The PREDIMED clinical trial from Spain is discussed elsewhere for the outstanding effects of extra virgin olive oil (EVOO) on breast cancer and diabetes. However, a secondary finding had to do with the intake of nuts. According to a separate paper on this topic, over a period of almost five years, there were 323 total deaths in a group of about 7,000 Spanish men and women aged 55 to 80 years (Guasch-Ferré 2013). Of these, there were 81 deaths from heart disease and 130 from cancer.

But eating nuts regularly was linked to a lower chance of dying from any cause. Those participants who ate nuts more than three times a week had a **39% lower risk of death.** This risk reduction was primarily for deaths due to heart disease and cancer. Even more significant were the results in participants who were not only consuming nuts frequently but were also following a Mediterranean diet supplemented with nuts. This group had the lowest mortality risk, showing **an astonishing 63% reduction in total mortality** compared to the baseline of non-consumers of this important food category (Guasch-Ferré 2013).

While the health benefits of nuts and seeds are immense, it is important to consume them in moderation due to their high caloric content. A recommended serving is usually about one ounce per day. (I weighed out one ounce of walnuts, and it came to a small handful.) According to the Long meta-analysis (above) there was a dose-response curve with nut consumption. And therefore, if your weight will support it, it would probably be desirable to increase that to about one-and-a-half ounces per day. But moderation is key, as it will ensure that you can reap numerous benefits without overindulging.

AN OFTEN-OVERLOOKED FACTOR: NUT SKINS

Often overlooked, the *skins* of nuts like almonds and walnuts are also potent sources of antioxidants. These ingredients contribute to the overall health benefits of nuts and seeds, reinforcing their status as dietary superheroes in the fight against cancer and other diseases. So definitely go for raw or lightly roasted nuts with their skins attached, rather than blanched or heavily processed nuts. Peanuts are not actually nuts, but legumes. They do have some health benefits, as well, but it is not as strong as tree nuts.

There is also a big difference in the carb content of nut varieties. As a result, walnuts and almonds are low in net carbs, while cashews and pistachios are relatively high. My late friend, Robert Atkins, MD, strongly advocated the consumption of macadamia nuts, which have a very low "net carb" score (more fat, protein and fiber than carbohydrates). They are thus ideal for those on a low-carb or keto diet. But all tree nuts (and maybe even peanuts) convey profound health benefits.

WHOLE GRAINS & LEGUMES

Whole grains, key parts of most traditional diets, are rich in fiber, essential nutrients, and cancer-preventing compounds, offering substantial health benefits and playing an important role in cancer prevention when incorporated into the diet. Including whole grains and legumes in your traditional diet is vital in maintaining health and potentially preventing cancer. I celebrate these nutrient-rich foods for their high fiber content, essential nutrients, and compounds that may protect against cancer.

However, the question of grains is a bit complicated for people who struggle with type 2 diabetes or even prediabetes. As a T2D patient for the past ten years, I am cautious with the quantity of grains and legumes that I eat. I do eat small amounts of these and include them in dishes that also contain fats, fiber, and protein, which slows the entry of glucose into the bloodstream. A good example is tabbouleh, where some whole-grain bulgur wheat is mixed with copious amounts of parsley, mint, olive oil, and lemon juice.

Whole grains such as oats, barley, and einkorn (the original wheat) are nutrient powerhouses. They retain valuable nutrients often lost in refined grains, including dietary fiber essential for digestive health. Fiber-rich whole grains can help with weight management, a crucial factor in reducing cancer risk. These grains also contain B vitamins, iron, magnesium, and antioxidants. Researchers associate these compounds in whole grains like lignans and saponins with anticancer qualities.

Legumes, including lentils, chickpeas, and beans, are also essential to most traditional diets. Rich in fiber and protein, they also offer a variety of micronutrients. The fiber in legumes is mainly linked to a lower risk of colorectal cancer. They also contain bioactive compounds like isoflavones and protease blockers, which research suggests may stop cancer cell growth and promote normal cell death in cancer.

Combining whole grains and legumes in a diet provides synergistic nutritional benefits. Together they form a complete protein profile, which is especially valuable in plant-based diets. This combo also helps stabilize blood sugar levels, which is essential in preventing obesity and related cancer risks.

Aune Meta-Analysis of Whole Grain Consumption (2011)

This is another study from the prolific Dagfinn Aune, Ph.D., of Imperial College London. He performed a meta-analysis of 45 studies on the effect of whole grain consumption on disease states. Whole grains were significantly associated with a reduced risk of chronic diseases. A meta-analysis of 45 studies found that a daily increase of 90 grams of whole grains (about three servings, such as two slices of bread and one bowl of cereal) reduces the risk of coronary heart disease by 19%, cardiovascular disease by 22%, and total cancer by 15%. Moreover, all-cause mortality was reduced by 17% (Aune 2011, Aune 2016).

Higher whole grain intake also correlated with lower mortality from respiratory diseases (22% reduction), infectious diseases (26% reduction), and diabetes (51% reduction). These benefits were observed with whole grain intake up to 210-225 grams per day (seven to seven and a half servings), but with only minimal benefits from refined grains, such as white bread, or white rice. These findings therefore support dietary guidelines recommending increased whole grain intake to lower the risk of chronic diseases and premature mortality.

15. HERBS & SPICES

"Culinary spices and herbs contain polyphenols and other antioxidants. Although many other nutrients and foods have anti-inflammatory potential, spices, and herbs contribute to the Mediterranean diet's anti-inflammatory and overall health-protective role"
–Krystle Zuniga, Ph.D., Texas State University (2019).

Herbs and spices are not only essential for their flavor but are pivotal to The Moss Method for their health benefits. Commonly used herbs like basil, oregano, rosemary, thyme, and parsley, along with spices such as garlic, turmeric, and saffron, are known for their anti-inflammatory and antioxidant qualities. These qualities are essential to reducing chronic disease risks and enhancing lifespan (Martínez-González 2015).

Historically, herbs and spices composed much of humanity's medicine chest, reflecting a diet focused on natural, unprocessed ingredients that maximize health benefits. For instance, garlic is used worldwide for its heart and circulatory benefits, while rosemary and oregano are high in antioxidants that promote disease prevention. This tradition not only makes the diet appealing but also aligns with The Moss Method's emphasis on food as a fundamental part of health (Pérez-López 2016).

POWERFUL HERBAL INGREDIENTS

(With a nod to Simon and Garfunkel.)

- *Parsley (Petroselinum crispum):* Beyond being a garnish, parsley is abundant in antioxidants, particularly apigenin, which supports immune function and combats cancer. Apigenin's benefits include anti-inflammatory effects, support the removal of toxic compounds, improvement of cancer treatments, genetic influence on cancer development, hormonal balance, induction of cancer cell death, blocking tumor growth, and slowing of cancer cell spread (Kim 2016).

- *Sage (Salvia officinalis):* Known for its rich flavor and healthy qualities, sage contains carnosic acid and rosmarinic acid, potent antioxidants with qualities inducing normal cell death in cancer, particularly effective against prostate and colon cancers (Abdul Ghani 2023, Kiokias 2021).

- *Rosemary (Rosmarinus officinalis):* Used widely in Mediterranean cooking and traditional medicine, rosemary supports anticancer qualities, evidenced by its ability to reduce tumor size and improve the effectiveness of other treatments like vitamin D3 (González-Vallinas 2014, Moore 2016).

- *Thyme (Thymus vulgaris):* This herb is rich in thymol and carvacrol, which have shown potential against breast and colon cancer cells. Thyme enhances the effectiveness of chemo drugs, reducing their toxic side effects (Kubatka 2019, Fan 2015).

- *Oregano (Origanum vulgare):* We should also mention oregano, an herb that originated in Africa, was widely cultivated in southern Europe, and is now naturalized throughout much of the temperate zone. Oregano is most familiar as the dried green herb available in shakers at Italian restaurants all over the world. There is intriguing research from Slovakia on the use of oregano against a common line of breast cancer cells. They wrote: "Our results demonstrate, for the first time, a distinct tumor-suppressive effect of oregano in the breast cancer model" (Kubatka 2017).

Even a relatively small amount of oregano suppressed cancer formation in lab rats. The inclusion of just 0.3% oregano in the rats' feed suppressed tumor frequency by 55.5%, tumor incidence by 44%, and tumor volume by 44.5% compared to control animals (ibid.) This amount, by my rough calculation, equaled about half an ounce per day for a 150-pound person.

EMERGING RESEARCH ON CARDAMOM & GINGER

- *Cardamom:* Recent studies suggest cardamom, particularly the compound cardamonin, is effective against cancer stem cells, offering new paths for cancer treatment (Bhattacharjee 2013, Jia 2016).

- *Ginger:* Known for its main ingredient, gingerol, it has anti-inflammatory and anticancer effects, potentially enhancing the effectiveness of other anticancer agents (Lee 2008, Brahmbhatt 2013). I rarely make black tea without a generous piece of organic ginger (cleaned, peeled, and chopped). It is one of the most healthy things available in the supermarket.

Herbs and spices improve the flavor of dishes while providing substantial health benefits, particularly in cancer prevention. By integrating these ingredients into daily meals, The Moss Method not only promotes a diet rich in natural, unprocessed items but also uses the inherent healing qualities of these culinary elements to combat cancer effectively.

---

16. MAITAKE

Grifola frondosa, known in English as hen of the woods, or as maitake in Japanese, is a notable variety of mushrooms under study for its possible anticancer benefits. Maitake (the "dancing mushroom" in Japanese) has been the subject of both experimental and clinical research due to its possible effects on cancer and the immune system. Below is a summary of key findings from various studies:

EXPERIMENTAL EVIDENCE ON POLYSACCHARIDES

Maitake contains healthful chemicals called polysaccharides, particularly beta-glucans, which have shown anti-tumor qualities in lab studies. These compounds appear to work by stimulating the immune system, enhancing the activity of natural killer (NK) cells, and inducing programmed cell death in cancer cells (Kodama 2003).

Maitake D-fraction (MD fraction) appears to stop the growth of cancer through its stimulation of a class of white blood cells called natural killer (NK) cells:

> *"Maitake D-fraction hindered metastatic progress, lessened the levels of tumor markers, and increased natural killer (NK) cell activity in all patients examined. As a result, it appears to repress cancer growth and primarily exerts its effect by stimulating NK activity" (Kodama 2003, edited).*

In 2002, authors at the Department of Microbial Chemistry, Kobe Pharmaceutical University, reported on the results of a combination of maitake powder and MD fraction in patients with advanced cancer:

> *"Cancer regression or significant symptom improvement was observed in 58.3% of liver cancer patients, 68.8% of breast cancer patients, and 62.5% of lung cancer patients. The trial found a less than 10% to 20% improvement for leukemia, stomach cancer, and brain cancer patients" (Kodama 2002, edited).*

Research on this edible fungus began in 1984, with a publication on the effects of an extract by injection on various tumor types in mice (Suzuki 1984). About one-quarter of these reports came from the laboratory of Hiroaki Nanba, Ph.D., of Kobe Pharmaceutical University, Japan.

Nanba isolated the D-fraction from maitake by repeatedly treating the mushroom's fruiting body (the aboveground portion of the mushroom) with alcohols, acids, and alkaline substances. The D-fraction enhanced both arms of the immune response in normal mice. He concluded,

> *"Its administration may improve host defense against foreign germs and protect healthy individuals from infectious diseases" (Kodama 2003).*

I had the pleasure of interviewing Nanba in September 1994 when he came to the U.S. to present a paper at the New York Academy of Science seminar on *Cancer Prevention: From the Laboratory to the Clinic* (NYAS 1994, Nanba 1995).

[See a video of my discussion of maitake with Mike Shirota, president and CEO of the Mushroom Wisdom company, who accompanied Dr. Nanba to New York in 1994.]

MSKCC Phase I/II Human Trials

Oddly enough, at a time when Memorial Sloan-Kettering Cancer Center was mostly known for its hostility to anything "alternative," some scientists there developed an intense interest in maitake. In fact, a clinical study there showed in exquisite detail that a maitake extract could stimulate various parameters of the immune systems of breast cancer patients. There were increased immune cells and cytokines (hormone-like substances) essential for a robust immune response (Deng 2009).

Another clinical trial of maitake demonstrated its possible role in improving the immune function in patients with myelodysplastic syndromes (MDS), a group of cancers in which the bone marrow does not produce enough healthy blood cells (Chen 2010).

Maitake has been shown to activate various immune cells, including macrophages, natural killer cells, and T cells, as a result enhancing the body's immune response (Kodama 2003). Studies have also indicated an increase in immune-stimulating cytokines in response to maitake (Mayell 2001). While most researchers have focused on cancer, some suggest that maitake may also be helpful in fighting viral and bacterial infections due to its ability to stimulate the immune system (Kubo 1994).

These mushrooms are rich in various active compounds, demonstrating substantial anticancer activity (Ng 2002). In Japan, lentinan from shiitake mushrooms and the D-fraction from maitake mushrooms have both found their place in cancer treatment due to their immune-adjusting effects and possible anticancer qualities (Kodama 2003, Kobori 2007).

D-FRACTION DROPS

Since highly concentrated maitake D-fraction can be administered as drops under the tongue, *it is one of the few natural treatments given to people who can no longer eat solid foods.* It has thus been essential to patients and family members in dire situations. At the very least, it provides the relatives of standardized patients with the psychological comfort of "doing something" to aid the patient during extremely trying or tragic situations.

For many years, Memorial Sloan-Kettering Cancer Center (MSKCC) and Weill Cornell Medical School were actively involved in research on a beta-glucan extracted from maitake. This was found to stimulate the production of an immune-related protein, which promotes the growth of a type of white blood cells that fight infections.

Their research showed that taking maitake orally helped develop specific primitive cells in the bone marrow to become active myeloid cells necessary for the immune system. This process also improved the recovery of white blood cells in the blood, which are crucial for fighting infections, especially after damage to the bone marrow caused by chemo (Lin H 2010).

In a non-randomized clinical trial, maitake mushrooms were found to boost the immune system. Specifically, it improved the activity of neutrophils and monocytes, key types of white blood cells, in healthy ways. For patients with Myelodysplastic Syndromes (MDS), a form of blood cancer, maitake treatment notably increased their monocytes' response to E. coli bacteria and stimulated the production of reactive oxygen species, indicating a stronger immune response. Although four patients experienced a different type of white blood cell, other changes in blood protein levels were not important. This showed maitake's possible benefits for immune system support without side effects (Wesa 2015).

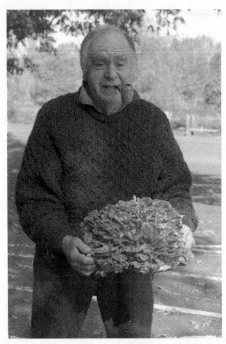

Sam Donato with his prize "hen of the woods" maitake mushroom, Colonial Park, Somerset, NJ, October 2015. Source: Martha B. Moss

Maitake sometimes grows in unexpected places, even in the U.S. My wife, Martha, took this picture of Sam Donato, posing with a maitake mushroom he found in Somerset, New Jersey, in October 2015. We had met Sam moments before in Colonial Park, where he had come with the declared intention of finding a "hen of the woods" mushroom. True to his word, he found this glorious specimen at the base of

216

an oak tree about 15 minutes later! He cherished its culinary value but seemed hardly aware of its medicinal usage.

---

17. HONOKIOL

Another important, but little-known, natural treatment is honokiol. Honokiol is a compound derived from the bark, seed cones, and leaves of trees belonging to the genus *Magnolia officinalis*. It is a botanical agent, but is definitely not a food factor. To get its beneficial effects, you will have to take it as a supplement. The label dose is one 250 mg capsule per day.

The unusual name, "honokiol," comes from one of particular species, *Magnolia honoki*, from which the compound was first isolated. This natural product has been used for centuries in traditional Asian medicine, particularly in China, South Korea, and Japan, for a variety of purposes including treating anxiety, neurological disorders, inflammation, and more.

Historically, magnolia extracts, containing honokiol and other related compounds like magnolol, have been used in traditional medicine practices for their wide-ranging drug qualities. The use of Magnolia and its extracts can be traced back to ancient texts, illustrating its long-standing significance in herbal medicine.

In modern research, honokiol has garnered attention for its potential anti-cancer qualities among other health benefits. Studies have suggested that honokiol can cause programmed cell death in cancer cells, stop the formation of new blood vessels that feed tumors, and improve the effectiveness of chemo, all without harm. Its methods of action include changing the signal networks involved in cell survival, reproduction, and death.

(Signal networks refer to the complex systems of communication within cells that use chemical signals to respond to changes and coordinate activities. These networks help cells process information and make decisions necessary for the organism's functioning and survival.)

There are at present over 1,200 PubMed-indexed articles on honokiol, indicating considerable research interest. Of these, almost one-third relate to cancer. According to scientists at the University of Southern Alabama:

According to the MSKCC website, honokiol has shown antitumor effects in the test tube against a very wide array of cancer types: leukemia, lung, bladder, prostate, melanoma, breast, glioblastoma, neuroblastoma, and oral cancer cell lines. In murine models, honokiol enhanced low-dose docetaxel treatment against prostate cancer growth and bone metastasis, and reduced breast tumor growth biomarkers.

According to researchers at The University of Kansas Medical Center, Kansas City, in combination with radiation therapy "honokiol is a potent blocker of colon cancer growth that attacks the stem cells" (Ponnurangam 2012).

Honokiol kills cell lines of oral squamous cell carcinoma (Huang KJ 2018).

Despite this, there are very few clinical trials of honokiol and none to my knowledge that addresses its clinical effects in cancer. So while this is a promising botanical agent, it lacks the kind of clinical data that would establish its effectiveness in cancer prevention.

Beyond its anti-cancer potential, honokiol has also been studied for its anti-inflammatory, antioxidant, anti-anxiety, and neuroprotective effects. Its ability to cross the blood-brain barrier makes it a compound of interest for neurological conditions as well.

18. LUTEOLIN

Luteolin, a pigment found in various fruits, vegetables, and herbs, is renowned for its anti-inflammatory, antioxidant, and anticancer properties (Luo Y 2017). Common sources include celery, thyme, green peppers, and chamomile tea. For example, celery contains 1 to 2 milligrams (mg) of luteolin per 100 grams, while thyme packs around 45.5 mg per 100 grams. However, getting enough luteolin from these foods can be challenging due to factors like food composition and individual digestion. Realistically, few people consume 100 grams (nearly four ounces) of these foods in one sitting.

Fortunately, luteolin supplements offer a more reliable and concentrated source, typically providing between 100 to 200 mg per capsule. Despite being less popular than turmeric—searched about 50 times more frequently on Google in the U.S.—luteolin is a potent compound with significant health benefits. It inhibits tumor growth by targeting essential cellular processes, including programmed cell death, cell cycle regulation, blood vessel formation, and cancer cell migration.

Luteolin works by modulating specific proteins within cells. These proteins often promote cell growth and prevent cell death. By decreasing their activity, luteolin halts cancer cell growth and encourages their destruction. Conversely, luteolin boosts proteins that promote normal, programmed cell death, helping eliminate damaged or unwanted cells. For instance, p21, a protein involved in controlling cell division, is enhanced by luteolin, further inhibiting cancer cell proliferation.

Moreover, luteolin's anticancer effects are amplified when combined with other chemotherapeutic agents, potentially offering more effective treatments with reduced side effects (Singh Tuli 2022). Beyond its anticancer capabilities, luteolin exhibits strong antioxidant properties, protecting cells from free radical damage in various models, including liver cells and nervous system disorders (Prasher 2022).

Luteolin also promotes the self-destruction of cancer cells by adjusting protein levels, facilitating natural cell death processes. This makes it a promising candidate for cancer treatment (Singh Tuli 2022). Additionally, luteolin influences cellular cleanup, aiding the regeneration of healthier cells by affecting molecules crucial for this process in cancer cells (Han M 2023).

Luteolin's multifaceted anticancer potential lies in its ability to interfere with various cell processes, promoting cell death, cleanup, and cycle regulation. Its antioxidant qualities further enhance its appeal as a cancer-fighting agent. While challenges like availability persist, ongoing research and development of luteolin extracts hold promise for making this powerful compound more accessible for cancer prevention and treatment.

19. LYCOPENE/TOMATO

Lycopene, a potent antioxidant found in tomatoes, is celebrated for its potential to change the networks that could help reduce the population of cancer stem cells, especially in conditions like breast cancer. Among its qualities, it has notable anticancer qualities and is particularly effective against prostate cancer due to its ability to interfere with key cellular processes involved in cancer's growth.

The best amount of lycopene to take can differ depending on your health goals. Supplements usually contain between 10 to 30 milligrams per day. However, lycopene is also naturally available through dietary sources, primarily tomato-based products, which are a practical addition to a balanced diet. The form and availability of lycopene are important. Supplements provide a concentrated dose, but lycopene from food is part of a natural mix that may improve absorption. This absorption is improved when tomatoes are cooked or processed, as heat breaks down the plant's cell walls, releasing more lycopene and making it available for absorption in the gut. Additionally, consuming lycopene with fats such as olive oil further improves its availability.

Lycopene's health benefits are many:

- *Anticancer Benefits:* Lycopene is associated with a reduced risk of prostate cancer. It stops the growth of cancer cells and may interfere with cancer's growth. Routine intake of lycopene has been linked with delayed growth and improved treatment outcomes in patients with locally advanced prostate cancer (Kapala 2022).

- *Antioxidant and Anti-inflammatory Properties:* Lycopene helps neutralize harmful free radicals and reduce cell damage from oxygen and inflammation, which are known contributors to cancer development (Aggarwal 2003, Goel 2008).

- *Circulatory System:* It may help improve lipid (fat) profiles and reduce blood pressure, supporting overall heart health.

THE UNEXPECTED BENEFIT OF SALSA

Chinese scientists carried out a fascinating study of tomato and tomato products and colorectal cancer (CRC). Their subjects were over 100,000 American adults. They looked at the impact of raw tomato, tomato juice, tomato catsup, or pure lycopene on the risk of CRC incidence or mortality. The bottom line was **that a higher consumption of tomato salsa was associated with a 20% lower risk of colorectal cancer incidence**, whereas there was no significant benefit associated with any of the other forms of tomato (Jiang Z 2023). They offer the following explanation for this unusual finding:

*"Tomato salsa, with its complex blend of ingredients, offers **synergistic interactions** among its bioactive compounds. It is not only a rich source of*

*antioxidant lycopene but also includes phenolic acids, flavonoids, and ascorbic acid. These ingredients interact to amplify the health benefits of salsa. For instance, fats in avocados and olive oil, common in salsa recipes, significantly boost lycopene's bioavailability. **The combined antioxidants provide stronger protection against oxidative stress and inflammation than any single compound alone**" (Jiang Z 2023, edited)*

This is in line with The Moss Method's emphasis on the power, indeed the necessity, of synergistic action when it comes to the natural or dietary approach to cancer prevention.

(See our discussion of The Power of Synergy, a key concept in The Moss Method.)

Incorporating lycopene into your diet is not only good for its health qualities but can also be a culinary delight. Opting for tomato-based dishes, *especially those of cooked and processed tomatoes,* combined with EVOO, enhances lycopene's more limited activity. Examples include not just salsa, but sauces, soups, and stews, where tomatoes are cooked down, releasing more lycopene due to the breakdown of cell walls. Pairing these dishes with olive oil not only improves flavor but also increases the absorption of lycopene into the body and adds the incredible power of EVOO to the mix.

Lycopene's integration into routine dietary practices offers substantial health benefits, particularly in cancer prevention and heart health. It is a valuable part of a balanced diet, contributing not only to reduced cancer risk but also to overall well-being. As research continues to uncover the full spectrum of lycopene's health benefits, it remains a key nutrient in search of a healthy lifestyle. However, as with any supplement, it should be used thoughtfully and in moderation, with an awareness of its interactions and side effects.

For those considering supplements, choosing high-quality products with verified purity and potency is crucial. It is important to be aware of potential interactions with drugs, particularly blood thinners, and the possible side effects of high intake, such as GI discomfort and changes in skin color. Consult healthcare providers before beginning supplement use, especially if you are on drugs that could interact with lycopene.

20. MILK THISTLE/SILYMARIN

Milk thistle (*Silybum marianum*), is a plant known for its liver-protecting effects. Silymarin is the active compound extracted from this plant's seeds, responsible for its medicinal benefits. It is known for its antioxidant, anti-inflammatory qualities, and potential anticancer effects, and is a valuable addition to your health regimen. It attacks cancer stem cells (CSCs) in various cancers and provides crucial support for liver health.

When considering the incorporation of milk thistle/silymarin into your daily routine, there are several important aspects to keep in mind:

- The recommended range typically includes around 550 milligrams (mg) of milk thistle extract per capsule, standardized to at least 80% silymarin content. The exact dosage may vary depending on your specific health goals.

- Milk thistle/silymarin is available in different forms, such as capsules or tablets. It is worth noting that the availability of silymarin can be influenced by factors like the extraction method and formulation.

- This powerful compound offers benefits, including liver protection and support against toxins. Its antioxidant and anti-inflammatory qualities help manage cell damage from oxygen and inflammation. Ongoing research is exploring its potential in the treatment of various diseases, including cancer.

- While milk thistle seeds or extracts can contribute to your overall health, they generally contain silymarin in lower concentrations compared to standardized supplements.

- When choosing silymarin supplements, opt for those with standardized extracts that explicitly mention their silymarin content. It is essential to consult with healthcare providers before starting supplements, especially if you are taking drugs. Follow the recommended dosage and administration guidelines, as indicated on product labels or as advised by your healthcare professional.

To maintain the potency of silymarin supplements, store them in a cool, dry place. Be vigilant about potential side effects, particularly GI discomfort, and promptly consult a healthcare provider if you experience negative reactions.

Be aware of the possible side effects, which may include *GI discomfort,* headaches, or allergic reactions. Additionally, *consider potential interactions with drugs such as blood thinners, diabetes drugs, and drugs that deliberately suppress the immune system, such as for organ transplant recipients.*

Incorporate milk thistle/silymarin creatively into your diet. Experiment with a smoothie by blending spinach, banana, berries, and milk thistle tincture. For a flavorful twist, use milk thistle powder when preparing dishes like roasted cauliflower with pesto. You can also enjoy an herbal tea infusion by steeping milk thistle seeds alongside chamomile and mint.

In summary, understanding the benefits of milk thistle, silymarin, and silibinin can improve your holistic wellness approach, aligning with a balanced diet and routine medical supervision, which are fundamental elements of The Moss Method. When using supplements, always favor quality, follow recommended dosages, and consider your individual health needs.

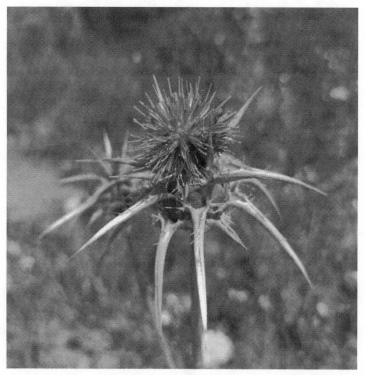

Milk thistle flowerhead (Silybum marianum) Source: Wikimedia Commons

THE QUESTION OF DIETARY SUPPLEMENTS

In The Moss Method, we favor obtaining one's anticancer plant chemicals directly from clean, traditional foods. However, we recognize that not everyone can sprout seeds, brew therapeutic teas, or whip up nutrient-packed smoothies. Often, we need to get important nutrients from concentrated sources or forms that our bodies can easily use, especially when these nutrients are hard to find in regular foods or when traditional ways of preparing them aren't practical.

The challenges go beyond simply finding these compounds in foods. For many, particularly those battling cancer, the disease can dominate their lives, leaving little energy or time for careful food preparation. This issue is particularly acute for the millions living in assisted living or long-term care facilities, where dietary choices are often limited. As of 2018, over 9.5 million Americans resided in such settings, and this group includes a significant number of cancer survivors (Sengupta 2022). Additionally, many individuals either lack access to a kitchen or choose not to cook, opting instead for lifestyle choices that do not favor traditional food preparation.

These practical challenges are compounded by personal and cultural dietary preferences, which develop over a lifetime. The American dietary landscape, for instance, is influenced by individual tastes and external pressures from friends, family, and the medical community. Despite a high uptake of dietary supplements — with 74% of U.S. adults taking them and 55% using them regularly (CRN 2023) — skepticism remains. This doubt is especially prevalent among healthcare providers who often rely on a drug-centric approach due to their medical training.

Yet, it's undeniable that supplements play a role in filling nutritional gaps, especially when adequate nutrition through diet alone is impractical. Mainstream medical practice has gradually embraced the use of supplements for specific lacks, such as iron for anemia and calcium and vitamin D3 for bone health, marking a shift from alternative to accepted medical practice.

MAINSTREAM MEDICAL USE OF SUPPLEMENTS

This movement reflects a broader acceptance and integration of supplements into nutritional health strategies, supported by evidence of their benefits across a range of conditions—from bone health and pregnancy complications to the restoration of the gut microbiome and beyond.

Examples of the conventional medically approved use of supplements include iron for anemia; calcium and vitamin D3 for bone health; folic acid for complications of pregnancy; vitamin B12 injections for deficiencies; probiotics to restore the gut microbiome, especially after antibiotics; psyllium husk for constipation; magnesium for muscle cramps and spasms; omega-3 fatty acids for heart health; chondroitin and glucosamine for osteoarthritis; and melatonin for insomnia. Some of these uses emerged from complementary and alternative medicine (CAM) before they became widely accepted among mainstream physicians.

THE CASE FOR SUPPLEMENTS: ENHANCING ANTI-CANCER DIETS

In The Moss Method, while I emphasize the superiority of whole foods, I also recognize that supplements serve as vital allies in the anticancer fight, especially when whole foods are not accessible or their nutrients are not adequately bioavailable. Curcumin, for example, presents a compelling case for supplements due to its enhanced purity and concentration over the turmeric rhizome.

The best dosage determination requires professional guidance. Talking with healthcare professionals ensures that supplement use is appropriately tailored to individual health needs, considering factors such as availability, health goals, and personal tolerance.

It is also crucial to remain vigilant for any negative reactions. The FDA's Safety Reporting Portal offers a way of reporting and seeking advice on issues related to supplement use.

RECOMMENDED SUPPLEMENTS IN THE MOSS METHOD

In The Moss Method, we make the case that the most powerful anticancer plant chemicals may already be in your kitchen. These include red grapes and peanuts (for resveratrol), soy milk (for isoflavones), cruciferous vegetables (for sulforaphane), green tea (EGCG), extra virgin olive oil (polyphenols), garlic (allicin), black pepper (piperine), apples (ursolic acid) blueberries (quercetin), and more. However, for most of these, there are serious availability issues.

But despite the general superiority of whole foods over supplements, in many cases, one must fall back on supplements. These will be discussed in several categories.

This section delves into specific supplements recommended under The Moss Method, including curcumin, EGCG from green tea, sulforaphane, and others, each chosen for their potential to contribute to anticancer efforts.

The integration of supplements into a clean, traditional diet is not merely a concession to practicality but a strategic improvement of the diet's anticancer potential. This approach, deeply rooted in The Moss Method, allows for a broader intake of essential anticancer compounds, especially when daily dietary habits cannot accommodate the full spectrum of these compounds due to various constraints.

We suggest augmenting your clean, traditional diet with the nutraceuticals discussed elsewhere in this book. These would include, at a minimum, using turmeric for its curcumin, green tea for its EGCG, broccoli and radish sprouts for their sulforaphane, and extra virgin olive oil (EVOO) for its polyphenols. These will greatly improve the anticancer potential of any clean, traditional food plan.

NOTE: in all cases, the manufacturer suggests taking one (1) capsule daily, or as recommended by a healthcare practitioner. A few exceptions are noted below.

- **Curcumin:** A blend providing at least 40% curcuminoids (200 mg, i.e. milligrams) and 3% turmerones (15 mg) from turmeric (rhizome), 30% galactomannans (150 mg) from fenugreek (seed). (A possible substitute for organic turmeric powder.)

- **EGCG:** Decaffeinated green tea extract (leaf). With 98% polyphenols, 725 mg, 45% of which are EGCG. Each serving might contain a small amount of caffeine (max. of 3.6 mg). (A substitute for fresh and organic Japanese green tea, such as matcha, sencha, or shade-grown gyokuro.)

- **Sulforaphane:** In addition to vitamin C (as ascorbic acid) 100 mg, it should contain a broccoli seed extract standardized to 10% glucoraphanin, 385 mg; and white mustard seed extract providing 145 mg of myrosinase.

(This is a substitute for raw radishes, fresh broccoli, or, best of all, broccoli and radish seed sprouts.)

- **Pomegranate juice (powder):** Pomegranate is a powerhouse of anti-cancer stem cell chemicals. These include ellagic acid, ursolic acid, and luteolin, which cause a reduction in the production of the WA4 breast cancer cell line that contains a majority of cells with stem cell traits. Ellagic acid from pomegranate stops one of the key networks of inflammation in the human body and a marker of cancer stem cells.

- **Garlic:** About 1,200 milligrams (mg) of garlic bulb extract. Two capsules one to four times daily with the heaviest meals, or as recommended by a healthcare practitioner. (A substitute for raw or very lightly sauteed garlic consumed soon after crushing.)

- **Luteolin**: A supplement containing luteolin from Japanese sophora flower buds plus an extract of long pepper root. (A substitute for numerous botanical products, such as celery, broccoli, peppers, thyme, parsley, etc.)

- **Mushroom extracts**: A mixture of organic extracts of reishi, shiitake, maitake, turkey tail, and chaga fungi. Should have at least 20% Beta-glucans. A serving is generally two 500 mg capsules. (A substitute for a broth or soup made from either fresh or dehydrated forms of the same mushrooms.) Organic extracts of the fruiting bodies (not the mycelia) of such mushrooms as shiitake, maitake, turkey tail, reishi, and chaga. The label dose is two 500 mg capsules, or 1,000 milligrams per day, containing a minimum of 20% beta-glucans. Another good product is Maitake Mushroom D-fraction, the best-researched part of the anticancer mushroom, *Grifola frondosa*. (See my discussion of maitake mushrooms.)

- **Quercetin:** Each 30-milligram (mg) capsule should provide 35 quercetin (10 mg) from Japanese sophora concentrate (flower bud), and 30% galactomannans (8 mg) from fenugreek seed. It might also contain an additional 3 mg of quercetin for optimization. (A substitute for capers, onions, elderberries, apples, kale, tomatoes, etc.)

- **Resveratrol:** A blend from Japanese knotweed root, with 35% galactomannans (77 mg) from fenugreek seed and some quercetin 9 mg, providing 35% quercetin (3 mg) from Japanese sophora flower bud concentrate, and 30% galactomannans (2.7 mg) from fenugreek seed. (A substitute for organic red wine.)

- **Soy isoflavones:** Isoflavone concentrate standardized to 40% isoflavones (54 mg)] including genistein and daidzein. (A substitute for organic soy products, including a soy milk smoothie or soup base that provides 75 mg of isoflavones per each 8 fluid ounce (240 mL) serving.)

- **Feverfew:** One company offers a feverfew extract of *Tanacetum parthenium,* which equals the dose given in clinical trials. It consists of aboveground parts of the plant standardized to a minimum of 0.5% parthenolide. As a result, each capsule yields a minimum of 2.5 milligrams of parthenolide. Two capsules contain 5.0 mg, which slightly exceeds the clinical trial dose of 4.0 mg.

GENERAL CAVEATS & SAFE USE OF SUPPLEMENTS

- KEEP OUT OF REACH OF CHILDREN. There have been notorious instances in which children have been injured or even killed when parents have left out "alternative medicines" that they thought were perfectly safe. Treat these substances with the respect they deserve and keep them stored safely away from children.

The journey towards integrating supplements into an anticancer diet must always be navigated with caution, appreciating the potency of these compounds and adhering strictly to recommended dosages unless advised otherwise by a healthcare professional. This careful approach maximizes benefits while minimizing risks, ensuring that the supplement strategy aligns with the overall goals of The Moss Method.

- DO NOT EXCEED THE RECOMMENDED DOSE

- Do not purchase if the outer seal is broken or damaged.

- When using nutritional supplements, consult your physician if you are undergoing treatment for any medical condition or if you are pregnant or lactating. There can be unintended consequences.

If you or someone you know has experienced a serious reaction or illness from a dietary supplement, you can stop using the product and report the incident through the FDA's Safety Reporting Portal at www.safetyreporting.hhs.gov. You'll be prompted to start a new report and choose the appropriate category for submitting a voluntary report. It is important to provide as much information as possible to help the FDA evaluate the product.

If You Need Assistance: For questions about reporting on dietary supplements, you can contact the FDA at DSRSupport@fda.hhs.gov. For technical support with the Safety Reporting Portal, reach out to SRPSupport@fda.hhs.gov. Additionally, the FDA's toll-free information line (1-888-INFO-FDA or 1-888-463-6332) is available for further guidance on how to report issues with medical products, including dietary supplements.

PLANT CHEMICALS & PARTICULAR KINDS OF CSCS

I will now discuss plant compounds that counteract the most dangerous type of cancer cells, known as cancer stem cells (CSCs). CSCs are a small, resilient subset of cells within a tumor that drive its growth, spread, resistance to treatment, and recurrence. These cells are notoriously difficult to eradicate with conventional treatments, posing a risk for cancer relapse.

Targeting CSCs today is akin to the early days of cancer immunotherapy. This field was intensively studied for decades before becoming widely recognized. For instance, my Sloan-Kettering Institute boss, Robert A. Good, MD, Ph.D., was featured on the cover of *Time* magazine in 1973 for his work in immunotherapy. Yet it took another 40 years for this approach to gain universal acclaim and lead to Nobel Prizes, with public recognition only broadly emerging after the FDA approved the immune drug ipilimumab (Yervoy) in 2011 (Sharma 2011).

Cancer stem cells are similarly acknowledged by the scientific community as crucial targets in cancer treatment. However, despite numerous attempts, no effective drug or vaccine has been developed to target CSCs. This gap presents a unique opportunity for The Moss Method, as many of our Primary and Secondary Elements were chosen because they effectively target CSCs in numerous laboratory settings.

These elements, mainly non-toxic foods or *Generally Recognized as Safe* (GRAS) supplements, can be used in combinations without causing the severe side effects often associated with multiple drug therapies. Individually and together, natural food-derived compounds can safely and effectively target multiple CSC markers simultaneously.

Recognizing that research in this area is still in relatively early stages, we have incorporated these findings into The Moss Method. An abundance of laboratory data shows that these compounds are generally well-tolerated and beneficial. We apply the Precautionary Principle here, believing there is little to lose and much to gain by using these functional foods against the core of the disease.

(See our comments on the Precautionary Principle and its application to cancer prevention.)

While most clinical trials on plant chemicals do not specifically focus on CSCs, a growing number of studies provide strong support for the following recommendations. These are based on detailed examinations of CSC markers in various cancer types. Although this science is still developing, it highlights the potential benefits of including the functional foods recommended in The Moss Method in your diet.

For example, curcumin/turmeric has shown significant promise in colorectal cancer (CRC). A clinical trial in Leicester, UK, found that giving 2,000 mg (two grams) of curcumin per day more than doubled the survival time of patients with advanced CRC receiving standard FOLFOX chemotherapy (Howells 2019). *(See my detailed discussion of this clinical trial.)*

We know from other studies that curcumin targets CSCs, something that none of the drugs in FOLFOX (folinic acid + fluorouracil + oxaliplatin) can achieve.

This view aligns with the thinking of many academic scientists. Researchers at the University of Malaya, Kuala Lumpur, state:

> *"Despite advanced treatment strategies, [stage III or IV] colorectal cancer is rarely cured completely due to recurrences. Evidence shows that this is due to a small population of cells, called cancer stem cells (CSCs), in the tumor mass that have the self-renewal and differentiation potential to give rise to a new tumor population" (Ramasamy 2015, edited).*

Discoveries in the 1970s made the widescale exploration of cancer stem cells possible in the following decades. For example, monoclonal antibodies were invented by Georges J.F. Köhler and César Milstein in 1975, a breakthrough that earned them the Nobel Prize in Physiology or Medicine in 1984, along with Niels K. Jerne. Using these sophisticated molecular probes scientists were able to show that curcumin (alone or with chemo) can target and kill colon cancer stem cells (Yu Y 2009). Additionally, scientists have used fluorescent tracers like FITC and PE to label specific markers on CSCs. Pioneers such as Mohammed Al-Hajj and Sheila Singh utilized these techniques to detect and isolate CSCs in breast and brain cancers, respectively (Al-Hajj 2003; Singh 2004).

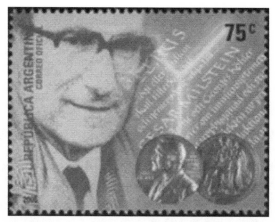

Cesar Milstein postage stamp from his native Argentina. Source: Author's collection.

TARGETING COLORECTAL CANCER STEM CELLS

All told, there are several dozen markers of cancer stem cells (CSCs), which vary among tumor types. The list is continuously evolving. For example, some of the markers of colorectal cancer stem cells include CD24, CD133, CD44, CD166, and EGFR. Scientists at Wayne State University exposed typical colorectal cancer cells to mainstream FOLFOX chemotherapy. The FOLFOX-surviving cells were then treated with various substances. They found that curcumin reduced the population of colon cancer stem cells by an impressive 80% to 90% (Yu Y, 2009; Nautiyal S, 2011).

Writing in the journal Translational Oncology, the Detroit authors concluded:

> *"Curcumin by itself or together with conventional chemotherapy could be an effective treatment strategy for preventing the emergence of chemo-resistant colon cancer cells by reducing/eliminating CSCs (Yu Y, 2009, edited)."*

Even if curcumin "only" kills 80 to 90% of colorectal CSCs, remember that it works in synergy with other compounds such as EGCG, quercetin, resveratrol, soy isoflavones, and sulforaphane, which also target a broad array of CSC markers. Together, these natural compounds may provide a powerful adjunct to conventional therapies, particularly for those currently undergoing cancer treatment, in consultation with their oncologists.

I agree with the curcumin researchers who more recently wrote:

> *"Combination therapy is now a leading aspect of cancer therapy. In comparison to single-agent therapy, combining anti-cancer medications improves effectiveness due to targeting important pathways synergistically or additively"* (Afshari, 2023).

Many cancer treatment researchers are pursuing combinations of curcumin, in either its native or modified form, with chemo drugs, including the classic FOLFOX. With our focus on prevention, however, we anticipate highly beneficial effects from the combination of dietary curcumin and other similarly effective plant chemicals. To us, a totally non-toxic approach based around innocuous dietary compounds is the only viable method of cancer prevention. That is the essence of The Moss Method.

THE SCIENTIFIC BASIS OF THIS APPROACH

This section on Nutraceuticals that Target CSCs is crucial for anyone concerned with preventing the occurrence or recurrence of specific types of cancer. We will distinguish these by their tissue locations such as breast, colon, or lung. Although an earlier draft of this book included detailed molecular mechanisms showing how each plant chemical interacted with particular cancer stem cells, I have chosen to omit these complex details to enhance clarity for our readers.

Nonetheless, despite the abbreviated nature of the listing of plant chemicals given below, it is important to realize that the science behind these recommendations is robust. I provided some indications of how this knowledge was obtained in the previous discussion of colorectal cancer.

(See my previous discussion of colorectal cancer stem cells.)

The complexity of the cancer stem cell markers, such as CD44, CD133, ALDH1, and EpCAM, is an obstacle for laypeople trying to understand this topic. These markers illustrate how intricate cancer research has become, with ongoing studies continuously uncovering new markers as scientists understand more about the variations between CSCs and normal stem cells (Singh 2004; Clarke 2006).

Highly technical details are pivotal for scientists but can be overwhelming for a general audience. The profound nature of the CSC breakthrough and the numerous studies supporting it are paving the way toward a more effective non-toxic approach to cancer. That said, we will not delve further into the granular details, as this book focuses on providing actionable information for cancer prevention that is accessible to anyone with an average high school education. We continue to follow Einstein's advice: "Make everything as simple as possible, but not simpler."

For those seeking a deeper dive into how these findings can be applied to specific cases, I recommend Myfanwy Webb's pioneering study in Integrative Cancer Therapies on how she used plant chemicals to target the CSCs in her own breast cancer (Webb 2020).

(Listen to my podcast discussion with Dr. Webb after publication of her paper.)

Also, many of the nutraceuticals mentioned in the lists below are reviewed in detail in the respective sections on the leading cancer-fighting plant chemicals.

(See my discussion of the leading Nutraceuticals of The Moss Method.)

For the sake of completeness, the present chapter also introduces a few new plant chemicals, providing information to allow you, should you wish, to incorporate these ingredients into your daily life.

Always remember Carl Sagan's memorable slogan, "The absence of evidence is not the evidence of absence." This means that a lack of current evidence linking a plant chemical to cancer prevention does not rule out future discoveries (Feres 2023). In other words, even if a particular substance isn't mentioned in the following lists, it is still a good idea to keep our 10 primary and 10 secondary elements in mind, because these have myriad health benefits, not all of which have yet been discovered.

LESSER-KNOWN NUTRACEUTICALS THAT TARGET CSCs

While most of the plant chemicals listed below should, by now, be well known to you, there are others that have hardly been mentioned that will show up in our discussion. Here is a brief description of a few of the lesser-known nutraceuticals that are at least mentioned in our lists.

- *Apigenin:* Found in parsley, celery, and chamomile, apigenin shows promise in disrupting a key process involved in bladder CSCs, offering a hopeful avenue for prevention (Ghanbari-Movahed 2023). The most concentrated source in the food supply is dried parsley. I buy this item by the pound and incorporate it into a wide variety of dishes.

- *Baicalein:* This is a plant chemical derived from the roots of the Chinese skullcap plant (*Scutellaria baicalensis*, known for its anti-inflammatory and antioxidant properties. It has gained attention in cancer research due to its

233

potential to inhibit tumor growth and induce programmed cell death in various cancer cells (Lin 2013).

- *Boswellia serrata (Frankincense):* This was among the gifts of the Magi in the New Testament. Now known for its anti-inflammatory qualities, boswellic acids are being studied as an alternative to traditional drugs, with potential in attacking specific aspects of cancer stem cells that drive their growth and survival (Ammon 2019).

- *Indole-3-carbinol (I3C):* Present in cruciferous vegetables, this compound (abbreviated I3C) may change how some CSCs behave, reducing their likelihood of survival and reproduction, as a result offering a natural means of lowering the risk of cancer (Semov 2012).

- *Mangosteen:* This tropical fruit has been researched for its xanthones contained in the pericarp, with antioxidant qualities that may offer health benefits, especially against multiple myeloma. (The pericarp is the part of a fruit that surrounds the seeds, typically consisting of three layers.) (Wu A 2022)

- *Ursolic acid:* A natural compound found in the waxy coatings of fruits such as apples, as well as in herbs like rosemary and thyme. It has anti-inflammatory and antioxidant properties. Ursolic acid can inhibit the growth of cancer cells and induce programmed cell death in breast, colon, and leukemia cancers. It also can suppress tumor spread and new blood vessel formation (Kang D 2022). (Dehydrated apple peels, a good source of fiber, is available for sale over the Internet. It has a mildly pleasant taste and aroma.)

- *Withaferin A:* Derived from the roots and sometimes the leaves of the evergreen shrub, *Withania somnifera,* better known by its Indian name, Ashwagandha. This is commonly included in teas and tinctures associated with Ayurvedic medicine. Withaferin A is being explored for its potential to counteract the growth and spread of CSCs, suggesting its value in natural prevention measures for pancreatic, ovarian, and breast cancer, as well as multiple myeloma (Xing 2023).

What follows is a listing of natural substances that target particular kinds of cancer stem cells, organized alphabetically by the anatomical location of the primary tumor. All of these listings are accompanied by reference to the articles listed in our annotated Bibliography. From there you can follow the link to the relevant PubMed listings and, in most cases, to full free texts of the articles in question.

Each of the given references, if pursued through PubMed, will provide an explanation of the CSC markers that are targeted by the plant chemical in question. Please note that these are not always identified in the research papers as CSCs, but the markers in question have subsequently been shown to be characteristic of CSCs.

We have given an illustration, above, of how this works in colorectal cancer. As one more illustration, let's look at the first such reference in the discussion of bladder cancer. The authors do not specify CSCs by name in the cited paper (Zhu 2013). But they show that apigenin targets the **PI3K/Akt pathway** and the **Bcl-2 family of proteins**.

We know from other studies that the PI3K/Akt pathway is commonly seen in CSCs, while the Bcl-2 family of proteins is also abundant in CSCs and helps these cells evade programmed cell death. But these pathways are blocked by apigenin, a plant chemical that is abundantly present in parsley, both fresh and dried. In my household we eat an abundant amount of parsley, not only sprinkling dried parsley flakes on many foods, such as omelets, but also as the main ingredient in tabbouleh salad, a wonderful source of many beneficial plant chemicals.

(See my Tabbouleh salad recipe.)

A similar analysis could be provided for the other research papers in these lists, demonstrating which plant chemicals target the markers of various site-specific CSCs, but this would take us far afield of our main purpose.

BLADDER CANCER

Exploring the use of natural plant compounds to counteract bladder cancer, particularly by attacking cancer stem cells (CSCs), represents a promising frontier in preventive strategies. These compounds, found in everyday foods, herbs, and teas, are being examined for their potential to disrupt the growth and spread of these resilient cancer cells.

- Apigenin (Zhu 2013, Xu 2016)
- *Berberine* (Zhuo 2017)
- *Chaga* (Abugomaa 2023)
- *Curcumin (*Wang 2017, Liang 2017, Zhang 2018)
- *EGCG (*Sun 2019)
- *Luteolin* (Lv 2022)
- *Resveratrol* (Zucchi 2023, Pandey 2019)

- *Silymarin* (Wu 2013)
- *Ursolic Acid* (Kornel 2023)

While these plant-based chemicals offer intriguing possibilities for research into bladder cancer prevention, it is important to remember that much of this study is still in the early stages. Further investigation, including clinical trials, will be necessary to fully understand their effectiveness and safety in a preventive context. But the exploration of these natural compounds reveals the growing interest in leveraging dietary and herbal substances as part of a broader strategy against cancer.

BRAIN CANCER

In the fight against brain cancers, particularly astrocytomas and gliomas, the potential of natural plant compounds is gaining significant attention. Scientists are exploring the ways in which these naturally occurring substances, found in everyday herbs, spices, and foods, could play a pivotal role in combating these devastating diseases. By targeting the cancer stem cells that fuel the growth and spread of brain tumors, these plant-derived agents may offer a promising avenue for both treatment and prevention.

The following natural compounds are being investigated for their potential contributions to defensive strategies against brain cancers, with a focus on their ability to disrupt the pathways critical to the survival and growth of cancer cells.

- *Curcumin* (Zhuang 2012, Gersey 2017)
- *EGCG* (Zhai 2021)
- *Resveratrol* (Castino 2011, Jhaveri 2019)
- *Sulforaphane* (Bijangi-Vishehsaraei 2017)

BREAST CANCER

In the quest for breast cancer prevention, the power of natural compounds found in our daily diet and supplements is gaining attention for their ability to attack cancer at its most fundamental level—cancer stem cells (CSCs)

These substances are being explored for their potential to disrupt the beginning, growth, and spread of cancer through various means. These are as follows:

- *Curcumin* (Calaf 2018)
- *EGCG* (Drenkhahn 2013)
- *Extra Virgin Olive Oil* (Cruz-Lozano 2019, La Rosa 2023)

- *Honokiol* (Sengupta 2017)
- *Luteolin* (Sun 2015)
- *Piperine* (Kakarala 2010)
- *Quercetin* (Li 2018)
- *Resveratrol* (Pandey 2011)
- *Soy Isoflavones* (Pan 2012)
- *Sulforaphane* (Prud'homme 2012)

These natural substances offer promising paths for research into breast cancer prevention. By focusing on the foundational cancer stem cells, these compounds reveal potential networks to shield ourselves from cancer through dietary and supplemental choices.

COLORECTAL CANCER

In the prevention of colorectal cancer, the role of natural plant compounds is coming into sharp focus. Researchers are delving into how these substances, present in common herbs, spices, and foods, might play a crucial role in stopping cancer at its source—by attacking the cancer stem cells responsible for the disease's growth and spread.

Below are some noteworthy natural agents and their contributions to the protective strategies against colorectal cancer:

- *Artemisinin* (Li 2007)
- *Ashwagandha* (Choi 2015, Kodura 2010, Bonandi 2021)
- *Curcumin* (Rhamasami 2015, Khan 2021)
- *EGCG* (Sharma 2019)
- *Honokiol* (He 2013)
- *Quercetin* (Wang 2019)
- *Resveratrol* (Sinha 2020)
- *Soy Isoflavones* (Patel 2018)
- *Sulforaphane* (Wang M 2024)
- *Ursolic Acid* (Liao 2023)

While these plant-based chemicals offer promising paths for research into colorectal cancer prevention, it's important to note that much of this exploration is still at the preliminary stage. Future, more in-depth studies and clinical trials will be critical in fully unraveling their potential for human health and safety.

FEMALE GENITAL TRACT

Exploring natural plant compounds for their potential to prevent cancers of the female genital tract, including uterine and cervical cancers, reveals a promising area of study. These compounds, found in everyday foods and herbs, are being researched for their natural abilities to stop cancer cells from growing and spreading, laying the groundwork for preventive strategies.

Here's a glimpse into several notable natural agents and their contributions to preventing these types of cancer:

- *Apigenin* (Luo 2019)
- *Berberine* (Chu 2014)
- *Curcumin* (Feng 2014)
- *EGCG* (Nagini 2019)
- *Luteolin* (Imran 2019)
- *Resveratrol* (Frazzi 2017)
- *Sulforaphane* (Cheng 2016, Shoaib 2023)

The ongoing research into these plant chemicals is vital, offering hope for new, natural prevention methods against uterine and cervical cancers. This exploration underscores the importance of diet and natural supplements as part of a broader strategy to reduce cancer risk.

KIDNEY & RENAL PELVIS CANCER

The journey into utilizing natural plant compounds for combating kidney and renal pelvis cancers is on the rise, marking a new approach toward tackling the elusive cancer stem cells (CSCs) associated with these diseases. Although this area of research isn't as advanced as it is for other cancers, certain plant-derived chemicals have already shown promise for their anticancer capabilities, potentially affecting CSCs as well.

Here's a snapshot of some natural substances and their contributions to fighting these types of cancer:

- *Apigenin* (Meng 2017)
- *Berberine* (Naveen 2016)

- *Curcumin* (Gong 2021)
- *EGCG* (Lyu 2022)
- *Luteolin* (Imran 2019)
- *Resveratrol* (Li 2017, Liu Y 2024)
- *Sulforaphane* (Li 2016)

While these plant compounds have yielded encouraging results in preliminary studies, it's important to note that their direct impact on CSCs in kidney and renal pelvis cancers remains to be fully elucidated. Ongoing research is vital to unlocking their full healing ability and understanding the means by which they act against these cancers. Such studies are crucial in judging whether these natural substances could be integrated into treatment strategies for kidney and renal pelvis cancers, potentially offering new healing options.

LUNG CANCER

In the pursuit of preventing lung cancer, particularly the most common type known as non-small cell lung cancer (NSCLC), the potential of natural compounds derived from plants is capturing the interest of researchers and health enthusiasts alike. These substances, found in foods and herbs that are part of our daily diets, are being explored for their protective qualities against the root cells responsible for cancer's beginning and spread, termed cancer stem cells (CSCs).

Here's a closer look at some of these promising natural agents and how they might shield us from lung cancer:

- *Apigenin* (Li 2021)
- *Artemisinin* Tong 2016)
- *Baicalein* (Gao 2010)
- *Curcumin* (Baharuddin 2016, Abdul Satar 2021)
- *EGCG* (Zhu J 2017)
- *Milk Thistle (Silymarin)* (Corominas-Faja 2013)
- *Quercetin* (Hsu HS 2011)
- *Resveratrol* (Eroglu 2020)
- *Soy Isoflavones* (Fu 2020)
- *Ursolic Acid* (Chen Q 2020)

These plant-based substances, with their distinctive abilities to counteract lung CSCs, offer new prospects for research into cancer prevention. While much of this knowledge is emerging, the emphasis on natural, dietary strategies reveals a proactive approach to reducing the risk of lung cancer. Further studies, including human trials, will be crucial in fully understanding their preventive potential.

MELANOMA

The exploration of natural plant compounds as a way to prevent melanoma, a serious form of skin cancer, is gaining ground in the scientific community. This new research focuses on how these natural substances can stop the growth and spread of cancer at its most elusive sources, the cancer stem cells (CSCs).

Here's a look at some key natural compounds and their promising actions against melanoma CSCs:

- *Berberine* (Shah 2022)
- *Curcumin* (Srivastava 2019, Xu 2018, Zheng 2018)
- *EGCG* (Fujiki 2018)
- *Parthenolide* (Sztiller-Sikorska 2020)
- *Quercetin* (Biswas 2022)
- *Resveratrol* (Gong 2020)
- *Soy Isoflavones* (Huang 2014)

These natural compounds, with their distinct action against melanoma CSCs, represent intriguing possibilities for research into melanoma prevention. Although this area of study is still developing, the early evidence shows the powerful role that diet and natural supplements might play in a broad strategy to prevent the most dangerous form of skin cancer. Further investigation, especially through clinical trials, is essential to fully understand their effectiveness and safety.

MULTIPLE MYELOMA

Exploring natural plant compounds offers promising directions in the prevention of multiple myeloma. These substances, found in our diets and natural remedies, have shown potential in preliminary studies for their protective effects against the development of cancer cells.

Here's a closer look with the specific references included:

- *Berberine* (HY Hu 2013)

- *Curcumin* (Mekkawy 2022)
- *EGCG* (Flood 2011, Shammas 2006)
- *Luteolin* (Zhou W 2014)
- *Mangosteen* (Joehrer 2021, Obolskiy 2009)
- *Resveratrol* (Geng 2018)
- *Sulforaphane* (Brunelli 2010, Jakubikova 2011)

These studies underline the potential of integrating specific natural compounds into strategies aimed at reducing the risk of multiple myeloma. While promising, it is crucial to continue research, particularly through clinical trials, to confirm their effectiveness and safety in humans. This ongoing exploration could lead to new preventive measures against multiple myeloma, showing the importance of natural substances in our diet and their role in cancer prevention

Role of Curcumin in Myeloma: The authors put particular emphasis on the role of curcumin. I was especially gratified to see this paragraph, which is fully in line with the thinking behind The Moss Method:

> *"The main reason for the incurability of multiple myeloma could be related to the presence of cancer stem cells (CSCs). They confer treatment resistance and are associated with recurrence and poor prognosis. Recently, curcumin has been demonstrated to be efficient against these cells, increasing normal cell death"* *(Andreazzoli 2024, edited, citing Mekkawi 2022).*

Role of Vitamin D in myeloma: Vitamin D plays a role in multiple myeloma (MM) management, with a lack that is common at diagnosis and linked to advanced disease stages. It also influences treatment outcomes, as seen with the standard drug bortezomib, whose effectiveness is enhanced by vitamin D.

Vitamin D's impact on the immune system is notable; supplements with calcitriol (0.25 µg daily) have been shown to improve lymphocyte count recovery and relapse-free survival after autologous stem cell transplantation (ASCT). Specifically, a randomized-controlled trial versus placebo demonstrated improved outcomes in these areas, showing vitamin D's possible role in improving the effectiveness of myeloma therapies and supporting immune adjustment. This evidence underscores the value of measuring and supplementing vitamin D levels in myeloma patients to maximize the benefits of treatment and immune response. This is also fully in line with The Moss Method.

NOTE: Role of EGCG in Myeloma

One cautionary note is the relationship between EGCG in green tea and bortezomib (Velcade), a boronic acid-base drug used in the treatment of MM. As the name implies, it contains the element boron, also found in borax and boric acid.

The data on its relationship with green tea is decidedly mixed. By promoting cell damage from oxygen and affecting specific cell networks, EGCG has shown its possibility to cause cancer cell death. Notably, its action against the glutamine metabolism crucial for MM cells' survival hints at new treatments, aligning with The Moss Method's emphasis on leveraging natural compounds in cancer therapy through an impact on metabolism.

EGCG's interaction with bortezomib (Velcade) presents a complex picture, underscoring the need for further research. Scientists at the University of Southern California (USC) wrote that their laboratory results indicated that green tea antioxidants such as EGCG may have the ability to negate the healing role of boronic acid-based drugs, including bortezomib (Golden 2009).

(This shows the importance of evidence-based integration of natural compounds into cancer treatment protocols, a principle central to The Moss Method.)

Some people regard this as–literally–a tempest in a teapot. Later in that same year, Chinese scientists reported the *exact opposite effect* of EGCG on bortezomib:

> *"The treatment of a myeloma cell line with EGCG from green tea stops cell reproduction and causes the programmed death of cancer cells, and there is a combined effect when EGCG and bortezomib (Velcade) are combined. These findings provided experimental evidence for the effectiveness of EGCG alone or in combination with bortezomib in multiple myeloma therapy" (Wang Q 2009, edited).*

There is also no mention of this interaction in the classic DeVita textbook. To this point, the conflict between EGCG and bortezomib has only been suggested based on laboratory studies and theoretical arguments. Unfortunately, a clinical trial at the Barbara Ann Karamanos Cancer Institute in Michigan, which might have settled the

242

issue, was terminated because of the low accrual of test subjects. So there is a strong supposition, but no proof, that EGCG is contraindicated in those taking the drug.

A contemporary summation of green tea's effect on cancer is captured in this journal article:

> *"Natural compounds in tea, like EGCG, have shown antagonistic effects against various cancers in studies. These effects may involve stopping cancer cell reproduction and growth through several mechanisms. This includes scavenging harmful free radicals, suppressing the spread of cancer cells, and potentially improving the body's immune response. Some studies also suggest these compounds might interact with other cancer drugs and adjust cellular signaling pathways."* (Li X 2022, edited).

This possible negative interaction of EGCG and bortezomib is an example of why we do not recommend The Moss Method as a self-help program for patients *who are currently undergoing active cytotoxic cancer treatment.* This should only be done with the active participation of licensed healthcare providers, such as board-certified oncologists and hematologists.

NON-HODGKIN LYMPHOMA

Exploring the potential of natural plant compounds in the fight against lymphoma, particularly non-Hodgkin lymphoma (NHL), opens up a promising avenue for cancer prevention and management. These compounds, found in common foods and herbs, are being studied for their ability to attack resilient cancer stem cells (CSCs).

Here's a brief overview of some key natural agents showing potential in this area:

- *Apigenin* (Ghanbari 2023)
- *Berberine* (Zhao 2021)
- *Curcumin* (Li 2018)
- *EGCG* (Wang 2015)
- *Luteolin* (Tsai 2016)
- *Resveratrol* (Bhaskara 2020)

It is important to note that while the influence of these plant compounds on CSCs in lymphoma is promising, the research is less developed compared to that in solid

243

tumors. Further studies are needed to fully understand how these natural substances can specifically attack CSCs in NHL. This ongoing research is crucial for uncovering new, effective ways to use plant compounds in lymphoma prevention and treatment, offering hope for new approaches to healing.

OVARIAN CANCER

The investigation into natural plant compounds provides a promising avenue for ovarian cancer prevention, emphasizing their potential role in halting the development and spread of cancer at its earliest stages by attacking cancer stem cells (CSCs). These naturally occurring substances, found in common dietary sources, are gaining attention for their potential to proactively disrupt cancer's foundational cells.

Here's an overview of several key natural agents and how they could contribute to preventing ovarian cancer:

- *Berberine* (Jin 2015, Cheng CS 2022)
- *Curcumin* (Liu X 2023, Yallapu 2015)
- *EGCG* (Bae 2017, Luo 2013, Lin J 2017)
- *Indole-3-Carbinol* (Firestone 2003)
- *Lycopene* (Sahin 2017, Holzapfel 2017)
- *Quercetin* (Chen S 2012, Wang 2018)
- *Resveratrol* (Tang 2013)

These plant-derived substances represent intriguing possibilities for research into ovarian cancer prevention. While these studies show the potential of diet and natural supplements in contributing to a wide-ranging strategy against cancer, further research is needed to fully understand their effectiveness in preventing ovarian cancer. The promise shown by these natural agents throws light on the path towards new dietary-based prevention strategies.

PANCREATIC CANCER

Delving into the potential of natural plant compounds for pancreatic cancer prevention reveals a very active field of study focused on halting the growth of this particularly challenging cancer at its source. These compounds, which are parts of many common foods and herbs, are being explored for their ability to disrupt the growth and survival of the most persistent cancer cells.

Here's a glance at several promising natural substances and their potential roles in pancreatic cancer prevention:

- *Apigenin* (Ujiki 2006, Tsouflas 2001, Rinkenbaugh 2016)
- Boswellia serrata (Frankincense) (Ammon 2019)
- *Curcumin* (Feng 2014)
- *EGCG* (Tang 2012, Kciuk 2023)
- *Luteolin* (Huang X 2015, Meerson 2021)
- *Resveratrol* (Florio 2023)
- *Sulforaphane* (Li 2016)

While these natural compounds offer hopeful prospects for pancreatic cancer prevention, it's important to emphasize that the research is in its initial stages. Further in-depth studies are necessary to fully ascertain their effectiveness and safety in a preventative context. The exploration into these plant chemicals opens up new paths for developing preventive measures against pancreatic cancer, pointing towards the importance of dietary choices in cancer prevention strategies.

PROSTATE CANCER

The exploration of natural plant compounds as a preventive strategy against prostate cancer is gaining momentum, particularly for their potential to attack the cancer's root cells, known as cancer stem cells (CSCs). These compounds, found in a variety of common foods and herbs, are being studied for their ability to disrupt the processes that allow these difficult cells to thrive and spread.

Here's a look at several promising natural substances and their contributions to preventing prostate cancer:

- *Curcumin* (Choi 2010, Sha 2016, Vatankhah 2022)
- *EGCG* (Tang 2010, Singh 2012)
- *Honokiol* (Crane 2009)
- *Luteolin* (Tsai 2016)
- *Lycopene* (Palozza 2010)
- *Piperine* (Makhov 2012, Samykutty 2013)
- *Resveratrol* (El-Benhawy 2021)
- *Soy Isoflavones* (Zhang L 2012)

- *Sulforaphane* (Li 2015)
- *Withaferin A* (Moustafa 2022)

These natural substances represent promising paths in the ongoing effort to prevent prostate cancer by directly attacking cancer stem cells. While research in this area is still unfolding, these compounds show the potential of diet and natural supplements in a broad cancer prevention strategy.

THE POWER OF SYNERGY

"The evidence for health benefit appears stronger when put together in a cooperative dietary pattern than for individual foods or food constituents."
— David R. Jacobs, Jr., Ph.D., University of Minnesota School of Public Health (2009, edited)

Scientific reductionism is a method of breaking down complex phenomena into simpler parts. For several hundred years it has stood as a pillar of research. Reductionism has been important in deciphering numerous processes, sparking discoveries and innovations. By dissecting systems into fundamental parts, scientists have constructed detailed maps of its intricacies.

However, reductionism's sharp focus can sometimes blur the interconnectedness and complexity of larger systems. This is particularly evident in the fields of nutrition and health, where the holistic approach offers invaluable insights. *Holism* judges the impact of whole foods and complex mixtures—typical of traditional diets—and recognizes the effects that these combinations yield (Brahmbhatt 2013). Such interactions often produce outcomes greater than the sum of their parts, suggesting a complexity that isolated parts do not capture.

Despite promising findings from laboratory and observational studies on these cooperative interactions, there remains a gap before these results can influence clinical practice. The rigor of randomized controlled trials (RCTs) often reverts focus to single parts, which, while necessary, may not fully represent the benefits of holistic solutions.

In both complementary and mainstream medicine, there has been an ongoing quest for "magic bullets"—single solutions to complex health issues. While early cancer research hoped for simple cures, recent decades have seen a shift towards targeted therapies that have improved outcomes.

Yet, the advantages of traditional dietary practices and their key parts extend beyond the contributions of individual nutrients. The synergy among various nutrients—and psychological factors—is crucial. For example, the collective effect of a diet or an approach like The Moss Method far exceeds the impact of its individual elements.

By focusing exclusively on single nutrients, we run the risk of overlooking the broader picture, that one's overall diet and lifestyle are paramount in preventing chronic diseases such as heart disease and cancer. As articulated by researchers at the University of Minnesota, the concept of food synergy underpins this perspective, suggesting that health benefits are more pronounced when the parts are considered within their dietary patterns rather than in isolation. Supplemental studies reinforce this view, indicating that while supplements can be helpful in states of deficiency, the greatest amount of use remains through food (Jacobs 2009).

Frontiers in Nutrition Article (2023)

A 2023 article in the journal *Frontiers in Nutrition* suggested a solution similar to The Moss Method. Traditional Asian and Mediterranean diets, a dozen authors pointed out, are full of unique plant-based compounds that studies suggest might help prevent cancer, in this case, cancer of the prostate. In countries like Japan, where people traditionally ate few Western foods, prostate cancer was formerly very rare. But as Western eating patterns become more common there, rates of prostate cancer are going up.

For over 60 years, they wrote, scientists have studied plant compounds, testing them to see if they could stop prostate cancer cells from growing. They found that these compounds affect many different processes within cancer cells. However, there was a problem: The amounts of these compounds that killed cancer cells in the lab were higher than what one can generally get from food.

For example, curcumin in turmeric is only about 3-5% of the total weight and even that small amount isn't absorbed very well when people eat it. Yet we also know that in the Mediterranean region (as well as in some Asian societies), people who ate lots of turmeric, as well as other nutraceuticals, had much lower rates of prostate and different kinds of cancer. This fact points to the synergy of compounds within the turmeric roots (the so-called curcuminoids) and chemicals in other foods included in the diet. Why not use a variety of plant chemicals together and see how well they work in combination?

In search of synergy, the same authors tested seven plant-based compounds in traditional diets on various prostate cancer cell lines (Gano 2023). The seven compounds they tested were quercetin, curcumin, genistein, indole-3-carbinol (I3C), another type of soy extract, resveratrol, and EGCG from green tea. The bottom line was this six-word conclusion: **"Synergy was observed with all combinations"** (Gano 2023).

All combinations. In other words, the good results were "super additive" no matter how they paired these compounds. Each of the many separate pairs did better when combined with another item, regardless of how researchers scrambled them. The combined effect of any two substances was more important than a mere addition of their individual effects.

The implication of this finding is huge. It points to the fact that these nutrients, when **taken together, improve each other's helpful health impact.** Just like food ingredients can create a harmonious dish, these individual ingredients similarly blend their health benefits for the person taking them. *Perhaps we perceive certain mixtures of flavors as enticing because unconsciously, our bodies perceive them to be healthy.*

As a side note, there is scientific interest in understanding how flavor preferences may be linked to the nutritional value of foods. Humans have evolved to seek out flavors that signal nutrient richness and to avoid those indicative of toxins or spoilage. Sweetness, for instance, often signals the presence of essential energy sources. Bitterness can indicate potential toxins. This evolutionary point of view suggests that one's attraction to certain flavors is not just for pleasure but also for survival (Drewnowski 1997, Beauchamp 2009).

A HOLISTIC REALITY: MISLEADING LABELS

Individual differences are key in how these dietary components are processed and work in the body, highlighting the importance of tailored approaches to nutrition and health.

Consider also the complexity of natural foods: green tea, for instance. While many think green tea is synonymous with one chemical EGCG, it contains numerous other ingredients, including quercetin, theanine, caffeine, and vitamins and minerals. These parts also vary greatly depending on freshness, variety, growing conditions, and brewing methods.

The Gyukuro green tea that I prefer, for instance, which has precise brewing instructions on the package, offers a vastly different sensory experience than the everyday supermarket tea bags. Whenever people tell me they "don't like green tea," it always turns out that their experience with it has been limited to some tepid tea bags from the supermarket.

In fact, according to independent testing, several commercial green teas contain very little EGCG. For example, the Republic of Tea Decaf People's Green Tea had only

8.6 mg of EGCG and 18.7 total catechins in a serving. This is about one-tenth of what Trader Joe's Organic Green Tea or Rishi Green Tea had (Cooperman 2024).

Among prepared green tea beverages, 12 ounces of the most popular brand of green tea with ginseng and honey contains just 8.9 mg of EGCG (Cooperman 2024). This is a tiny amount. What this green tea with ginseng and honey has in abundance though is added sugar. According to the manufacturer's own website, a 16-ounce bottle contains 68 grams of sugar, which equals 16 teaspoons of the sweet stuff. That's a mind-boggling amount, which can wreak havoc on people with diabetes or prediabetes, which is now almost half the U.S. population.

(See my discussion of the statistics on the prevalence of diabetes and prediabetes in the U.S.)

SYNERGY AMONG PLANT CHEMICALS

Having recognized the important roles of both detailed and broad approaches in understanding health and nutrition, let's look more closely at the synergistic action of plant chemicals. This exploration will show how combining different ingredients, characteristic of The Moss Method, can lead to stronger effects for preventing and treating cancer. These examples show that working together, these parts can achieve better health results than they would on their own. To paraphrase Aristotle, the whole is greater than the sum of its parts.

Scientists are paying more attention to how different plant chemicals work better together than alone. This idea of synergy, where the total effect is greater than each part by itself, is key to The Moss Method. This approach uses synergy to boost the effectiveness of our strategies against cancer. Researchers have used this method to study how plant chemicals can fight cancer (Chou T-C 1984).

KEY COMBINATIONS

Here, arranged alphabetically, are some of the evidence-based examples of synergy among anticancer nutrients. Their existence helps explain why The Moss Method has a much greater impact on cancer than what is seen with studies of any particular plant chemical:

- *Apigenin and Curcumin*: These two compounds, primarily found in parsley and turmeric, bind to tubulin in cancer cells, inhibiting their ability to reproduce. This mechanism is similar to the action of two standard anticancer drugs, paclitaxel (Taxol) and docetaxel (Taxotere), which are derived from the Pacific yew tree (Choudhury 2013). (Tubulin is a protein that forms microtubules, essential for cell structure, transport, and division.)

- *Berberine and Silymarin*: This combination has shown potential in improving lipid metabolism and enhancing liver health, suggesting benefits for conditions like non-alcoholic fatty liver disease (Fogacci 2019).

- *EGCG and Caffeine:* In green tea, their combination can improve metabolism and fat burning, indicating a cooperative effect that one could potentially use for weight management. (Kelly 2008)

- *Curcumin, EGCG, and Resveratrol*: This trio attacks head and neck cancer cells more effectively together than separately, suggesting a cooperative method that enhances their individual anticancer qualities (Piao 2016).

- *Curcumin and Ursolic Acid*: Studies have pinpointed a synergistic effect of curcumin and ursolic acid. The synergistic targets involve NF-κB, Akt, androgen receptors, and programmed cell death pathways (Besasie 2024).

- *EGCG, Resveratrol, and Gamma-Tocotrienol in Breast Cancer*: This combination's effectiveness underscores how various antioxidants can combat cancer cells more effectively than individually (Hsieh 2008).

- *EGCG, Resveratrol, and Vitamin E in Breast* Cancer: This combination exemplifies how antioxidants can work together, potentially enhancing each other's capacity to neutralize cancer-promoting cell damage from oxygen (Hsieh 2008).

- *EGCG and Curcumin Against Various Cancers*: Their combined effectiveness in leukemia, breast, and lung cancer shows how these plant chemicals may interact at the molecular level to disrupt cancer cell reproduction (Somers-Edgar 2008, Ghosh 2009, Saha 2010, Zhou D 2010, Zhou D 2013).

- *EGCG and Red Guajillo Peppers against Cancer*: The addition of red pepper increases the anticancer activity of green tea, showing the potential of combining spices and teas for enhanced healing effects (Hanau 2014).

- *EGCG and Sulforaphane in Antioxidant Synergy:* Their cooperative effect boosts antioxidant capacity and adjusts anti-inflammatory genes, demonstrating how different plant chemicals can improve each other's effectiveness in neutralizing harmful oxidative processes (Zhang 2019).

- *Garlic and Vitamin C:* The combination of garlic and vitamin C has been studied for its potential to improve heart health by reducing blood pressure and arterial stiffness (Mumtaz 2020).

- *Ginger and Turmeric:* Both are known for their anti-inflammatory qualities. Combined, they may offer enhanced benefits for reducing inflammation and pain, potentially benefiting conditions like arthritis (Zhou 2022).

- *Lycopene and Olive Oil:* Olive oil enhances the absorption of lycopene from tomatoes, a prime example of how dietary fats can increase the availability of certain plant nutrients, thereby potentiating their health benefits (Lee 2000).

- *Lycopene and Vitamin E in Prostate Health:* Found in tomatoes and nuts, respectively, these compounds work together to improve prostate health, demonstrating the potential of dietary parts for health benefits (Linnewiel-Hermoni 2015).

- *Omega-3 Fatty Acids and Curcumin in Cancer Cell Apoptosis:* Their combined effect dramatically increases normal cell death, underscoring the potential of dietary parts to work together in disrupting cancer cell survival methods (Swamy 2008).

- *Omega-3 Fatty Acids and Polyphenols:* Found in fish oil and certain plant-based foods such as EVOO. These compounds may work together to reduce inflammation and cell damage from oxygen, potentially benefiting heart health and brain function (Scoditti 2014).

- *Probiotics and Prebiotics (Synbiotics):* The combination of probiotics and prebiotics is known as synbiotics. They can have a cooperative effect on gut health, enhancing the survival and effectiveness of good gut bacteria. *Synbiotics* are found in certain foods that offer both good bacteria and fiber to stimulate their growth (Yadav 2022).

- *Quercetin and Curcumin Against Cancer Cell Reproduction:* Their cooperative blocking of cancer cell growth suggests a cooperative interaction that disrupts key networks in cancer cells (Srivastava 2019).

- *Quercetin and EGCG in Prostate Cancer:* Together, they stop cancer stem cell traits, invasion, and migration, indicating a cooperative effect on key networks involved in cancer's growth (Tang 2010).

- *Quercetin and Resveratrol in Cancer Prevention:* The combination boosts each other's anticancer effects, indicating a potential for enhanced effectiveness in cancer prevention strategies (Li 2019).

- *Red yeast rice and a Taiwanese mushroom, Antrodia cinnamomea.* These powerfully synergize against androgen-refractory prostate cancer cells (Yao CJ 2023).

- *Resveratrol and Curcumin in Anti-Inflammatory Responses:* Their interaction enhances anti-inflammatory effects, which could be crucial in preventing inflammation-related cancers (Zhang 2019).

- *Soy Isoflavones and Curcumin in Prostate Health:* Compounds like genistein suppress PSA production in prostate cells, suggesting a cooperative effect on prostate cancer prevention (Ide 2010, Tang 2010).

- *Sulforaphane and Soy Isoflavones in Breast Cancer:* Their synergy is a powerful example of how combining plant chemicals can lead to more effective anticancer strategies than when used alone. This combination was nearly three times more effective than expected for additive effects, illustrating the power of cooperative interactions in enhancing anticancer effectiveness (Paul 2018).

- *Sulforaphane and Maitake Mushroom Extract:* In Phase II Enzyme Induction, this blend causes enzymes that provide a natural defense against environmental threats, showcasing how combining plant chemicals can strengthen the body's process of removing toxic compounds (Slider 2015).

- *Sulforaphane, Quercetin, and Green Tea Extract.* These three have super-additive effects on pancreatic cancer cells (Apari 2014).

- *Turmeric and Black Pepper:* Piperine in black pepper enhances the absorption of curcumin from turmeric. This classic combination perfectly illustrates how certain food combinations can dramatically improve nutrient uptake (Heidari 2023).

- *Vitamin C and Iron Absorption:* Consuming vitamin C with iron-rich foods improves iron absorption, revealing the importance of food pairings in maximizing nutrient uptake (Diaz 2003).

- *Vitamin C and Plant Pigments:* Pigments found in fruits and vegetables can improve the absorption and effectiveness of vitamin C, which is important for immune function and skin health (Colunga 2020).

- *Vitamin D3 and Calcium in Bone Health:* Research suggests combining vitamin D3 and calcium is more effective in promoting bone health and preventing osteoporosis than either nutrient alone (Khammissa 2018).

SYNERGY IN PROSTATE CANCER

I want to focus on a paper from a dozen scientists in Australia on the effects of plant chemicals on prostate cancer cells. The authors considered seven substances from foods and supplements: quercetin, curcumin, genistein, resveratrol, indole-3-carbinol (I3C), EGCG, and another product of soy digestion. They studied each of these seven alone and in all possible paired combinations (Gano 2023).

In two types of prostate cancer cells, I3C showed the most important synergy when combined with five different plant chemicals, especially curcumin and quercetin. Genistein had the most substantial cooperative effect with EGCG from green tea. In another cell type, the highest synergy was with resveratrol (from grapes/berries) when combined with soy and green tea factors. This study showed a strong synergy between these highly active plant chemicals.

These examples show how combinations of plant chemicals work together in special ways that can help prevent and treat cancer. They show us both how these combinations work and why they're important for health and fighting cancer. This information helps us see the complex ways plant chemicals can work against cancer and points to new areas for research on diet and cancer treatments. By learning more about how these chemicals work together, scientists in the future can come up with better ways to prevent and treat cancer.

Our knowledge about how plant chemicals work together is still growing, but what we know so far tells us it's important to look at how different parts of one's diet interact for a full picture of their health benefits. This way of thinking helps us better understand how food can prevent and treat diseases, including cancer. It points out why we need to think about how each person's body might react differently, find the right amounts of these chemicals to use, and consider the big picture of nutrition science. As we learn more about the combined power of plant chemicals, we see new ways to improve health through what we eat and how we live. Combining detailed scientific research with a broad, holistic view lets us unlock more of the potential benefits of plant chemicals for health and well-being.

NEGATIVE INTERACTIONS

You should also be aware of some potentially negative interactions:

- *Resveratrol and Curcumin* are potent anti-inflammatory agents and antioxidants. There is some evidence suggesting these two compounds might work cooperatively. However, both can also potentially increase the risk of

254

bleeding if taken in high doses, especially for individuals on anticoagulant therapy (Shaito 2020).

- *EGCG and Iron:* EGCG can bind to iron and stop its absorption. This effect might be more pronounced if combined with other compounds that have similar effects (Zwolok 2021).

- *Soy Isoflavones and Hormonal Drugs:* Soy isoflavones might have estrogenic effects. While not directly interacting with the other plant chemicals in The Moss Method, its use might be of concern in hormone-sensitive conditions. You should discuss this with your doctor. This is a huge topic of debate, but we agree with the conclusions of a 2022 meta-analysis:

> *"The consumption of soy isoflavones can reduce the risk of breast cancer in premenopausal and postmenopausal women" (Boutas 2022).*

- *Allicin and Blood Thinners:* Allicin, found in garlic, has blood-thinning qualities. This fact could potentially interact with other natural blood thinners like high-dose fish oil or vitamin E (Izzo 2001).

- *Quercetin and Enzymes:* Quercetin can influence the activity of certain enzymes and transporters involved in drug metabolism (Mohos 2020). While specific interactions with the other plant chemicals listed are not well-documented, it is something to be mindful of, especially when you are taking more than one agent at a time.

Generally, when one consumes the compounds in question as part of a balanced diet, there is little likelihood of negative interactions. However, the potential for interaction increases when one takes these substances in supplemental form, especially at high doses. **It is important to remember that "natural" doesn't always mean "safe in any amount", and interactions can be complex.** Be sure to involve your primary care physician or cancer specialists (oncologists) in discussing nutraceutical and supplement use.

THE SUPERIORITY OF WHOLE FOODS

"Whole foods" are foods that are consumed in their natural, unprocessed, or minimally processed state. They are free from additives or artificial substances and typically include fruits, vegetables, whole grains, nuts, seeds, and unprocessed meats and dairy products. Whole foods are rich in essential nutrients such as vitamins, minerals, fiber, and antioxidants in their natural form.

In contrast, the opposites of whole foods are processed or refined foods and dietary supplements. Processed foods often undergo modifications from their original state, including the addition of sugars, salts, fats, preservatives, and artificial ingredients. This processing can strip away helpful nutrients and fiber and often leads to a higher calorie density with lower nutritional value. Refined foods, such as white bread or white rice, have been processed to remove certain parts of the original grain, resulting in a loss of nutrients and fiber.

The extreme forms of processed foods are fast foods, which function within their own milieu, called Fast Food Culture (Trichopoulou 2001). In Fast Food Culture, portions, whole meals, and indeed entire diets, have been manipulated for commercial reasons, with little regard for the ultimate effect on the health of the population. Unwholesome foods and choices are driven by intense advertising campaigns and by the manipulation of ingredients to bring about a state of quasi-addiction in many individuals. This is supported by the frantic pace of life of so many individuals in so-called "rich" countries.

Dietary supplements, while useful in certain contexts, are concentrated forms of nutrients or other compounds intended to supplement the diet, not replace it. They come in various forms like tablets, capsules, powders, or liquids, and can include vitamins, minerals, herbs, amino acids, and enzymes. Supplements can be helpful in specific situations, such as a lack of nutrients, but they lack the complex mixture of nutrients and other compounds found in whole foods. For instance, the fiber and plant chemicals present in whole foods not only contribute to nutrient absorption but also offer additional health benefits such as improved gut health and reduced disease risk.

In the context of eating for health, a diet rich in whole foods is generally preferred over one reliant on supplements or processed foods. Whole foods provide a balanced array of nutrients in forms that the body can use, along with other non-nutritive substances that contribute to overall health. This approach aligns well with holistic health strategies, emphasizing the role of diet in maintaining health and preventing disease.

(See my discussion of a closely-related phenomenon called The Food Matrix.)

FUNCTIONAL FOOD EXTRACTS

"Functional food extracts" refer to concentrated forms of bioactive compounds that are derived from whole foods and retain some of the complex mix of nutrients and plant chemicals found in the original food source. These extracts are designed to provide health benefits beyond basic nutrition, attacking specific health concerns or improving overall health. They often include a range of compounds such as vitamins, minerals, antioxidants, fiber, and other plant nutrients. Examples include green tea extract, rich in antioxidants, or turmeric extract, which contains curcumin.

In contrast, isolated chemicals derived from food are singular, specific compounds that have been extracted and purified from their food source. Unlike functional food extracts, these isolated chemicals do not contain the broader range of nutrients or compounds found in the whole food. An example is ascorbic acid (vitamin C) derived from oranges, which contains only the vitamin C without the additional plant pigments, fibers, and other compounds present in the whole fruit.

Functional food extracts maintain a broader spectrum of the original food's nutrients and plant chemicals, whereas isolated chemicals are singular compounds. They offer a cooperative combination that can provide a range of health benefits, potentially more effective due to the combined action of multiple parts. Isolated chemicals, while helpful, may not provide the same broad spectrum of effects.

Especially important in the context of The Moss Method, the presence of multiple compounds in functional food extracts may improve the availability and effectiveness of certain nutrients, whereas isolated chemicals, being singular, might not be absorbed or used by the body as effectively in the absence of other supporting nutrients.

Isolated chemicals, due to their concentrated nature, may present a greater risk of side effects or interactions, especially at high doses. Functional food extracts, being closer to the natural food state, are generally considered safer, although they can still have side effects if not used properly.

Isolated chemicals can be useful in high-dose healing methods or in cases of the lack of specific nutrients. But studies comparing the effects of isolated plant chemicals with those of whole foods often demonstrate the superiority of whole foods. For example, a study compared the levels of two chemicals associated with cancer spread treated with EGCG: a crude green tea extract (GTE), or a broad nutrient mixture. The results indicated that the nutrient mixture, similar to the combination suggested in The Moss Method, was most effective, outperforming isolated EGCG:

> *"These results suggest the enhanced effectiveness of nutrients working in synergy to change complex networks" (Roomi 2010, edited).*

Elsewhere, some of the same authors concluded:

> *"Most investigations on anticancer methods of polyphenols (antioxidants) were conducted with individual compounds. However, several studies have indicated that anticancer effectiveness and scope of action can be further enhanced by combining them cooperatively with chemically similar or different compounds" (Niedzwiecki 2016, edited).*

Such findings emphasize the significance of plant chemicals in nutraceuticals, particularly their cooperative interactions. While reductionist approaches offer detailed insights into specific parts, a holistic viewpoint is essential to capture the full complexity of these foods and their impact on health.

The idea behind these studies is that combining nutrients that fight cancer in similar or helpful ways can work better together than alone. This synergy means their combined effect on cancer is greater than the sum of their individual effects. By targeting different aspects of cancer at the same time, these mixtures can more effectively slow cancer growth.

For instance, combining green tea with onion, which is rich in quercetin, notably enhances the availability of EGCG. D. James Morré found that it was greatly enhanced by just 5% by weight of guajillo chili peppers (Morré 2006, Hanau 2014). *(See my discussion of the role of guajillo peppers.)*

These interactions improve how well the body absorbs and uses green tea's ingredients, called catechins, boosting their cancer-fighting abilities. The example of green tea shows that whole foods—which contain a variety of nutrients and compounds—are generally better than single, isolated chemicals. This supports the holistic approach of The Moss Method, using complete diets and plant ingredients for better health and wellness.

ENHANCED COOPERATIVE INTERACTIONS

Take a simple traditional meal, for example: a salad dressed with extra virgin olive oil (EVOO) and lemon, grilled fish, a glass of red wine, and perhaps an apple with cheese for dessert. The mix of olive oil (rich in healthy fats and antioxidants) and lemon (which has vitamin C) helps your body absorb more antioxidants. This not only makes the meal tastier but also more nutritious. The antioxidants found in olive oil and red wine help reduce cell damage from oxygen, which can prevent chronic diseases like heart disease and certain cancers (Carluccio 2003).

Another great pairing is legumes (like beans or lentils) with whole grains (such as barley or rice). This combo provides complete protein and many different types of dietary fibers, which improve gut health and lower the risk of energy-related disorders, a step toward diabetes and heart disease (Anderson 2009). These fibers help keep your gut healthy, and are important for a strong immune system and proper metabolism. The nutritional benefits increase if you sprout the grains and legumes and eat them raw.

Remember that sprouts begin to lose their nutritional and enzymatic benefits if heated above 118°F (48°C), because heat breaks down enzymes and reduces the vitamins, minerals, and plant nutrients that are sensitive to heat, lowering their health advantages and changing their natural state. Therefore, to best use sprouts in hot dishes, simply sprinkle them on top or gently mix them in to warm them slightly.

These examples show a traditional way to maintain health: It's not just about eating individual 'superfoods' or separate nutrients, but about how different foods work better together. Combining various foods and food groups enhances overall health benefits, showcasing the best of food synergy (Bach-Faig 2011).

THE IMPORTANCE OF SYNERGY IN CANCER PREVENTION

The Moss Method reveals the importance of synergy, which is how different plant chemicals in foods work better together than alone, especially in a traditional diet. Although traditional diets are supported by strong indirect evidence for their effectiveness, direct evidence from detailed studies like randomized controlled trials (RCTs) is often lacking.

While some studies on supplements like melatonin, vitamin C injections, and curcumin show promise, they typically have limitations such as small size or potential flaws that make some experts skeptical. Also, standardizing ingredients like green tea for research is challenging because its chemical makeup varies depending on where and how it's grown.

Despite these challenges, a wide range of studies strongly support the effectiveness of traditional diets in preventing cancer. For example, traditional diets, which include a variety of plant-based foods such as fruits, vegetables, grains, olive oil, and red wine, are proven to help reduce cancer risk due to their combined effects.

(See also our comments on the potential dangers of high-carb foods such as fruit juices.)

This synergy among different dietary ingredients is key. However, it's harder to find strong evidence for the cancer-preventing benefits of individual parts or specific chemicals within these diets.

A notable exception is the 2019 Howells clinical trial, where 2,000 milligrams per day of purified curcumin, when combined with standard FOLFOX chemotherapy showed significant survival benefits. But clear results from trials on single ingredients are rare.

(See my discussion of the Howells clinical trial and the NCIs criticism of it.)

This shows the advantage of eating a varied diet over focusing on single foods or nutrients. The overall benefit of traditional diets comes from the combined actions of many parts working together (Howells 2019).

SHIFTING VIEWPOINTS: THE IMPORTANCE OF FOOD SYNERGY

The concept of food synergy calls for a shift in viewpoints from isolated nutrients to the complexity of whole foods and their patterns of use. This approach recognizes that food is more than just a sum of its nutrients; it is a symphony of parts that can impact health when combined with a balanced diet. This point of view is crucial for understanding nutrition science, guiding daily dietary choices, and informing health policies (Jacobs 2003). The latter are guidelines or principles that govern actions aimed at promoting health.

Synergy occurs when the combined effect of multiple agents or elements exceeds the sum of their individual effects. For instance, plant chemicals like soy isoflavones or sulforaphane show potential in attacking cancer stem cells (CSCs). Still, their power is amplified when combined, exemplifying the concept of 2+2 equaling more than 4.

IMPLICATIONS FOR PUBLIC HEALTH

Understanding food synergy enriches our knowledge of nutrition science and has practical applications in one's eating habits and public health guidelines. It encourages a focus on whole foods and various balanced diets, which naturally embodies this synergy. This understanding can lead to more effective dietary guidelines and public health strategies, promoting a healthier society by moving away from single-nutrient guidelines towards a holistic view of nutrition.

Is such an approach safe to do? Since I am mainly speaking about the use of foods that are *Generally Recognized as Safe* (whether or not officially designated by the FDA as GRAS), basic safety can be assumed. The real question is whether or not it is safe NOT to use this approach. Here I apply my version of the Precautionary Principle.

POMI-T

A prime example of the power of powders is POMI-T, a commercial product. It is a simple and convenient way of obtaining four powerful anticancer plant chemicals at the same time. The label dose is two 500 milligrams (mg) capsules per day taken with meals. However, the manufacturer's website states about the recommended dose:

> *"Pomi-T is not a drug so there is no specific dosage and it is designed to be taken as part of a healthy balanced diet. The daily dosage depends on the food intake for that day. For example, a day with a good diet including plenty of dark green vegetables, berries, fruit, and teas would only require one tablet, whereas, on an average day then 2-3 would be better. Men within the Pomi-T trial took 2 tablets a day."*

(See our discussion of the POMI-T Trial (2014).

It is remarkable that this mixture of safe nutrients can attack numerous hallmarks of cancer. By contrast, toxic drugs might *in the future* attack one, two or even three of the key markers of cancer cells, but most likely at great financial cost and damage. For example, there are some examples of three or even four drug regimens in conventional chemo, such as the famous FOLFOX regimen of oxaliplatin, folinic acid, and 5-FU for colorectal cancer (de Gramont 1997). But such combo regimens become increasingly toxic and difficult to administer, not to mention the fact that, when it comes to attacking cancer stem cells (CSCs), such drugs do not yet exist.

261

However, many studies show that non-toxic plant chemicals already attack the hallmarks of cancer, including CSCs, rendering them inoperative. Without delving into the maze of these CSC markers, let's just say that the ingredients in POMI-T all attack cancer cells via different mechanisms, but in cooperative ways (Shoaib 2021). It's an illustration of the concept of synergy among natural agents.

(See our discussion of the power of synergy, a key concept in The Moss Method.)

This approach leads to a lot of overlap and cooperative action among different compounds. Indeed, compounds found in plants are known for their wide-ranging abilities to block cancer's growth and spread. They can prevent cancer cells from renewing themselves, moving, invading other tissues, forming groups, and resisting chemo. Moreover, they can trigger cancer cells to self-destruct and turn into less harmful types. These actions touch on almost all the major traits of cancer identified by Hanahan and Weinberg.

[See my extended discussion of the Hallmarks of Cancer.]

Here then is a plausible explanation of why the POMI-T clinical trial was so positive in its effects. The four substances in the formula, at the very least, attack four of the main signs of cancer stem cells.

(This multi-targeted approach, applied more broadly, can potentially lead to a better blocking of cancer's growth than is currently available.)

It is particularly relevant to the question of cancer prevention, where one is dealing with a relatively small number of abnormal cells. Results suggest that combining compounds like this could offer a cooperative effect by covering a broader spectrum of the molecular processes driving cancer. This is a key element of The Moss Method.

LIFESTYLE FACTORS

Moving from understanding the cooperative effects of whole foods on health, let's now examine some lifestyle factors. This shift reflects a broad approach to well-being, focusing on physical activity, stress management, and community interactions as key to disease resistance and overall health. It is not just about the nutritional content of meals but also how we live our lives. These lifestyle choices play a role in health, enhancing the benefits of a balanced diet. This section explores these factors in detail, emphasizing their importance in a holistic health strategy.

While scientific reductionism has helped us identify the specific pathways through which compounds like berberine and resveratrol combat cancer, The Moss Method also recognizes the importance of a holistic lifestyle. Regular physical activity, stress management, and a nutrient-rich diet work together to create an internal environment that resists cancer development. This is an example of what scientists call organicism, and lay people call holistic medicine.

For example, I will examine how physical activity, stress management, and community interactions shape well-being and influence resistance against diseases like cancer. This is a holistic approach, considering not just what we eat but also how we live, interact, and find balance in the modern world. I will address some of the most difficult and contradictory questions in considering any traditional diet, including the role of red meat, alcoholic beverages, coffee, and chocolate.

But I will start with an issue that is so fundamental that people often overlook it in their quest for health, which is the not-so-simple question of water.

THE GLOBAL WATER CRISIS & ITS IMPACT ON CANCER

The global water crisis represents one of the most important public health issues of our time. It affects billions of people worldwide and poses specific challenges for cancer survivors who need to vigilantly manage their long-term health.

The crisis is characterized by both scarcity and contamination of water resources. According to the United Nations, over two billion people live in countries experiencing high water stress, and around four billion face severe water scarcity during at least one month of the year. But even for people in advanced, reasonably well managed countries, the quality of water is of paramount importance. This is especially so for cancer survivors, who need to avoid contaminants that could potentially trigger a recurrence of their disease (UNESCO 2022).

IMPORTANCE OF CLEAN WATER IN CANCER PREVENTION

Cancer survivors often face a compromised immune system, making them more susceptible to both communicable and non-communicable diseases. Waterborne contaminants such as chlorine, fluoride, and industrial chemicals can interact with cells in ways that may contribute to cancer recurrence. Ensuring access to clean and safe water is crucial in the daily lives of cancer survivors aiming to prevent the disease.

STRATEGIES FOR SECURING CLEAN WATER

Home Filtration Systems

Installing a home water filtration system is one of the most effective ways for cancer survivors to ensure they are consuming clean water. Technologies such as carbon block filters, reverse osmosis, and UV filtration can remove or significantly reduce harmful contaminants:

- *Reverse Osmosis:* Effective in eliminating pesticides, heavy metals (like arsenic and lead), and germs from water.
- *Carbon Block Filters:* These are useful for removing organic compounds and chlorine byproducts, which are known cancer-causing substances.

Selecting a filter that is certified by the National Sanitation Foundation (NSF) or similar government or non-profit bodies ensures it meets rigorous safety standards.

Bottled & Distilled Water

For those who may not have access to reliable filtration systems, bottled or distilled water presents a viable alternative. Distilled water, having been boiled and condensed from vapor, is free from impurities and microbial contaminants, making it one of the safest options for immunocompromised individuals such as cancer survivors. I routinely drink both filtered water and also a sparkling mineral water that I prefer, the German Gerolsteiner. This contains a mixture of six minerals that I find very pleasing.

Staying Informed & Advocacy

Cancer survivors should stay informed about their local water quality by reviewing environmental reports and testing their water routinely. This knowledge can help in making informed decisions about necessary home modifications for water treatment.

Additionally, advocacy for better local water treatment policies and practices can help improve the overall quality of available tap water, benefiting the entire community.

For cancer survivors, the management of environmental risks, including waterborne contaminants, is essential in preventing recurrence. Effective strategies include installing certified filtration systems, opting for bottled or distilled water, and actively participating in community advocacy to improve local water standards. These measures not only provide immediate health benefits but also contribute to the long-term well-being of survivors.

ALCOHOL: A TWO-EDGED SWORD

Alcohol, particularly red wine, has been a part of many traditional diets, enjoyed in warm social settings and fulfilling meals. However, the health implications of alcohol drinking are detailed and complex.

The Dietary Guidelines for Americans define moderate drinking as up to one drink per day for women and up to two drinks per day for men (USDA 2020). In this context, a "drink" is a five-ounce glass. A typical bottle of red wine contains about 25 ounces, which is around 5 glasses.

Benefits of Alcohol?

A surprising finding is that moderate use of alcoholic beverages might actually decrease the incidence of some cancers, such as multiple myeloma (MM). In the National Institutes of Health (NIH)-AARP Diet and Health Study, which started in 1995-1996 and included nearly 500,000 people, there were 1,312 cases of MM by the end of 2011. They found that people who drank more often were less likely to get MM (Santo 2019).

Specifically, those who had two drinks a day had a statistically significant 30% lower risk. ("Statistically significant" means that the result was not likely due to chance.) For people who drank even more, the risk also seemed to go down, but those findings weren't as clear-cut. This large study suggested that drinking a moderate amount of alcohol might lower the risk of developing myeloma (ibid.)

265

Prostate Cancer & Red Wine

Harvard researchers studied alcohol intake among over 5,000 men diagnosed with localized prostate cancer. They found that men who drank red wine in moderation had a lower risk of developing a deadly form of the disease. Specifically, moderate drinkers had a 16% lower risk of advanced prostate cancer compared to non-drinkers. Among men who had prostate cancer, moderate red wine drinking was associated with *a 50% lower risk of the cancer advancing to a dangerous stage and a 26% lower risk of death*. These findings suggest that moderate red wine use might have protective effects against advanced prostate cancer (Downer 2019).

But the use of alcohol, even red wine, comes with complexities related to the presence of alcohol, including potential health risks such as a disruption of one's sleep patterns, and an increased risk of liver disease. So it is a two-edged sword.

Red Wine: The Science

It's worth briefly reviewing what the science shows regarding wine's health benefits. While acknowledging that alcohol abuse is a serious danger, a 2023 scientific review also concluded:

> *"Wine differs from other alcoholic beverages and its moderate consumption not only does not increase the risk of chronic degenerative diseases but is also associated with health benefits particularly when included in a Mediterranean diet model" (Hrelia 2023).*

A detailed analysis of the data on wine is beyond the scope of this discussion. However, we will point out a few key points, based on studies involving tens of thousands of participants. When it comes to heart disease and the risk of dying in general, red wine *does* appear to have considerable benefits:

- At all levels of intake of alcohol, wine drinkers were at a significantly lower risk of dying of any cause than were non-wine drinkers (Grønbaek 2000)
- For middle-aged women, moderate alcohol consumption decreased the risk of ischemic heart disease (IHD) by 40% to 60%, with the higher dose actually performing better (Stampfer 1988).
- Drinking a moderate amount of wine (up to half a liter per day) was linked to a 13% lower risk of major heart issues, such as heart attacks and strokes,

266

among over 11,000 patients who had recently had a heart attack (Levantesi 2013).

That's the good news. But the other "edge of the sword" is alcohol's generally negative effect on cancer:

> *"There is a strong scientific consensus that alcohol drinking can cause a dose-related increase of cancer risk." There is a "clear pattern of links between alcohol consumption and the development of cancer of head and neck, esophagus, liver, breast, colon and rectum" (Hrelia 2023).*

Although the trend is towards total avoidance of alcohol, we favor the traditional Italian view that the moderate consumption of red wine (especially if it is organic) is a reasonable health choice:

> *"The 'Mediterranean way of drinking' is the regular, moderate consumption of wine, mainly with food. This increases one's lifespan, reduces the risk of heart disease and does not appreciably influence the overall risk of cancer. However, heavy alcohol drinking is associated with digestive, upper respiratory tract, liver and breast cancers; therefore, avoidance or restriction of alcohol consumption to two drinks per day in men and one drink per day in women is a global public health priority" (Giacosa 2013, edited).*

BEST WINES FOR RESVERATROL

Leroy L. Creasy, MS, of Cornell University, Ithaca, who first discovered resveratrol in wine in 1991, performed a comparative study of its variable content in wine. He found that Pinot Noirs from the nearby Finger Lakes contained relatively high amounts of resveratrol. One wine in particular, Konstantin Frank's *Fleur de Pinot Noir,* came out first among all the wines he tested. This had about 50% more resveratrol than the more common Pinot Noirs from the U.S. West Coast or Burgundies from France.

This finding was ascribed to the humid climate in the Finger Lakes. The Frank winery no longer offers *Fleur de Pinot Noir,* but it does produce similar wines, such as *Old*

Vines Pinot Noir 2021. If you are into wine, their vineyard is well worth a visit, as is the entire wine region of New York's Finger Lakes.

A study in a newsletter devoted to Pinot Noir found that the resveratrol content of wines from various wine-producing regions was as follows:

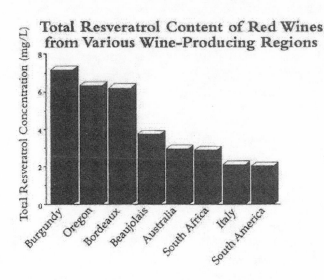

Comparison of resveratrol content in red wines. *Source: Gaffney (2019)*

Pinot Noir grapes are the primary variety used in the classic red wines of Burgundy and are nearly synonymous with red wine in Oregon. While some believe the anticancer effects of wine are solely due to resveratrol, this view overlooks the complexity of fine, aged red wines.

This complexity arises from the vintage and "terroir"—a French term describing the unique environmental conditions like soil, climate, and topography that shape the character of wine from a specific location. Researchers employing advanced "molecular fingerprinting" techniques have analyzed the myriad natural compounds in red wines, revealing that wine reflects a molecular diversity influenced by the grapes, yeast, winemaking process, and environment (Roullier-Gall 2014).

For those interested in a natural source of resveratrol without alcohol, non-alcoholic wine is available. Several prominent brands are *Wander + Found,* which offers Pinot Noir; *Fre,* which produces a Cabernet and a Red Blend; and *Ariel,* which has a Cabernet. These all have less than 1% alcohol content. Whether the alcohol in wine adds anything of value to one's health is still being debated. The answer is probably, No.

Researchers continue to include red wine in traditional diets because of its cultural significance, potential health benefits, and social aspects. Still, excessive alcohol use can negate these benefits. It is crucial to practice moderation and consider individual health conditions when including alcohol in the diet.

THE QUESTION OF RED MEAT

One of the most controversial issues when one considers diet is the topic of red meat. To be clear, in scientific terms, red meat is defined as meat that contains myoglobin, a protein found in the muscle tissues of mammals, which gives such meat its red color.

"Red meat" in scientific reports includes most mammalian sources including beef, pork, lamb, veal, mutton, horse, venison, and goat. Pork is often marketed as "the other white meat," but in scientific terms, it is classified as a red meat.

There are a lot of strong opinions on the health value of red meat, but often these do not reflect a fair summation of the experimental facts.

(For this discussion, I am leaving aside all ethical and environmental aspects of this question, and considering only the health implications for humans, particularly regarding cancer prevention.)

Many authors of health books recommend that cancer patients eliminate red meat from their diets. For example, here is a quotation from the blog of my friend and colleague, Keith I. Block, MD, on the topic of the keto diet. Referencing his own book, he writes:

> *"Anyone familiar with* Life Over Cancer *knows that I recommend our patients significantly reduce, or better still, eliminate, red meat from their diet" (Block 2012).*

Others simply restrict their intake to a total of one pound or less per week. Here is a quotation from Walter Willett, Ph.D., who is widely considered the dean of cancer epidemiologists in the U.S.:

> *"Given our findings and previous work by others, a limit of about one serving per week of red meat would be reasonable for people wishing to optimize their health and wellbeing"* (Brownstein 2023).

There are at present over 1,800 articles in PubMed referencing red meat and cancer. This breadth of research almost guarantees that there will be considerable disagreement within the research community on this (or almost any other topic). However, this question is particularly heated, because of overlapping scientific, ethical, and philosophical concerns over animal rights.

No single study can answer all the questions about red meat and cancer and it would be easy to get lost in a morass of conflicting claims. However, I will analyze one paper that particularly impressed me, the results of which align with many other papers of this type.

Annals of Internal Medicine (2019)

When it comes to such a controversial topic as eating red meat, there is always a danger of subjectivity and bias. Even basing oneself on scientific papers is no guarantee against prejudice. After all, there are more than 37 million citations in the PubMed database, dating back to the late 18th century (Fearon 1783, Rush 1786). If you try hard enough, you can find justification for almost any point of view in the scientific literature.

So we have to choose our points of reference with special care. I have tried to do that with a close study of a systematic review published by an international team of authors in 2019. This paper checks all the boxes of a high-quality study. It appeared in one of the highest-impact journals in the world, the *Annals of Internal Medicine*. It had 20 distinguished authors from 13 separate institutions in 8 countries. Together they produced a systematic review, or study of studies, that analyzed data from over six million people across 56 other independent studies (Han MA 2019).

These 20 researchers investigated the link between eating red meat and the risk of developing or dying from cancer. They aimed to understand how changes in meat eating could influence cancer outcomes (Han MA 2019).

For technical reasons, they did not recommend how much red meat one could safely consume. But they found that *cutting back by three portions of red meat per week* would lead to *a very minor decrease in the risk of dying of cancer* over one's lifetime.

That small benefit was mainly seen when the reduction was in *processed meats* like conventional sausages or bacon. These typically have added chemicals, such as nitrates and nitrites, and sugar as well.

Specifically, reducing one's red meat consumption by three servings of unprocessed meat per week was associated with the likelihood of 7 fewer deaths from cancer per 1,000 people. The results were *not statistically significant* in regard to the overall incidence of cancer or specific types of cancer. In other words, even this tiny reduction may have been due to chance.

In summary, while this *Annals of Internal Medicine* meta-analysis suggests that consuming less red and processed meat may have a small impact on cancer risk, the evidence supporting these findings was far from robust. This indicates that the decision to reduce meat intake for cancer prevention has to be made with a look at other health goals and personal dietary choices. Even eliminating red meat entirely is unlikely in and of itself to add very much to one's chances of survival from cancer.

PROCESSED MEAT REDUCTION

By processed meat, the authors meant meat that has been preserved by smoking, curing, salting, or adding preservatives, for example, hot dogs, sausage, ham, and cold-cut deli meats (Han MA 2019). There was a slightly greater reduction in overall cancer deaths and specifically prostate cancer deaths with a cutback in processed meat eating.

Although the study suggests that reducing meat intake by three servings per week may have a slight benefit in lowering cancer deaths and incidence for certain types of cancer, the overall benefit was very small. Plus, the certainty of the evidence was deemed to be low, showing the need for further research to clarify these associations.

The reader can take away from this study what they wish. For me, I conclude that the additional risk of cancer from eating red meat is very small. I choose to follow Professor Willett's guidelines and eat up to a pound of red meat per week. I avoid all preserved meats as well as any high temperature grilling of meat (which itself can form harmful chemicals). I also follow common sense guidelines for the prevention of colon cancer: I limit my use of alcohol, do not smoke, eat high-fiber foods every day, exercise, watch my weight, and periodically use a home screening test. (Colonoscopies are generally not recommended once you pass the age of 75.)

Critics of red meat frequently cite two scientific reasons for avoidance:

1. The presence of nitrates and nitrites in processed meat, and

2. The presence of cancer-causing chemicals that are produced in well-done or charbroiled meat.

One can concede both of these points and yet still conclude that red meat eaten in moderation is harmless I cancer. I agree that heavily processed meat containing the typical amounts of nitrite and nitrates are probably harmful. (My first published article, in the Nation, was on precisely this topic.) This caveat applies to most packaged or smoked, heavily salted, fermented, and/or cured meats.

The scientific consensus is also that one should avoid high-temperature cooking and eating barbecued, blackened, or charred meat. I agree with that. There are many journal articles suggesting that these cooking practices generate certain harmful chemicals, which are normally viewed as a health concern (Helmus 2013).

WHAT'S WRONG WITH A PLANT-BASED DIET?

Given the previous discussion on disordered metabolism and its implications, it's important to address common dietary recommendations. Plant-based diets are often promoted as healthy and beneficial for preventing various chronic diseases, including cancer. However, they can be problematic for individuals with diabetes or prediabetes, conditions that affect about half the population. Managing carbohydrate intake is crucial for these individuals, even when the carbohydrates come from seemingly healthy foods like fruits, root vegetables, and grains.

For instance:

- *Fruits:* While fruits are rich in vitamins, fiber, and antioxidants, they can also contain high levels of natural sugars. For example, a medium banana contains about 27 grams of carbs, which can significantly raise blood glucose levels. Similarly, grapes and cherries, while nutritious, are high in sugar content and can impact blood sugar control.

- *Root Vegetables:* Root vegetables like potatoes, beets, and carrots are nutritious but also high in starches. A medium potato has approximately 37 grams of carbs, which can lead to spikes in blood sugar levels, especially in individuals with insulin resistance or diabetes.

- *Grains:* Whole grains provide fiber and essential nutrients, but they are also dense in carbohydrates. A cup of cooked brown rice has around 45 grams of carbs. For those managing diabetes, even whole grains need to be consumed in moderation to prevent blood sugar spikes.

For individuals with diabesity—a term that encompasses both obesity and diabetes—managing the intake of these "healthy" carbs is crucial. Consuming high-carb foods without restraint can lead to elevated blood glucose and A1c levels. The American Diabetes Association (ADA) recommends maintaining an A1C level below 6.5% to reduce the risk of diabetes-related complications.

Incorporating these foods into a diabetic-friendly diet requires balance and portion control. Pairing carbohydrates with high-fiber foods, healthy fats, or proteins can help mitigate blood sugar spikes. For example, combining a small apple with a handful of almonds balances the fruit's carbs with the fats and proteins in the nuts, leading to a more gradual increase in blood sugar.

A BALANCED APPROACH

While plant-based diets can offer numerous health benefits, they need to be tailored to individual metabolic needs. For individuals with diabetes or prediabetes, moderation and careful monitoring of blood sugar responses are key. Consulting a healthcare provider or dietitian can help create a personalized eating plan that considers these metabolic challenges while still providing the nutritional benefits of a plant-based diet.

COFFEE & CHOCOLATE

Coffee and chocolate present fascinating health benefits worthy of exploration, particularly in cancer prevention. Coffee, a globally revered beverage, is celebrated for its energizing qualities and its composition of bioactive compounds. Notably, research has indicated that regular use of coffee, ideally without added sugar or cream, may offer protective effects against certain types of cancer, such as liver and colorectal cancer (Yu 2011). Population-based studies have also suggested an inverse relationship between coffee intake and the incidence of liver cancer, *revealing its potential role in cancer risk reduction.*

There are two essential compounds in coffee believed to confer these benefits. These have strong antioxidant qualities, which help to protect cells from damage and may reduce cancer risk. Their method of action involves neutralizing dangerous free radicals and reducing chronic inflammation, essential processes in preventing cancer development.

Dark chocolate, marked by its high cocoa content, is rich in plant pigments and antioxidants. These are natural substances found in dark chocolate (and other foods) and are known for their antioxidant qualities, which can help protect cells from damage. These compounds, particularly EGCG, have been studied for their health benefits, including cancer prevention. As potent antioxidants, they combat cell damage from oxygen, a key contributor to cancer beginning (Steinberg 2003).

The pigments in dark chocolate neutralize reactive oxygen species, reduce DNA damage, and stop the reproduction of cancer cells. They also promote normal cell death in cancer cells. For optimal health benefits, it is advisable to *choose dark chocolate with a high cocoa content, minimal processing, and low sugar content* (Andújar 2013).

Coffee and chocolate's inclusion, *in moderation and with minimal processing*, can improve the diet's health-promoting qualities. These foods represent unconventional but valuable additions to a dietary approach focused on cancer prevention and overall wellness. But they also contain caffeine theobromine (derived from two Greek words meaning "food of the gods"). Theobromine is in the class of chemicals called "alkaloids." Although food-derived, many alkaloids have drug-like qualities.

PHYSICAL ACTIVITY

Physical activity is a fundamental part of traditional lifestyles, intertwined with the principles of The Moss Method. This lifestyle emphasizes the importance of incorporating physical activity into daily routines for overall well-being, potentially reducing cancer risk by lowering stress levels and promoting positive mental health. Of course, people have their favorite forms of exercise, and I have no desire to interfere with those.

The Moss Method is a model for utilizing physical activity in cancer prevention. Exercise is crucial in adjusting energy-related problems, balancing hormones, and reducing chronic inflammation, all linked to cancer development and growth.

Routine exercise improves insulin sensitivity. This phrase refers to the body's ability to effectively use insulin, which is important for adjusting blood sugar levels and can influence cancer risk. *As a result, routine exercise is a key factor in cancer prevention, especially for cancers associated with insulin resistance, such as breast and colorectal cancer.* Enhancing insulin sensitivity disrupts harmful signal networks that could promote cancer cell growth.

Additionally, physical activity manages chronic inflammation by increasing anti-inflammatory substances and reducing signs of inflammation.

The age-old traditional lifestyles naturally incorporate physical activity, as part of daily life, contrasting with the sedentary habits now prevalent in many societies. Daily activities like walking to the market, gardening, or participating in community events exemplify this approach, offering a sustainable way to integrate exercise into your life.

Even mild, enjoyable activities can impact energy-related health and cancer risk. Including movement embodies a holistic approach to well-being that complements dietary choices, forming a wide-ranging cancer strategy aligned with The Moss Method.

Routine physical activity is one of the most effective ways to improve energy-related health, impacting multiple cancer-related networks. It enhances insulin sensitivity, decreases inflammation, and adjusts one's hormones (Friedenreich 2016).

The Moss Method extends beyond dietary choices; it encourages a lifestyle that emphasizes physical activity and social interaction which are vital in enhancing overall well-being.

Following a traditional diet, including judiciously chosen supplements, while engaging in physical activity builds a cooperative relationship, essential for promoting overall health. The nutrient-rich profile of a traditional diet, abundant in fruits, vegetables, whole grains, and healthy fats, provides the necessary fuel for physical activities.

This relationship is meaningful for muscular strength and recovery time, which are crucial for those engaging in routine exercise. This diet has anti-inflammatory qualities, making a more effective physical activity regimen easier (Fernández-Elías 2015).

In addition, physical activity bolsters the energy-related benefits of one's diet. Exercise improves insulin sensitivity and heart health, enhancing the diet's heart-healthy fats and high fiber content. This harmonious interplay effectively reduces the risk of chronic diseases like obesity, type 2 diabetes, and heart disease, illustrating the holistic approach, where diet and physical activity are essential to a lifestyle that fosters vigorous health (Swift 2014).

FOREST BATHING

I would like to suggest something that is low stress, appropriate for all age groups, and has proven helpful effects. This is frequent walking in the woods. In Japan this is called shinrin-yoku, which translates as "forest bathing." It is "bathing" only in the sense that it involves immersing oneself in the natural environment of a forest, taking a mindful walk through the woods to soak in the atmosphere through all five senses. Some people call this "vitamin N," where N stands for nature immersion therapy. At the Nippon Medical School in Tokyo there is even a Department of Forest Medicine (Li Q 2022).

Professor Qing Li has summarized the health benefits of shinrin-yoku or forest bathing:

- An increase in natural killer (NK) activity, the number of NK cells, and the levels of anti-cancer proteins within cells, suggesting a preventive effect on cancers.

- A reduction of blood pressure and heart rate showing preventive effect on hypertension and heart diseases.

- A reduction of stress hormones, such as urinary adrenaline and noradrenaline and salivary/serum cortisol contributing to stress management.

- An increase in the activity of parasympathetic nerves and reduces the activity of sympathetic nerves to stabilize the balance of the autonomic nervous system.

- An improvement in sleep (ibid.)

There are at present over 100 papers indexed in PubMed on the topic of forest bathing. Almost all of them report positive health effects from the practice. Needless to say, it costs nothing, takes little time, and can be engaged in by almost anyone, regardless of their age or health status.

A clinical trial in China showed lower levels of heart disease-associated factors in participants after their forest experience. Moreover, forest bathing led to a decrease in pro-inflammatory blood chemicals (Mao GX 2012).

In another trial, forest bathing showed heart and metabolism benefits. Participants reported reductions in anxiety and depression (Yao 2022).

(See my conversation with Ben Moss on the Japanese practice of "forest bathing," and its positive effects on the immune system on YouTube.)

SOCIAL RELATIONSHIPS

The cultural context of your daily life is also critical. Social relationships impact the risk of death, as shown by Julianne Holt-Lunstad, Ph.D., and her Utah colleagues (2010). They examined 148 studies with over 300,000 participants. *There was an extraordinary 50% increased likelihood of survival for people with strong social relationships.* All types of social engagement proved beneficial, but the results were staggering when they looked at a complex measure of social integration. There was a 91% improvement. The most robust predictor of survival was a "complex measure" that judged multiple parts of social integration. This concept included marital status, the size of one's social network, and the degree of participation.

Keep this in mind as you proceed: not only is it helpful to be married, but as one gets older, it is effortless to lapse into a state of social isolation. However, there is an intrinsic value to cultivating close friends and broader circles of friendly acquaintances. As the title of a study of Eastern European village life once put it, "Life is With People" (Zborowski 1962).

In traditional societies, meals are often family-centered and social events, which promote mindful eating and solid social bonds linked to improved mental health (Fischler 1988, Dunbar 2017). The emphasis on seasonal and local foods supports both nutritional health and sustainability. At the same time, the act of cooking is a mindful, creative process that contributes to mental wellness (Kabat-Zinn 1990).

THE ROSETO EFFECT

Named for Roseto, Pennsylvania, a town in the Lehigh Valley founded by Italian immigrants from the original Roseto in southern Italy, the Roseto Effect exemplifies the impact of social and cultural factors on health. This unique case study revealed a notably low incidence of heart disease among its residents, put down to their robust community bonds and lifestyle rather than diet alone.

In the 1960s, researchers discovered that despite dietary similarities, Roseto had a lower heart disease rate than nearby towns and half the national average rates. This finding helped to establish that stress can contribute to heart disease. Investigators linked this discrepancy to the town's close-knit community structure, with strong social ties and shared meals contributing to reduced stress. It improved overall well-being (Wolf 1989).

However, these protective factors waned as Roseto's residents integrated more into mainstream American culture. The community-centric lifestyle shifted towards individualism, and heart disease rates rose to match those in surrounding areas. But this change, reflecting alterations in diet, social structures, and cultural practices, showed the importance of lifestyle factors in maintaining health (Egolf 1992).

The Roseto Effect is a powerful testament to the holistic nature of the traditional lifestyle. It suggests that its health benefits derive from its nutritional aspects and the encompassing cultural practices, such as communal dining and strong social networks.

The psychological benefits of this lifestyle go beyond its nutritional aspects. The rituals surrounding mealtime, including leisurely dining, mindful eating, and nurturing strong social relationships, collectively foster a wide-ranging approach to well-being. Embracing these practices offers a valuable model for enhancing mental health and managing stress in contemporary lives.

There is the French or Spanish use of la *siesta*. These are cultural traditions dating back to ancient Rome. A related concept is the *passeggiata*, with its casual strolling, friendly chatting, and people-watching, another ancient Roman practice. One is reminded of the poet Ovid's advice to "see and be seen".

Practices such as the siesta and the passeggiata offer both psychological and general health benefits (Milner 2009). However, it has been seriously undermined by modern day employment practices (Mozaffarian 2018). Nowadays, the passeggiata has, in a sense, been replaced by the lineup of cars getting highly processed meals from a drive-thru window.

The Moss Method is not just about nutrition but a synergy of dietary practices, physical activity, and socio-cultural factors, forming a holistic model for well-being. Understanding The Moss Method within a cultural context allows us to appreciate that its benefits extend beyond just nutritional aspects.

PSYCHOLOGICAL FACTORS

Adopting a health-focused lifestyle like The Moss Method is about changing your diet but also about developing new habits such as how you prepare and eat your food. Making these changes can be easier with specific techniques, like setting clear, achievable goals (such as adding more fruits and veggies to your meals or using olive oil instead of butter) and keeping track of what you eat. This way, you can see your progress and stay on track. These methods have been proven to help people change their eating habits successfully (Michie 2011).

Having support from family and friends can also make a big difference. Eating together, joining cooking classes, or learning about healthy eating in groups can make it easier and more fun to stick to these new habits. Studies have shown that getting this kind of support and education in a group setting can help people keep up with their new healthy eating habits over time (Schroeder 2017).

Foods rich in omega-3 fatty acids, antioxidants, and healthy fats are good for your brain. They can help lower the risk of mood disorders like depression and anxiety due to its anti-inflammatory effects and positive impact on brain chemicals (Sánchez-Villegas 2013).

In traditional cultures, meals are often relaxed and social, which can help reduce stress. Taking a short rest after lunch can also lower stress and blood pressure (Mesas 2022). Eating mindfully and enjoying each bite is another essential part of this lifestyle, which can help you feel more relaxed and overall happier (Kabat-Zinn 1990).

The Moss Method, with its dietary richness, is also pivotal in strengthening social bonds, mainly through shared dining experiences. As illustrated with the Roseto Effect, communal meals can foster a sense of warmth and togetherness. The research has revealed the substantial mental and physical health benefits of strong social connections. These bonds help reduce life's stresses, enhancing emotional well-being and lowering the risk of chronic diseases. For individuals battling cancer, shared meals and the sense of community can be especially helpful by providing emotional support (Dunbar 2017).

SOCIO-ECONOMIC ASPECTS OF THE MOSS METHOD

"Science will only fulfill its promises when the benefits are equally shared by the really poor of the world."
—*Cesar Milstein, MD, 1984 Nobel Laureate in Medicine or Physiology, co-inventor of monoclonal antibodies*

The socioeconomic benefits of The Moss Method include affordability, long-term economic benefits, and environmental sustainability, all of which contribute to its viability and appeal.

While The Moss Method might initially appear more expensive due to its focus on fresh produce and quality ingredients, it often turns out to be more economical in the long run than the Standard American Diet (S.A.D.) The Moss Method's emphasis on whole foods and home cooking can help save money consumers would otherwise spend on dining out and processed foods, which are staples of the S.A.D (Rao 2013).

Adhering to The Moss Method can actually lower medical expenses and drug costs due to improved overall health. This improvement contrasts with the S.A.D., often associated with chronic conditions such as obesity and [t2] diabetes, leading to higher healthcare costs over time (Finkelstein 2009).

The Moss Method also aligns with environmental sustainability principles, promoting eco-friendly agricultural practices by emphasizing fresh, locally sourced produce. In contrast, the S.A.D., reliant on mass-produced foods, often neglects local producers, negatively affecting local economies (Low 2011). This approach to diet minimizes ecological footprints, as sustainable agriculture typically uses less water and fewer chemicals, enhancing soil health and biodiversity. It is essential to consider local substitutions to reduce environmental costs associated with long-distance food transportation, as noted by Professor Joan D. Gussow of Columbia University (1995).

When judging the actual costs of a program, it is essential to consider more than just the immediate expenses. The Moss Method presents itself as a cost-effective lifestyle choice, providing health benefits and economic savings in the long term.

The Moss Method offers more than just a healthy eating pattern; it is a broad lifestyle approach that values cultural heritage, community, and a balance between physical and mental well-being. By adopting The Moss Method, individuals benefit their health and contribute positively to their communities and the environment, embodying a sustainable and responsible way of living.

CANCER TREATMENT & THE MOSS METHOD

The primary goal of this book is the prevention of the occurrence and recurrence of cancer. I have deliberately left the question of how to treat *existing cancers* out of the discussion. In other words, I am *not* recommending The Moss Method as a substitute for conventional care for any disease, including cancer.

However, that said, there is considerable literature on the topic of complementary medicine and treatment. PubMed returns almost 400 results in a search of "phytochemicals" (i.e., plant chemicals) and "cancer therapy." And this is hardly an exhaustive sample of the relevant articles. Many papers mingle the topics of prevention and treatment. There is also a body of literature on the use of botanical substances for chemo- or radioprotection, i.e., the use of substances to protect healthy cells from the damaging effects of radiation therapy, while still targeting cancer cells (Moss 2006).

While it is clearly not a focus of this book, the topic of treatment has repeatedly come up in our consideration of natural methods of preventing cancer. It certainly strengthens the case for prevention by knowing, for example, that the addition of four capsules of curcumin per day more than doubled the survival of patients with advanced colorectal cancer who were receiving multidrug chemotherapy (Howells 2019).

If one phytochemical could do that for people with very advanced existing cancers (where they are dealing with billions of malignant cells), what effect might a more concerted use of natural agents have in a much earlier stage of the disease?

For all these reasons, and more, I would be remiss not to inform readers about some instances in which ingredients of The Moss Method have been used together with conventional medical procedures in particularly beneficial ways. But, needless to say, decisions on such combined usage need to be made in consultation with one's oncologists, since negative interactions are also possible and need to be identified and avoided.

Vitamin C and Pancreatic Cancer (2018)

This was a test of intravenous vitamin C (IV-C) as an additive to the standard treatment for locally advanced pancreatic cancer. Cancer patients received radiation and a standard chemo drug gemcitabine (Gemzar). But they also got a drip containing vitamin C. In such patients, there was less radiation damage to normal tissues. The 16

University of Iowa co-authors showed that IV-C increased overall survival (OS). It went from an average of 12.7 months (the prior institutional average) to 21.7 months, for a gain of 9 months (in very sick patients). As to progression-free survival (PFS) it went from 4.6 months to 13.7 months, for a gain of 8.1 months.

The Iowa authors called IV-C "an optimal agent for improving treatment of locally advanced pancreatic cancer" (Alexander 2018). This, admittedly, was a trial of the intravenous form of vitamin C, not the oral route. But since vitamin C was, in a sense, the "flagship" of the complementary medicine Armada, I feel it is at least worth mentioning here.

The Lyon Diet Study (1999)

In the late 1990s, French scientists, who were studying survivors of heart attacks, decided to look at diet's possible impact on cancer incidence and deaths. As part of that study, 605 heart attack survivors were randomized to follow either a Mediterranean or a control diet.

Four years later, these people's cancer rates were then examined. In the Mediterranean diet group, the cancer rate was **less than half** that of the standard diet control group. There was a **56% reduction in total deaths** and **a 61% reduction in cancer incidence.** These startling results were not due to chance (de Lorgeril 1998, de Lorgeril 1999).

Vitamin D and Chemo (2007)

In a study of 250 patients with advanced prostate cancer, researchers in Oregon tested the effectiveness of a high-dose oral vitamin D formula used alongside the standard chemo drug docetaxel (Taxotere), compared to a placebo with docetaxel. The treatment involved administering docetaxel weekly for three weeks of a four-week cycle, with either 45 micrograms of vitamin D or a placebo given the day before each chemo session.

The primary aim was to determine if patients would experience a 50% reduction in prostate-specific antigen (PSA) levels within six months—a sign the cancer was responding to the treatment.

The results were encouraging: 58% of the patients treated with vitamin D saw the desired decrease in PSA levels, versus 49% of those who received the placebo. More importantly, the vitamin D group had a 33% better survival rate than the placebo group. This improvement increased the median survival time to 24.5 months for the vitamin D group, compared to 16.4 months for the placebo group, marking a significant gain in life expectancy.

Additionally, fewer severe side effects were reported in the vitamin D group, indicating that this treatment not only prolongs life but also enhances its quality by reducing the discomfort associated with chemo. These findings support the inclusion of vitamin D in the treatment protocols for advanced prostate cancer, pointing to its potential to substantially improve survival outcomes without additional damage. Further studies are necessary to verify these results (Beer 2007).

Diet and Blood Clot Study (2007)

Dietary ingredients can help reduce some dangerous side effects of cancer treatment. Venous thrombosis is one such side effect, which includes deep vein thrombosis (DVT) and pulmonary embolism (PE). Both conditions involve blood clots in the deep veins that can break loose and travel to the lungs, creating a potentially deadly situation. A study by the University of Minnesota over 12 years with 15,000 adults showed that eating more fruits and vegetables can lower the risk of these clots. Specifically, the study found that the risk of deep vein thrombosis was reduced by 27% to 53% in those who ate the most fruits and vegetables compared to those who ate the least (Steffen 2007).

According to the same study, eating fish at least once a week also reduced the risk of VTE by **30% to 45%**. However, people who ate the most red and processed meat had double the risk of VTE compared to those who ate the least. Overall, this study suggested that eating more fruits, vegetables, and fish, and less red and processed meat, can lower the risk of blood clots (ibid.)

Greek Lung Cancer Study (2021)

Greek researchers looked at how a traditional diet affects people with lung cancer. This study involved 30 patients with either small-cell (SCLC) or non-small cell lung cancer (NSCLC) in advanced stages. These patients were divided into two groups: one followed their usual diet with general nutrition advice, while the other group was given a tailored traditional Greek dietary plan (Gioxari 2021).

The study focused on various health measures, including blood tests, body measurements, and levels of certain vitamins. One key finding was that patients who followed the traditional Greek diet had a lower score on a scale that measures lung cancer-related inflammation (called the advanced lung cancer inflammation index) compared to those who didn't follow the diet. This is important because higher inflammation is often linked to worse outcomes in cancer.

Additionally, the Greek diet group saw a decrease in their platelet count, which is a type of blood cell involved in clotting. Interestingly, both groups maintained their body mass index (BMI) and body fat levels, but the group following their usual diet had higher blood sugar levels compared to the traditional Greek diet group.

In summary, this study suggests that a personalized traditional Greek diet for three months could positively affect important health markers in patients with advanced lung cancer. The final results of this ongoing study are expected to provide more insights into how diet influences inflammation, antioxidant levels, and overall nutrition in lung cancer patients (ibid.)

Olive Oil and Chronic Lymphocytic Leukemia (2022)

Greek researchers investigated the possible benefits of unrefined extra virgin olive oil (EVOO), rich in oleocanthal (OC) and oleacein (OL), for patients with early-stage chronic lymphocytic leukemia (CLL). These phenolic compounds, known for their anti-inflammatory, antioxidant, and neuroprotective qualities, mimic the enzyme-blocking activity of ibuprofen and display potent antioxidant activities. Before this study, their effects on humans remained untested.

The study was conducted in two phases: initially, 20 CLL patients were divided into two groups, with Group A consuming 40 milliliters daily of high OC/OL EVOO and Group B consuming low OC/OL EVOO for three months. After a 9-12 month interval, a second phase involved 22 patients, all-consuming high OC/OL EVOO for six months.

Results indicated that high OC/OL EVOO improved blood markers related to normal cell death during the first phase. The second phase showed reductions in white blood cell and lymphocyte counts—markers often elevated in CLL—along with increases in normal cell death and decreases in cancer cell survival proteins.

This pioneering study suggests that EVOO high in oleacein and oleocanthal, two natural phenolic compounds, could be good for CLL patients by promoting cancer cell death and improving energy-related health (Rojas Gil 2022). As an interesting side note, oleocanthal is chemically similar to ibuprofen, a common non-steroidal anti-inflammatory drug (NSAID), and has some of the same anti-inflammatory and sensory properties (Parkinson 2014).

Capecitabine and Olive Oil (2023)

In a study spanning November 2022 to May 2023, 45 patients with advanced colorectal or breast cancer were randomized into three groups to judge the impact of extra virgin olive oil (EVOO) on chemo side effects. The groups received the following treatments for comparison:

- Unrefined EVOO combined with the chemo drug capecitabine (Xeloda).
- Processed, extra light olive oil (ELOO) with capecitabine.
- Capecitabine alone.

The double-blind study ensured neither the patients nor their doctors knew the specific oil type received, thanks to identical packaging (Andayani 2023).

Results indicated benefits for those receiving EVOO. Only 13% of the EVOO group experienced hand-foot syndrome (HFS)—a painful chemo side effect—compared to 67% in the ELOO group and 80% in the control group. Furthermore, there were no severe cases of HFS in the EVOO group, whereas these occurred in 20% of the ELOO group and 40% of the control group. Additionally, the EVOO group showed reductions in the inflammatory marker hs-CRP.

These findings suggest that incorporating unrefined EVOO into the chemo regimen with capecitabine can substantially reduce the risk of HFS and decrease inflammation, supporting the broader health benefits of a Mediterranean diet rich in natural foods.

The Wayne State Ovarian Cancer Clinical Trial (2018)

Led by a Distinguished Professor from Wayne State University, Detroit, this trial explored the effectiveness of combining plant-derived chemicals with standard cancer treatments. Specifically, it investigated the impact of EGCG (a compound in green tea) and I3C (a compound in cruciferous vegetables), used either separately or together, alongside conventional therapies. (Kiselev 2018)

The trial grouped patients into five treatment categories:

- *Standard treatment alone, with and without chemo:* These groups saw the least benefit, demonstrating shorter survival times and faster disease progression.
- *Standard treatment plus I3C:* This combination allowed patients to live longer compared to standard treatment alone and slowed the advancement of the disease.

- *Standard treatment plus I3C and EGCG, with long-term chemo:* This regimen was the most effective, significantly delaying disease progression further than any other group.

The most substantial benefits observed were an extension of survival by up to 16 months and a delay in disease progression by up to 26 months over standard chemo alone.

These results underscore the potential of natural substances like I3C and EGCG to enhance the efficacy of standard cancer treatments, suggesting they not only extend survival but also better manage disease progression. This trial robustly supports incorporating these supplements into treatment plans for improved patient outcomes. We believe, however, that these results could have been made even better if they had adopted even more of the measures included in The Moss Method.

(While the results are promising, any modification to treatment plans incorporating elements like I3C and EGCG should always occur under strict medical supervision to adequately manage risks and potential side effects.)

The Howells Trial of Curcumin and FOLFOX Chemo (2019)

This clinical trial at the University of Leicester, UK, represented a milestone in curcumin research. This trial tested the combination of curcumin with mainstream FOLFOX chemo in treating colorectal cancer patients. FOLFOX stands for folinic acid (FOL) + fluorouracil (F) and oxaliplatin (OX). When curcumin was added to these, the combination was dubbed CUFOX. The results of this trial indicated improved survival rates and reduced tumor growth for patients receiving curcumin alongside chemo (Howells 2019).

Specifically, there was a median overall survival of 502 days in the curcumin group, a substantial improvement compared to 200 days in the FOLFOX-alone group. The major problem with this trial was its small size. It involved just 28 patients, showing the need for larger clinical trials to judge curcumin's effectiveness further.

Curcumin's anticancer effects, while needing further clinical validation, present a promising avenue in cancer prevention and treatment. Its ability to interact with various cancer-related networks makes it an addition to cancer care strategies, transcending its traditional culinary use and contributing to the globally inclusive approach to nutrition in The Moss Method.

The trial, a randomized albeit small study, aimed to evaluate the safety, effectiveness, and impact on quality of life when combining curcumin with standard chemo. The findings, published in the *Journal of Nutrition,* revealed that adding 2 grams of oral curcumin daily to the chemo regimen was not only safe and well-tolerated but also resulted in a notable extension of life.

Patients who received the combined curcumin and FOLFOX therapy (called CUFOX) experienced a significant increase in overall survival. The median survival extended from 200 days with FOLFOX alone to 502 days with the addition of curcumin. This substantial improvement underscores curcumin's potential as a life-prolonging adjunct to conventional chemotherapy, without increasing side effects or negatively impacting patients' quality of life. This groundbreaking research opens new paths for enhancing cancer treatment protocols with natural products, offering hope for better outcomes in the fight against metastatic colorectal cancer (Howells 2019).

*The National Cancer Institute's PDQ website states that **"the differences in survival rates were not statistically significant"** (PDQ 2024).*

However, this is untrue. To explain why, I must get a little technical. In statistics, the "P-value" indicates the likelihood that an observed result is due to chance, and not to the treatment in question. In the Howells study, the P-value for overall survival (OS) is given in the paper as 0.004. This means there was a mere 0.4% chance that the observed difference in overall survival between the two treatment groups (CUFOX and FOLFOX) occurred due to random variations rather than being real effects of the curcumin treatment. This falls well below the usual cut-off point for statistical significance.

Put another way, in the early 20th century, statisticians set a stringent standard that even a one-in-twenty chance of a result being due to happenstance would not generally meet the criteria for statistical significance (Fisher 1925). In the Howells study, the odds of the result being due to luck were just one in 250. This strongly suggests that the observed improvement in overall survival with the CUFOX treatment was overwhelmingly likely due to a truly beneficial effect of curcumin. Therefore, it is patently false to state that the differences in overall survival rates were not statistically significant.

However, the NCI/PDQ website offers its own explanation for the positive results. They imply that the difference in overall survival rates may have been due to an imbalance between the two groups in the percentage of patients who had two or more metastatic sites. They speculate this might have influenced the outcomes. While this is a possibility, they fail to mention that the percentage of patients in the CUFOX group who had dangerous peritoneal metastases was 22.2% versus 0% of those in the FOLFOX group (see Table 1 in the Howells 2019 paper).

All these questions could have been answered in a larger phase III randomized trial. Unfortunately, that never happened, and there is no indication that any such trial is planned or underway.

(I have attempted to protest to the authors of this PDQ section over their mischaracterization of the trial, but as of this writing I have not heard back from them.)

The Mt. Sinai Study of Genistein and Chemo (2019)

In a notable clinical trial, researchers explored the effects of genistein—a compound derived from soy and known for its anticancer properties—when used alongside standard chemo treatments (FOLFOX or FOLFOX-Bevacizumab) for patients with advanced colorectal cancer. The study found that adding genistein extended the time patients lived without their cancer getting worse to a median of 11.5 months. Importantly, it did not lead to an increase in side effects. By the sixth treatment cycle, over 60% of the patients showed a positive response. Based on these promising results, the authors from Mt. Sinai Hospital, New York, suggested that genistein deserves more extensive research in larger trials (Pintova 2019).

BROAD-SPECTRUM PLANT CHEMICAL STRATEGIES

Using a broad approach to healing, especially with plant chemicals, fits well with the complex nature of cancer stem cells. This method aims to use the many beneficial substances in plants to target different parts of cancer stem cells, which might help overcome their resistance to single-target treatments.

Using many plant-based agents together is based on the idea that one alone can't handle all aspects of cancer stem cells. For example, combining curcumin from turmeric, sulforaphane from broccoli, and resveratrol from grape skins can address different aspects of cancer stem cells, like inflammation and self-renewal, all at once, each in its own way.

- *Curcumin* is noted for its anti-inflammatory effects and ability to change genes involved in cancer's growth (Moon 2024).
- *Sulforaphane* has been shown to stop an enzyme important in the control of gene expression in cancer (Dickinson 2015).

- *Resveratrol* interferes with signals among cancer cells and can cause normal cell death (Jang 2022).

Despite many promising lab studies, translating these findings into effective clinical treatments has been slow. The primary challenges include:

- *Availability:* Many plant chemicals have poor dispersion in the body when taken orally, which significantly reduces their possible healing ability. Advanced delivery systems, such as nano formulations, are being explored to overcome this hurdle.

- *Complexity of Dosage Formulation:* Determining the best doses that can be safely combined without causing side effects is complex and requires more clinical trials.

- *Regulatory Hurdles:* Dietary supplements and natural products face significant challenges for approval by government bodies such as the FDA.

The possible role for natural compounds to play a significant role in cancer treatment, particularly in targeting CSCs, remains high despite these challenges. Future research directions include:

- *Enhanced Delivery Systems:* Using technology to improve the delivery and effectiveness of plant chemicals.

- *Combination Therapies:* Exploring the effects of combining many plant chemicals with traditional cancer therapies.

- *Genetic and Molecular Studies:* Understanding the specific interactions between natural compounds and the networks in CSCs can aid in formulating more effective therapies.

While the road to integrating plant-based chemicals into standard cancer treatment protocols is filled with challenges, the possible benefits are too significant to ignore. By continuing to explore the complex nature of CSCs and the broad abilities of plant chemicals, new methods that harness the power of natural compounds can be developed, offering hope for more effective and less invasive cancer treatments.

HEALING RECIPES

Cookery may seem like an unlikely way to fight a disease as severe as cancer. Nor am I suggesting them as an alternative to conventional care. However, I have carefully formulated these recipes to correspond to the scientific underpinnings of The Moss Method. This chapter includes recipes for a mushroom soup, a purple smoothie, a green smoothie, a salad, and salad dressing. The inspiration for the last two comes from the work of my friend Jim Duke, Ph.D. (1929-2017) of the U.S. Department of Agriculture.

Traditional diets, with their array of leafy greens, garlic, olive oil, fruits, tomatoes, fatty fish, fermented foods, nuts, whole grains, legumes, and a wide range of herbs and spices, represent the paragon of natural, wholesome nutrition.

These elements, backed by substantial scientific research, contribute to cancer prevention, heart health, and overall well-being. Embracing a traditional diet goes beyond mere food choices; it embraces a lifestyle that cherishes the natural bounty and wisdom of balanced, holistic nutrition.

Incorporating the key plant chemicals into one's daily meals is not just a nod to a rich culinary heritage. It is also a proactive step towards nourishing and fortifying our bodies against modern health challenges, which is epitomized by Fast Food Culture. A traditional approach emerges not just as a diet but as a path to health and wellness, combining the pleasures of taste with the science of increasing lifespan and well-being.

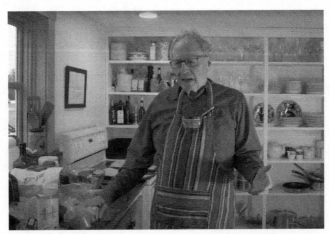

Dr. Moss in his kitchen in Maine making seed crackers.

290

THE MOSS METHOD GOLDEN MILK

Yield: 2 servings (1 day)

We have already written about the benefit of taking turmeric powder over a pure supplement of curcumin alone.

(See my discussion of a Revealing Clinical Trial of Turmeric Vs. Curcumin.)

The insight of a 2019 clinical trial at the University of Newcastle, NSW, Australia, opened up new possibilities for incorporating turmeric into the diet in ways that maximize its health benefits. A practical application of these findings is the creation of turmeric-based dishes and drinks, such as the Turmeric Latte or The Moss Method *Golden Milk*, which combines these nutritional elements deliciously, making it an ideal vehicle for enhancing curcumin's availability and, by extension, its excellent effects on health.

For maximum effect, this should be taken twice per day, perhaps with the morning and evening meals. This is how curcumin is typically given in clinical trials (Howells 2019).

The Moss Method *Golden Milk* is a creamy, health-promoting drink that is easy to make.

Ingredients:

- 2 cups of unsweetened organic soy milk. Edensoy contains 75 milligrams (mg) of naturally occurring isoflavones per 8-ounce portion. (Other brands either do not reveal the amount of isoflavones or contain about one-third as much.)

- 2 teaspoons of ground organic turmeric powder. You can adjust the amount of turmeric to taste. It is important to make the drink delicious, so you will want to consume it often!

- 1 teaspoon of ground ginger or (our favorite) chopped fresh ginger. Ginger contains anticancer elements, such as 6-gingerol and 6-shogaol, and at least 160 other "potential resources for health" (Zhang M 2021).

- ¼ teaspoon of ground black pepper. Black pepper contains piperine, which slows the absorption of curcumin into the system, as a result increasing its availability by as much as 2000% (Shoba 1998).

- 1 teaspoon of ground cinnamon. "Cinnamon as a whole and/or its active parts had anticancer activity in different types of cancer" (Dutta 2018, edited).

- 2 teaspoons of vanilla extract. You can easily prepare vanilla extract, as I do, by steeping vanilla beans in a pint of organic vodka, at least 70 Proof. This will be ready in a few weeks but will take several months to reach peak flavor.

- 1 tablespoon *of almond (or other nut) butter and your choice of sweetener.*

Instructions:

Combine the soymilk, turmeric powder, ginger, black pepper, and cinnamon in a saucepan and heat for about 4 minutes until hot but not boiling, whisking frequently.

1. Add vanilla and almond butter. Continue to whisk until hot but not boiling.

2. Adjust the flavors as needed by adding more sweetener, vanilla, turmeric, or ginger.

3. Serve immediately, reserving half for your evening portion.

Because of availability issues, it is best to consume this product at different ends of the day.

This recipe balances spiciness and sweetness, creating a comforting and healthy drink. It takes more work than popping a couple of pills, but it also conveys a very complex and promising mixture of healing compounds from the East.

SUPER HEALTHY SMOOTHIES

Smoothies offer a convenient and pleasant way to incorporate many nutraceuticals and functional food extracts into your daily regimen.

Scientific interest in smoothies has been slow to develop. However, in the last few years, some researchers have begun to explore the value of smoothies as a new delivery method of nutrients for a variety of health conditions, including some affecting cancer patients.

In one study from Southern Italy, scientists explored how smoothies made with sweet oranges (*Citrus sinensis*) and a type of grape (*Vitis vinifera*) could counteract some of the side effects of chemo. They found that these smoothies are rich in helpful compounds that can protect heart cells against damage caused by a chemo drug known for its cell damage from oxygen.

By scientifically analyzing smoothies, the research showed that a specific mixture of orange and grape in a 1:1 ratio effectively reduces heart cell damage without affecting the drug's ability to kill breast cancer cells. This suggests that incorporating such fruit smoothies into chemo protocols might offer a natural way to safeguard the heart in cancer patients undergoing treatment (Pepe 2020).

At the same time, scientists from Saudi Arabia and Egypt have shown that the addition of a pomegranate product could be added to a strawberry yogurt smoothie with excellent results. It enhanced their health-promoting qualities, including their antioxidant activity, which was even higher than that of ascorbic acid (vitamin C) in some tests.

This antioxidant effect helped reduce the growth of lung cancer cells and increased the activity of caspase-3, an enzyme that helps cells die off in a controlled way, which is a natural method of stopping cancer. This suggests that the smoothies might help fight cancer. Additionally, these smoothies were able to kill various harmful bacteria and fungi, showing they could also make foods safer to eat (Alsubhi 2022).

In line with these findings, I offer several recipes of my own, which could be of real benefit to people concerned with the occurrence or recurrence of cancer. I frequently have a version of one of these as a mid-afternoon snack, but feel free to experiment and work these into your schedule however you like. However, if you are battling T2D as well as cancer you will have to pay special attention to the potential impact of fruit on your blood sugar.

RWM PURPLE SMOOTHIE

Yield: 2 servings (1 day)

My RWM Purple Smoothie is delicious and has a robust scientific basis. It is low in net carbs but also contains blockers of many of the hallmarks of cancer. It also blocks some of the ways cancer stem cells grow and survive. We suggest repeating this three times per week and doing the same with RWM's Green Smoothie (recipe below).

Although my emphasis is on health, the reality is that most people won't repeatedly take anything that tastes bad, even if it is good for them. So I designed this to taste good.

Please adhere to the following recipe. In parentheses, I have given the brands of the products I currently use. But feel free to do comparison shopping.

You might improve this recipe with other ingredients, such as fresh or frozen fruit if you are sure that you are in the minority of people who do not have an issue with elevated blood sugar. One possibility is a grape skin powder. Be careful however to add only healthy whole food ingredients.

This recipe is for about a cup and a half. You can refrigerate half of this and drink them at different times of the day, such as four hours apart.

Drink the purple and the green smoothies on alternate days. Take a break on Sundays.

Choice of Blender: Because you will make smoothies almost daily, it is worth investing in a good quality product. I use a professional-level steel-and-glass 1.25-liter food blender. We will explain the reason for using these ingredients in the section following this recipe.

Ingredients:

- 1 cup unsweetened organic soy milk (preferably chilled).
- 1 teaspoon organic **maqui** berry powder
- 1 teaspoon **pomegranate** juice powder
- 2 small scoops of acerola cherry powder
- A 3.5-ounce pack of frozen unsweetened pure **açai**
- ½ cup of organic raspberries or **blackberries** (fresh or frozen)
- ½ cup of ice cubes or chipped ice. (You can dilute the drink with more soy milk or cold water if it is too thick.)

Instructions:

In the jar of the blender, place all ingredients and blend on high for 1-2 minutes or until you have completely pulverized the solid or frozen ingredients.

Tip: Be sure to give the mixture a stir **before** blending in order to avoid a back-spray of powder.

Nutritional Profile:

This recipe has been created with both cancer and T2D or prediabetes in mind. We have seen other purple smoothies online that contain 50 grams of net carbs! My Keto Purple Smoothie contains just 16 grams of carbs, with five grams of fiber, and so *9 grams of net carbs.* This is about half the net carbs of a Granny Smith apple.

As to its anticancer agents, it contains isoflavones from soy milk, colorful plant pigment anthocyanins, antioxidants from the maqui berry powder, ellagic acid from the blackberries, punicic acid from the pomegranate powder.

A Note on Soy: A daily dose of 75 milligrams (mg) of soy is similar to the amount that investigators typically use in clinical trials. For example, a 2023 clinical trial tested 50 mg in food and 100 mg in a supplement per day (Rajaram 2023).

RWM GREEN SMOOTHIE

Yield: 2 servings (1 day)

The RWM Green Smoothie packs a wallop, addressing many of the hallmarks of cancer and cancer stem cells (CSCs). It is a mixture of soy milk, avocado, broccoli sprouts, baby greens, and possibly some fruit as a source of nutrients and as a sweetener.

It is not easy to create a green smoothie that does not have a lot of carbs. The reason is that broccoli sprouts lend a slightly sulfurous taste and smell to this mixture; however, from a health point of view, it is probably the single most important element in the mix. The way around this problem is twofold. You need to add enough sweetener to the mix to hide the sulfurous taste. But it is equally important to serve the beverage very cold. This "hack" helps to mask the undesirable taste and smell. By doing these two things, you can make this second smoothie as delightful as the first. Well, almost.

If you are prone to high blood sugar you should consider using monk fruit, or some other natural sweetener. More fruit is another option but it will add to the carbohydrate load. If you are not in that half of the population struggling with prediabetes or "T2D," this will not harm you and will certainly improve the taste.

If you wish, you can drink this all at once, but it would be better to divide it in half and leave at least 4 hours between drinks.

Ingredients:

- 1 cup (8 oz.) organic unsweetened soy milk
- 1/2 kiwi fruit, peeled and quartered
- 1/2 medium-sized organic Hass avocado
- 1/2 medium-sized Granny Smith apple, cored and cubed
- 1 teaspoon of organic turmeric powder

- 1 cup raw fresh spinach (or arugula). Wash the greens, even if the label states that they are prewashed

- 1 ounce radish sprouts, do **not** heat above 158°F (70°C), as this will destroy the sulforaphene. (By the way, this is not a typo; there actually are two such compounds, sulforaphane and sulforaphene, with nearly identical spellings.)

- Ice cubes, to taste.

Instructions:

1. Blend the sprouts, avocado, kiwi, spinach, Granny Smith, and green apple with the soy milk.

2. Fold in the turmeric powder and sweetener (so they don't fly around) and blend again with the ice cubes until completely liquified.

3. Serve while still cold.

Nutritional Profile:

By my calculation, this Green Smoothie contains 324 calories, and 29 grams of carbs minus 11 grams of fiber, for a total of 18 grams of net carbs. If you drink half of that you will get 9 grams of net carbs per cup.

Soy: See the scientific note following the Purple Smoothie Recipe. This note explains the need to choose **organic unsweetened soy milk**.

Spinach (Spinacia oleracea): Spinach is the subject of over 4,000 scientific studies! We underestimate its power because of its familiarity. But it is indeed (to quote Mexican researchers) "one of the most perfect foods." Research has shown spinach is an amazing storehouse of helpful plant chemicals: there are approximately **100 chemical compounds** found in spinach (Gutierrez 2019).

Researchers are studying natural compounds in spinach called glycol-glycerol-lipids, which may help fight cancer. These compounds can block the development of new blood vessels that tumors need to grow and spread, offering a potential way to control or slow down cancer (Maeda 2011). This trait matches with Hanahan & Weinberg's Hallmark #7, which refers to cancer cells' ability to create blood vessels to access nutrients and eliminate waste products.

Studies also demonstrate that spinach-derived compounds selectively stop DNA activity, which is involved in cancer cell reproduction and survival.

One study found that spinach extracts showed cytotoxic activity against various cancer cell lines, including lung, breast, and liver cancer cells.

Additionally, spinach's overall plant chemical profile, including its antioxidants, has been studied for various health benefits, such as anti-inflammatory and anti-obesity effects, which can be indirectly related to cancer prevention. These findings suggest that spinach, with its unique blend of bioactive compounds, offers a promising path for developing new anticancer therapies.

(It is important to note that spinach is high in oxalates, which can contribute to the formation of kidney stones in susceptible people. This ingredient is something to consider for those who have a history of kidney stones or are at risk. Such people can substitute baby kale for the spinach in this recipe.)

COOPERATIVE INTERACTIONS

Sulforaphane and Soy Isoflavones in Breast Cancer: Their synergy is a powerful example of how combining plant chemicals can lead to more effective anticancer strategies than when used alone. This combination was nearly three times more effective than expected for additive effects. (Paul 2018)

Other instances of synergy in a green smoothie include:

- Genistein (soy milk) and quercetin (apple peel powder) (Hsieh 2009)
- Genistein (soy milk) and EGCG (Matcha tea) (Gano 2023)
- Ginger and isoflavones (soy milk) (Hsieh 2009)
- Green tea and apple extract (Nguyen M 2023)
- Indole-3-carbinol (broccoli sprouts) and quercetin (apple peel powder) (Gano 2023)
- Resveratrol (red grapes and grape skin powder) and EGCG (Matcha tea) (Gano 2023)

Creating smoothie recipes that are both delicious and packed with plant chemicals attacking cancer stem cells is a wonderful idea.

TIPS FOR SYNERGY & FLAVOR

- *Balance Sweet and Tart:* The natural sweetness of fruits like bananas and berries can balance the tartness of ingredients like pomegranate juice or yogurt.
- *Use Fresh When Possible:* Fresh ingredients often provide better flavor and more potent plant chemicals.

- *Experiment with Spices*: Cinnamon, ginger, and turmeric add health benefits and improve the flavor profile.

- *Adjust Consistency*: Depending on preference, adjust the thickness of the smoothie with more or less liquid (water, almond milk, soy milk).

Remember, balancing health benefits with taste is key to a successful smoothie. Encourage experimentation to find the perfect blend for individual palates. These recipes are just starting points. You can tweak the recipe according to your personal preferences and the availability of ingredients.

RALPH'S MUSHROOM SOUP

This powerful mushroom soup is nothing like the bland "cream of mushroom" of our childhood. This recipe relies on decades of research and development on the effects of various fungi on cancer. It contains five healing mushrooms, little known in the West but familiar to many Asian patients, especially in China and Japan. At the start of the U.S. "War on Cancer," there was a single, solitary paper on mushrooms and cancer (Lin JY 1974). Now, such articles appear three times per week—dare we say, like mushrooms after the rain? (Singh 2016).

Ingredients:

- 1 tablespoons olive oil

- 1 large onion, diced

- 2 carrots, peeled and sliced

- ½ head green cabbage, chopped

- 5 cloves of garlic, crushed and peeled

- 3 tbsp. (1.6 oz.) dried (= 1 lb. fresh) shiitake mushrooms (*Lentinus edodes*)*

- 3 tbsp. (1.6 oz.) dried (= 1 lb. fresh) maitake mushrooms (*Grifola frondosa*)

- 3 tbsp. (1.6 oz.) dried (= 1 lb. fresh) oyster mushrooms (*Pleurotus ostreatus*)

- 3 tbsp. of wild harvested raw fine chaga mushroom powder (*Inonotus obliquus*)

- 3 quarts purified or spring water

- 6 oz. fresh parsley

- 2 tbsp. "Herbs de Provence" (summer savory, parsley, sage, rosemary, thyme, lavender flowers)
- Salt or tamari sauce

Instructions:

Heat olive oil in a large pot or Dutch oven over medium heat. Add onion, carrots, and cabbage, and cook until softened, about 5 minutes.

1. Add garlic and cook for another minute, stirring frequently.
2. Add dried mushrooms and water. Bring to a boil
3. Boil the ingredients thoroughly until all of the dehydrated mushrooms are very soft— approximately 30 minutes. This is crucial, as it releases healthful chemicals from behind the rigid mushroom cell walls.
4. Turn heat down to simmer and add parsley and herbs de Provence. Simmer for an additional 5-10 minutes.
5. Add salt or tamari to taste.
6. Remove from heat and let the soup cool.
7. Strain the solids out, reserving the broth. The essential nutrients will be retained in the broth and the mushrooms will be tasteless.

Divide the soup into daily portions of 4 ounces. Refrigerate seven for the week ahead and freeze the rest.

(You must familiarize yourself with the benefits and risks (such as allergic reactions) associated with these ingredients, especially the mushrooms. There are many articles and videos online with this information.)

HEALING MUSHROOM BROTH

For an alternate preparation, try this broth.

Ingredients:

- 1 to 2 tablespoons olive oil
- 1 medium onion, chopped
- 2 carrots, chopped
- 2 celery stalks, chopped

- 4 garlic cloves, minced
- 1 tablespoon dried shiitake mushrooms
- 1 tablespoon dried maitake mushrooms
- ½ teaspoon dried reishi mushrooms (optional, due to higher cost)
- 8 cups (2L) vegetable broth or water
- 1 bay leaf
- 1 sprig fresh thyme or ¼ teaspoon dried thyme
- Pinch of salt and pepper to taste

Instructions:

1. Heat olive oil in a large pot or Dutch oven over medium heat. Add onion, carrots, and celery, and cook until softened, about 5 minutes.

2. Add garlic and cook for another minute, stirring frequently.

3. Add dried mushrooms, bay leaf, thyme, and vegetable broth or water. Bring to a boil, then reduce heat and simmer for 30 minutes to 1 hour, or until the broth is flavorful and fragrant.

4. Strain the broth through a fine-mesh sieve to remove the solids.

5. Season with salt and pepper to taste.

Tips:

- For a richer flavor, sauté the dried mushrooms with the vegetables for a few minutes before adding the broth.

- You can use other dried (or fresh) healthful mushrooms like lion's mane or portobello, adjusting the quantity based on taste and availability.

- To make the broth more filling, add tofu cubes, cooked whole grains, or noodles (if you tolerate carbs well).

- Store leftover broth in the refrigerator for up to 3 days or freeze it for longer storage. Ideally, have one cup of the broth per day.

Additional notes:

- If you are concerned about affordability, remember that dried reishi mushrooms can be pricier. Adjust the quantity or explore alternatives based on your budget.

- Consider buying your mushrooms from reputable companies for quality and consistency.

- Consult your healthcare professional before consuming healing mushrooms, especially if you have any underlying health conditions or take drugs.

Enjoy this delicious and healthy broth with the possible benefits of various healthful mushrooms! Remember, this is just a starting point, and you can experiment with different flavors and ingredients to create your own personal favorite healing mushroom broth.

RWM'S SUPERIOR SEED CRACKERS

Yield: 12-16 crackers

The biggest complaint we hear about the low-carb diet is the lack of bread, rolls, and crackers from the diet. However, it is possible to substitute a healthy, low-carb cracker for bread in most situations. There are various commercial products available (e.g., look for "low carb" or "paleo" seed crackers). I make my own, which are better tasting and more nutritious than most.

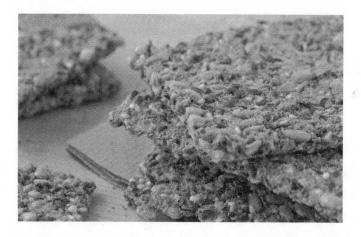

Watch a video of me explaining and demonstrating my process of making these seed crackers. – Editor's note: This link works only in PDF or Kindle edition. Paper book readers please visit YouTube and search for Ralph Moss and Seed Crackers.

You will need:

- 2 baking sheets
- Parchment paper
- Pizza cutter or sharp knife
- Measuring cups and spoons
- Firm spatula

Main Ingredients: All organic, whenever possible:

- 1/3 cup sunflower seeds
- 1/3 cup pumpkin seeds
- 1/3 cup flax seeds (golden is preferable)
- 1/3 cup chia seeds
- 1/3 cup sesame seeds (unhulled, hulled, or black seeds)
- 1/3 cup dehydrated onion
- 3 teaspoons sea salt or to taste
- You can also add some psyllium husks (to aid digestion and elimination), nigella or black (cumin) seeds (a popular Mideast general remedy), and/or caraway seeds (for flavor). Adding guajillo pepper chili powder could improve the impact of your green tea.
- Water (sufficient to make a slurry of the mixture)

You can also add any or all of the following ingredients:

- Fresh herbs, such as summer savory, mint, oregano or thyme
- Parsley flakes, dehydrated
- Paprika (plain, hot, or smoked)
- Red pepper flakes

Instructions:

Preheat the oven to 325°F (165°C).

1. Add to a large mixing bowl, the sunflower, pumpkin, flax, chia, sesame seeds, and the dehydrated onions for a total of two cups of solids. Mix well.

2. Add about one and a third cups of water until one has a slurry (the amount of water varies based on the weather and location.) Let this stand for 10

minutes. By doing this, the flax and chia seeds will soften and release some slippery compounds that let the whole mixture stick together. More water (or more seeds) may be needed as you proceed. The mixture should be consistent and spread quickly with no remaining water in the bowl.

3. Cut a piece of parchment paper to exceed the baking sheet's dimensions slightly. Spread the mixture to all the corners of the sheet so that you have a reasonably even mixture—thick enough to cover the parchment but thin enough to spread evenly. (Too thick and you wind up with seed cakes, which do not crackle when broken in half, too light and you get burnt-tasting little crackers.)

4. Bake for 30 minutes (half the baking time).

5. Remove from the oven and peel the entire sheet of seeds off the parchment paper while turning it over onto a fresh piece of parchment paper on the second baking sheet.

6. Cut the half-cooked sheet of cooked seeds into about 12 pieces using a pizza cutter or knife. The "crackers" should still be slightly moist on the side facing up. Return the baking sheet to the oven for another 20 to 30 minutes. Important: You will need to keep a close eye on it until it is cooked through and crispy—but not burnt. (This is where the "art of baking" comes in.)

7. Remove from the oven and place the cracker pieces on a cooling rack or platter until completely cool.

Store in a tin or a Zip-Lock bag in the refrigerator. If they get soggy, put them back in a 250°F (120°C) oven for five to ten minutes.

Once you get the hang of it, you can double the recipe to process two sheets simultaneously. Your family will probably grow to love these so they will be much in demand.

LOW-CARB SPROUTED SEED CRACKERS

Yield: 12-16 crackers

You will need:

- 1 Baking sheet
- Parchment paper

- Rolling pin
- Pizza cutter or sharp knife
- Measuring cups and spoons
- Firm spatula

Ingredients:

- 1 cup sprouted almond flour (made from ground sprouted almonds)
- ½ cup ground flaxseeds
- ¼ cup chia seeds
- ½ teaspoon salt
- 1 cup water
- Optional seasonings: garlic powder, onion powder, rosemary, or thyme for flavor

Instructions:

Preheat the oven to 325°F (165°C).

1. Line the baking sheet with parchment paper.

2. In a large bowl, combine the sprouted almond flour, ground flaxseeds, chia seeds, salt, and any optional seasonings you'd like to add. Mix well to ensure an even distribution of ingredients.

3. Add water to the dry ingredients and mix until a thick dough forms. Let the mixture sit for 5-10 minutes, allowing the chia and flax seeds to absorb the water and create a gel-like consistency. This will help bind the crackers together without the need for eggs or other binders.

4. Spread the dough onto the prepared baking sheet. Place another piece of parchment paper on top of the dough, and use a rolling pin to spread the dough evenly across the sheet, aiming for a thickness of about 1/8 inch (3 mm). Remove the top piece of parchment paper.

5. Score the Dough with a knife or pizza cutter into squares or rectangles, depending on your preferred cracker size. This makes it easier to break the crackers apart after baking.

6. Bake in the preheated oven for 30-40 minutes, or until the crackers are crispy and lightly golden. The baking time may vary depending on the thickness of the crackers and individual oven differences.

7. Cool crackers completely on the baking sheet. Once cooled, break them along the scored lines into individual crackers.

8. Store crackers in an airtight container at room temperature for up to a week, or in the refrigerator for longer storage.

These crackers are versatile and can be customized with various herbs and spices to suit your taste. They pair well with cheese, and dips, or can be enjoyed on their own as a low-carb snack. Enjoy experimenting with this recipe and the different flavors you can create!

Nutritional Profile:

To determine the carb content of a 1 oz (approximately 28 grams) serving of homemade low-carb sprouted seed crackers, we need to consider the ingredients used in the recipe. Since homemade recipes can vary widely in their specific ingredients and proportions, providing an exact number can be challenging without specific nutritional analysis. However, I can make an educated estimate based on the typical carb content of the main ingredients used:

- *Sprouted Almond Flour:* Almond flour, even when made from sprouted almonds, is low in carbs. Per ounce, almond flour contains about 3 to 5 grams of net carbs (total carbs minus fiber).

- *Ground Flaxseeds:* Flaxseeds are very high in fiber and low in net carbs. Per ounce, ground flaxseeds contain about 0.5 to 1 gram of net carbs.

- *Chia Seeds:* Chia seeds are also high in fiber. Per ounce, they have about 2 grams of net carbs.

Considering these are the main ingredients and assuming the crackers are composed primarily of these three ingredients, I can estimate the net carb content for a 1 oz homemade cracker. The calculation will also depend on the proportion of each ingredient used and the total yield of the cracker batch from the recipe provided.

If we roughly estimate based on the ingredients mentioned:

- The majority of the cracker's weight comes from almond flour, flaxseeds, and chia seeds.

- Assuming an even distribution and the addition of negligible carbs from seasonings or water, the estimated net carbs for a 1 oz serving of these crackers might be around 3 to 8 grams, considering the fiber content and the mixture of ingredients. This is a rough estimation and the actual carb content could vary.

For the most accurate nutritional information, especially if you're following a strict low-carb diet, it might be helpful to use a nutritional calculator where you can input the exact amounts of each ingredient used and calculate based on the specific yield of your recipe.

HIGH VITAMIN C LOW-CARB FRUIT SALAD

Yield: 2 servings

This fruit salad maximizes your vitamin C intake without compromising on taste. It's packed with antioxidants, fiber, and is perfect for a refreshing snack or a light dessert. It is also conscious of the fact that fruits are relatively high in carbs. So we have designed it to fulfill your vitamin C requirements without raising your blood sugar excessively.

Ingredients:

The fruit in this recipe can be fresh or frozen.

- 1 cup strawberries, halved
- 1 cup blackberries
- 1 medium avocado, cubed
- ½ cup raspberries
- 2 scoops (8 grams) of acerola cherry powder (buy it online)
- Juice of 1 lemon
- Mint leaves (optional)

Instructions:

Rinse the strawberries, blackberries, and raspberries under cold water. Halve the strawberries if large and keep the berries whole or as preferred.

1. Peel and stone the avocado. Cut into medium-sized cubes. Drizzle some lemon juice over the avocado to prevent browning.

2. In a large bowl, combine the halved strawberries, whole blackberries, raspberries, and cubed avocado.

3. Sprinkle a heaping scoop (4 grams) of acerola cherry powder evenly over the fruit. Pour the rest of the lemon juice over the fruits to help distribute the acerola powder smoothly.

4. Toss all ingredients gently with a spoon or salad utensils until the fruits are evenly coated with the lemon juice and acerola powder.

Chop the mint leaves roughly and sprinkle them over the salad to add a refreshing flavor.

Tip: For best flavor integration, let the salad chill in the refrigerator for about an hour before serving. Alternatively, serve immediately if preferred fresh and crisp.

Nutritional Profile (Per 1 Cup Serving):

- Vitamin C: Approximately **215 mg**

- Net Carbs: Approximately 9.4 grams (fits in well with a low-carb diet)

- Fiber: Approximately 7.9 grams (excellent as a prebiotic)

This salad not only delivers fantastic taste but also a significant boost in daily vitamin C, aiding in immune function, skin health, and overall well-being. The addition of acerola cherry powder, one of the world's best sources of vitamin C, ensures that each serving is packed with this essential nutrient, making it a smart choice for those looking to enhance their dietary intake.

Smoothie Equivalent

The same ingredients can be used as a smoothie, with a cup of either high-isoflavone organic soy milk or probiotic-rich organic grass-fed kefir.

TABBOULEH SALAD

Yield: 4 servings

Ingredients:

- 1 cup bulgur wheat (or quinoa for a gluten-free option)

- 1.5 cups boiling water

- 1 cup finely chopped fresh parsley (contains apigenin and luteolin)

- 1/2 cup finely chopped fresh mint (contains rosmarinic acid)

- 2 medium tomatoes, diced (contains lycopene)

- 1 cucumber, diced (contains beneficial cucurbitacins)

- 3 green onions, finely chopped (contains quercetin)

- 1/4 cup extra virgin olive oil (contains oleocanthal and hydroxytyrosol)
- 1/4 cup fresh lemon juice (contains vitamin C)
- 1-2 cloves garlic, minced (contains allicin)
- Salt and freshly ground black pepper to taste

Instructions:

1. Place the bulgur in a large bowl and pour the boiling water over it. Cover and let it soak for about an hour, or until the water is absorbed and the bulgur is tender. If using quinoa, cook according to package instructions.

2. While the bulgur is soaking, finely chop the parsley, mint, tomatoes, cucumber, and green onions.

3. Once the bulgur is ready, fluff it with a fork and let it cool slightly. Add the chopped parsley, mint, tomatoes, cucumber, and green onions to the bowl with the bulgur.

4. In a small bowl, whisk together the olive oil, lemon juice, minced garlic, salt, and pepper. Pour the dressing over the salad and toss well to combine.

5. Taste and adjust the seasoning with more salt, pepper, or lemon juice as needed.

6. Let the salad sit for at least 30 minutes before serving to allow the flavors to meld. Serve at room temperature or chilled.

This Tabbouleh salad is not only delicious but is packed with beneficial phytochemicals that align with the principles of The Moss Method.

JIM DUKE'S CANCER PREVENTION SALAD

In 1974, my friend James A. Duke, Ph.D., chief of the Medicinal Plant Resources Laboratory of the United States Department of Agriculture (USDA), published his famous cancer prevention herbal salad recipe. Duke's salad was in turn inspired by the work of Jonathan Hartwell, Ph.D., of the National Cancer Institute (NCI), in a lifetime of work summarized in his classic monograph, _Plants Used Against Cancer_ (Hartwell 1982, Graham 2000). Both of these gentlemen were pioneers, far ahead of their time. Incidentally, I dedicated my book, _Herbs Against Cancer_, to Jonathan Hartwell, and Jim Duke was on the advisory board of my newsletter, The Cancer Chronicles.

Duke's salad, reprinted in his popular book, *The Green Pharmacy: The Ultimate Compendium Of Natural Remedies From The World's Foremost Authority On Healing Herbs* (Duke 1998), contained the following ingredients: Garlic, onions, red pepper, tomatoes, red clover flowers, chopped cooked beets, fresh calendula flowers, celery, fresh chicory flowers, chives, cucumbers, cumin, peanuts, poke salad, purslane, and sage. Duke's Salad Dressing consisted of flaxseed oil, evening primrose oil, garlic, rosemary, a dash of lemon juice, and a dash of hot pepper.

I have modified his recipe to be lower in carbs (such as by removing the beets) and contain some ingredients that have come to the fore since Dr. Duke formulated his salad.

Yield: 2 servings

Ingredients:

- 4 cups spinach or dark green and red lettuce leaves
- ½ cup sprouts (broccoli, mung, or chickpea)
- ½ cup parsley chopped
- ½ cup onion, chopped
- 1 avocado, diced
- ½ cup cucumber, chopped
- ½ cup peanuts or raw walnuts
- ½ cup, when available, red clover, calendula, and chicory flowers
- 1 can of tuna packed in olive oil - optional

> *"Avocado fruit extract is effective in stopping cancer cell growth compared to normal cells. Avocado fruit is rich in plant chemicals, which play an important role in blocking the growth of cancer cells. Therefore, some experts suggest that the fruit extracts are appropriate complementary treatments for esophageal and colon cancers"* (Vahedi Larijani 2014, edited).

On the other hand, in the massive Nurses' Health Study, eating avocado was associated with a 21% increased risk of breast cancer (Ericsson 2023). My theory is that the harm comes from the estrogen stimulating? Blocking? Pesticides. We therefore recommend that women only consume organic avocados.

SUPER-HEALTHY SALAD DRESSING

Ingredients:

- 1/3 cup extra virgin olive oil
- 1/3 cup red wine vinegar (infused with herbs, especially summer savory - optional)
- 1/3 cup spring or filtered water
- 1 tablespoon lemon juice
- 2 crushed raw garlic cloves
- 1 teaspoon "Herbs de Provence' (a mix of summer savory, parsley, sage, rosemary, thyme, and lavender)
- 1 teaspoon sweet paprika or guajillo chili powder.

Instructions:

Whisk or blend to emulsify.

ORANGE MUSTARD

Yield: Approximately 2 Tablespoons

I was wracking my brain trying to figure out how to get more turmeric (and therefore more curcumin) into the average person's diet. Then I realized that in America, at least, there already are two common foods that contain a considerable amount of turmeric. The first is curry powder. Whenever I make a curry, I use an equal amount of turmeric in addition to whatever quantity of curry powder I am using in the recipe.

The other food is more surprising. You probably will not have to buy it, since most of us already have it in the refrigerator. It is yellow mustard! That all-American mustard that we associate with hot dogs, picnics, and baseball games. The bright yellow color of that "hot dog mustard" comes from a once-exotic Indian spice, turmeric.

Yellow mustard is made from the seeds of the mustard plant, vinegar, water, and spices, especially turmeric. The mustard seeds themselves do contribute to the flavor but are not responsible for the color. It is turmeric that imparts to yellow mustard its distinctive color, making it visually appealing and adding a mild spicy flavor.

Here is the recipe that I came up with:

- 2 tablespoons of organic yellow mustard.
- 1 teaspoon of ground organic turmeric powder.
- 1 teaspoon or so of water to thin out the mixture

According to testing by an independent laboratory, one teaspoon of ground organic turmeric powder contains **67.6 milligrams (mg) of curcuminoids** (Cooperman 2024). The turmeric already in yellow mustard contributes ~**30 mg** of curcuminoids. So we can estimate that this mixture contains about **100 mg** curcumin and related compounds. Even if you took just a small amount of this mixture per day it would provide a substantial amount of this healing substance. This is a way to avoid taking yet another cumbersome pill.

SPICY STIR-FRY WITH SPROUTS

Yield: 2 servings

Ingredients:

- 2 tablespoons of olive oil (healthy fat to aid absorption of nutrients)
- 1 large onion, finely chopped (high in quercetin)
- 1 red bell pepper, sliced (for a sweet flavor and resveratrol)
- 1 teaspoon of chili flakes or fresh chili pepper, finely chopped (adjust to taste)
- 2-3 cloves of garlic, minced
- 1 tablespoon of fresh turmeric root, grated (or one teaspoon of turmeric powder)
- Salt and black pepper, to taste
- A sprinkle of crushed red grapes or a small amount of red wine (for additional resveratrol) (optional)
- 1 cup of fresh broccoli sprouts (rich in cruciferous compounds)
- Fresh herbs like cilantro or parsley for garnish (optional)

Instructions:

1. Wash and chop the onion, red bell pepper, and chili pepper; mince the garlic; and grate the turmeric root. If using fresh chili, remove seeds for less heat.

2. In a large skillet or wok, heat the olive oil over medium heat. Add the chopped onion and red bell pepper. Sauté until the onion becomes translucent and the pepper softens.

3. Add the minced garlic, grated turmeric, and fresh or dried chili to the skillet. Stir well to combine. Cook for another minute until fragrant.

4. Season with salt and black pepper to taste. Sprinkle some crushed red grapes or a bit of red wine for an additional resveratrol boost.

5. Cook for another minute, then remove from heat.

6. Fold in the sprouts and serve immediately to avoid overheating.

7. Garnish with fresh herbs if desired.

Tips:

- For a complete meal, serve this stir-fry with a protein source like grilled chicken, tofu, or fish.

- Adjust the amount of chili to suit your taste for spiciness.

- Serve with a cup of green tea to enhance the effect.

This recipe is both healthful and tasty, and incorporates various ingredients known for their possible anticancer qualities while also being enjoyable to eat.

ROASTED CHICORY ROOT COFFEE

Yield: 1 serving

Ingredients:

- 2 tablespoons roasted chicory root (ground) [I favor Micro Ingredients™ Organic French Chicory Roasted]

- 1 cup water

Instructions:

1. Bring 1 cup of water to a boil.

2. Add 2 tablespoons of ground roasted chicory root to the boiling water.

3. Reduce the heat and let it simmer for about 5-10 minutes.

4. Remove from heat and strain the liquid through a fine mesh strainer or coffee filter into a mug.

5. Enjoy your chicory root coffee as is, or add milk and sweetener to taste.

Tips:

- For a New Orleans-style coffee, you can blend your roasted chicory root with ground coffee in a ratio of 1:2 (one part chicory to two parts coffee) and brew as usual.

- Adjust the amount of chicory root used to make the coffee stronger or milder according to your taste preferences.

SAMPLE MEAL PLAN #1

Designing a meal plan incorporating berberine, curcumin, EGCG, luteolin, mangosteen, resveratrol, and sulforaphane to **attack cancer stem cells (CSCs)** can be health-conscious and delicious. Here's a suggestion for a daily meal plan with minimal reliance on supplements:

Breakfast: Green Tea and a Fruit Bowl

- *Green Tea (EGCG):* Start with a cup of freshly brewed green tea for its EGCG content.

- *Fruit Bowl (Mangosteen juice, Resveratrol):* Prepare a fruit bowl featuring mangosteen and grapes, which are good sources of xanthones (from mangosteen) and resveratrol (from grapes). Find mangosteen at Asian and farmers markets. The juice is available at many whole food stores.

Lunch: Turmeric-Infused Vegetable Stir-Fry

- *Turmeric-Infused Vegetable Stir-Fry (Curcumin):* Create a stir-fry with a variety of vegetables like broccoli, cauliflower, and carrots. Use turmeric and black pepper in the seasoning to improve curcumin absorption.

- *Side of Broccoli Sprouts (Sulforaphane):* Include a side of fresh broccoli sprouts, a rich sulforaphane source.

Snack: Celery with Nut Butter

- *Celery Sticks (Luteolin):* Snack on celery sticks containing luteolin, with a smear of nut butter for added protein and flavor.

Dinner: Grilled Chicken or Fish with a Side Salad

- *Grilled Chicken or Fish:* Opt for lean proteins like chicken or fish for dinner.
- *Side Salad (Resveratrol, Luteolin):* Accompany it with a side salad that includes red grapes and a variety of leafy greens, both of which contribute to the intake of resveratrol and luteolin.

Supplements:
- Since it is challenging to include berberine in your diet, consider a berberine supplement, as this compound is not commonly found in Western diets.

Remember, while these foods and compounds have shown potential in attacking CSCs, they should be considered as part of *The Moss Method*. However, one should seek and use mainstream medical care whenever necessary.

SAMPLE MEAL PLAN #2

Here is another meal plan focused on **attacking cancer stem cells (CSCs)** incorporating curcumin, EGCG, extra virgin olive oil (EVOO), luteolin, quercetin, resveratrol, soy isoflavones, and sulforaphane.

Breakfast: Soy Yogurt Parfait and Green Tea

- *Soy Yogurt (Isoflavones):* Begin with soy yogurt, adding fresh fruits like berries (which also provide quercetin). It is very important to avoid the vast majority of commercial yogurts, which either contain sugar outright or else jams or fruit compotes that add greatly to the glycemic load. Sugar-added yogurt can have up to 30 grams of carbs per serving.
- *Green Tea (EGCG):* Accompany your breakfast with a cup of green tea for its EGCG content.

Mid-Morning Snack: Fresh Fruit or Vegetable Juice

- *Fresh pressed juice (Quercetin, Luteolin):* A juice made from apples, grapes, and some celery (for luteolin).

Lunch: Broccoli Salad with Olive Oil Dressing

- *Broccoli Salad (Sulforaphane):* Prepare a salad with fresh or lightly steamed broccoli high in sulforaphane.
- *Olive Oil Dressing (EVOO):* Add extra virgin olive oil (EVOO) to your salad dressing drizzled over the broccoli salad.

Afternoon Snack: Nuts and Berries

- *Nuts and Berries (Resveratrol, Ellagic acid):* A small serving of nuts and berries, particularly grapes or blueberries, for a dose of resveratrol.

Dinner: Turmeric-Infused Stir-Fry with Tofu

- *Turmeric-Infused Stir-Fry (Curcumin):* Prepare a vegetable stir-fry with a turmeric-based sauce. Use a variety of vegetables like bell peppers and carrots.

- *Tofu (Soy Isoflavones):* Include tofu, which is rich in soy isoflavones, as your protein source. Add radish sprouts at the last minute, but do not let them get heated above 158°F (70°C).

Evening Tea: Herbal Tea

- *Herbal Tea (*Quercetin*):* Finish your day with an herbal tea that includes ingredients like elderberry organic red tea, known for its quercetin content.

Supplements: Optional

- If specific nutrients are challenging to obtain routinely from the diet, such as luteolin, you may consider a supplement. However, always consult with a healthcare professional before incorporating any supplements, especially for individuals with health conditions or those on drugs.

SAMPLE MEAL PLAN #3

AN IMMUNE CHECKPOINT BLOCKADE MENU

This menu functions as an "immune checkpoint blockade" (ICB), using several natural immune checkpoint blockers. Asian researchers have shown that half a dozen natural agents also act as ICIs in the lab. This fact may be surprising, but the agents in question will be familiar to readers of this book. *The plant chemicals are colorful anthocyanins, apigenin, curcumin, EGCG, luteolin, resveratrol, and silymarin.* The following menu incorporates these compounds into a single meal. It can be both healthy and tasty (and more affordable than taking supplements).

Starter: Green Tea and Mixed Berry Salad

- *Green Tea (EGCG):* Start with a cup of freshly brewed green tea, rich in EGCG.

- *Mixed Berry Salad (Anthocyanins, Resveratrol):* Prepare a salad with a mix of blueberries, blackberries, and red grapes. These are excellent sources of the colorful plant pigments anthocyanins and resveratrol.

Main Course: Turmeric-Infused Grilled Chicken with Colorful Vegetables.

- *Turmeric-Infused Grilled Chicken (Curcumin):* Marinate chicken in a mixture of olive oil, lemon juice, garlic, and a generous amount of turmeric, then grill.

- *Pigment-Rich Vegetables (Apigenin, Luteolin):* Serve with a side of vegetables such as celery (rich in apigenin) and broccoli (rich in luteolin).

Dessert: *Mixed berries* with unsweetened yogurt or kefir and chopped almonds or walnuts.

These sample meals are an enjoyable way to incorporate potent plant chemicals into a routine diet. It is important to remember that while scientists have studied these ingredients for their health benefits, they are only one part of The Moss Method, and should be combined with a healthy lifestyle including physical activity, social interaction, and standard medical care when necessary. Also, for individuals with specific health conditions or those on drugs, it is always advisable to consult with a healthcare professional before making changes to one's diet, especially when incorporating specific supplements or plant chemicals. This caveat is doubly so if you are already on commercial immune checkpoint blockers since you do not want to inadvertently trigger side effects through cooperative effects.

THE MOSS METHOD & PLANT CHEMICALS IN TARGETING CSCs

Following The Moss Method means preventing cancer with a focus on CSCs using natural and nutritional elements in treatment plans. This method targets the root causes of cancer, especially the fact that it is driven by CSCs. A secondary goal is to help overcome the side effects of mainstream treatments, but that should only be attempted with the active participation of one's doctors.

Using natural compounds to target multiple markers of cancer stem cells is very promising. I believe a multi-targeted approach is needed, but using toxic drugs to accomplish this might not work due to their harm and expense. Plant chemicals are a better fit, but they're often overlooked because there's no financial incentive to pursue this approach.

FUTURE DIRECTIONS

The Moss Report (and themossreport.com website) have played a role in spreading information and sparking discussions about how natural products might be used in cancer treatment, especially in how they interact with cancer stem cells (CSCs). Through our podcasts, articles, and expert interviews, *The Moss Report* has helped bridge the gap between mainstream and natural approaches by focusing on three key areas:

1. *Educating Patients and Practitioners*: We provide easy-to-access, scientifically-supported information that examines how plant chemicals can be used safely and effectively in cancer treatment.

2. *Revealing Cutting-Edge Research:* We feature the newest studies and trials from across the globe that demonstrate how natural compounds could help enhance cancer treatment outcomes.

3. *Advocating for Integrative Practices:* We support a comprehensive approach to cancer treatment that combines traditional medicine with proven natural therapies, aiming to boost treatment success and ensure patient safety.

As we continue to uncover the complexities of cancer stem cells and their processes, the focus of future research and clinical trials will likely pivot toward more personalized and precise interventions. This includes:

*   *Personalized Plant Chemical Profiling:* Leveraging genetic, metabolic, and other data to predict individual responses to specific plant chemicals, improving the outcome of treatments.

*   *Advanced Formulations:* Developing more sophisticated formulations that improve the availability and targeted delivery of plant chemicals.

*   *Regulatory Advancements:* Working with government agencies like the FDA to establish clearer networks for the approval of natural compounds as legitimate elements of cancer therapy protocols.

The integration of plant-based chemicals into cancer care, particularly by targeting CSCs, offers a very promising addition to mainstream approaches. The Moss Method can also play a crucial role in educating and informing the public and healthcare professionals about the scientific advancements and practical applications of these natural therapies into cancer care especially in the context of prevention.

IN CONCLUSION

As I reflect on my career, from generating articles and press releases for MSKCC to developing The Moss Method, my goal has shifted from merely reporting advancements to actively contributing to the understanding and prevention of cancer. This book is a testament to the progress we've made and a guide for those seeking to minimize cancer risks through informed, practical approaches.

While the occurrence of cancer often brings personal despair, I have always aimed to show the positive strides made in research and treatment. This record of scientific advancement and the practical applications now available to the public offers not just knowledge but hope—demonstrating the power of evidence-based approaches to combating cancer.

The Moss Method's integration of reductionist and organicist perspectives offers a comprehensive approach to cancer prevention. By understanding the specific mechanisms of plant chemicals but also embracing a holistic lifestyle, individuals can create a powerful defense against cancer. This demonstrates once again that, when it comes to preventing cancer, the whole is indeed greater than the sum of its parts.

###

A GLOSSARY OF TECHNICAL TERMS

Aside from this glossary, here are two other glossaries of cancer-related terms:
The ACS Online Glossary, Understanding Research Terms (for Non-Scientists)
The NCI Dictionary of Cancer Terms

5-Lipoxygenase (5-LOX): An enzyme in the body that helps produce inflammatory substances, with blockers of 5-LOX being studied for their potential anti-inflammatory and anticancer effects.

Activating invasion and metastasis: Cancer cells acquire the ability to break away from their original location and form new tumors in different parts of the body. We call it cancer's "spread."

Alkaloids: Naturally occurring organic compounds that contain basic nitrogen atoms. Alkaloids are often found in plants and are known for their wide range of drug effects and toxic qualities.

Allicin: A compound in garlic noted for its heart benefits, antimicrobial qualities, and possible anticancer effects, particularly attacking cancer stem cells.

Anthocyanins: Water-soluble plant pigments responsible for the red, blue, and purple colors in many fruits and vegetables, especially berries, with possible antioxidant and health benefits. They reduce DNA damage and help protect against genetic changes leading to cancer.

Antioxidants: Substances that can prevent or slow damage to cells caused by harmful free radicals, often found in fruits and vegetables.

Apoptosis: The dominant form of programmed cell death, by which a body naturally eliminates damaged or unnecessary cells, including potentially cancerous ones. In this work, we call it "normal cell death".

Availability: This is the proportion of a substance (such as a drug, vitamin, or nutrient) that enters the blood circulation and becomes available to the attacked tissue after it is administered. Also called bioavailability.

Ayurvedic medicine: A traditional Indian healing system that uses diet, herbal treatments, and yogic breathing to maintain or restore health by balancing the body's three doshas—Vata, Pitta, and Kapha, which are believed to be the vital energies governing physiological functions.

Berberine: A compound extracted from several plants, including the barberry bush, used in traditional medicine, and noted for its possible benefits in treating various ailments, including energy-related and infectious diseases.

Beta-glucan: A fiber derived from various sources, including mushrooms, oats, and yeast, with immune-boosting and potentially anti-cancer qualities.

Bilberry: A dark blueberry known for its high content of anthocyanins and possible health benefits, especially for eye health.

Body Mass Index: BMI is a numerical calculation using height and weight to estimate a person's body fat, categorizing them as underweight, normal weight, overweight, or obese.

Bortezomib: A prescription drug sold as Velcade, used in multiple myeloma treatment, attacking specific proteins within cancer cells to stop their growth.

Boswellic acids: Compounds derived from *Boswellia* resin, known for their anti-inflammatory qualities and possible role in stopping 5-LOX.

C3 Complex: A curcumin supplement combining three curcuminoids for improved absorption and effectiveness.

Cancer Stem Cells (CSCs): A small group of cancer cells within a tumor believed to be responsible for the growth and spread of cancer and often resistant to standard treatments.

Cancer survivor: Someone diagnosed with cancer, regardless of their current treatment status.

Carbohydrates: A nutrient found in foods like bread, grains, fruits, and vegetables, which the body uses for energy.

Carcinogen: A substance or agent capable of causing or promoting cancer development in living tissue.

Carcinogenic: Having the possibility to cause cancer.

Catechin: A type of natural antioxidant found in various plants, such as tea leaves and cocoa beans, that helps protect cells from damage.

Chemoresistance: The ability of specific cells, like cancer stem cells, to withstand standard cancer treatments such as chemo and radiation, making them challenging to eliminate.

Chronic inflammation: A long-term, persistent inflammation in the body that can silently cause tissue damage and contribute to diseases like cancer.

Colony forming units: A measure used in microbiology to estimate the number of viable microorganisms in a sample, with each unit potentially growing into a visible colony.

Complex carbohydrates: In whole grains, these nutrients can disrupt the preferred energy use of cancer cells.

Cryoablation, Focal: A minimally invasive procedure used to treat prostate cancer, where cold temperatures are used to freeze and destroy cancer cells.

Curcumin: A compound in the yellow rhizome turmeric that helps kill cancer cells and repairs DNA, showing its versatility in cancer treatment.

Cytotoxic chemotherapy: A type of cancer treatment that kills cells, particularly rapidly dividing cancer cells, but also can affect healthy cells. Also called chemo.

Deep vein thrombosis: Deep vein thrombosis is the formation of a blood clot within a deep vein, typically in the legs.

Diabesity: A term combining diabetes and obesity, often used to describe their interconnected nature in public health. The diabetes and obesity epidemic refers to the widespread increase in cases of diabetes and obesity, often related to lifestyle factors like diet and physical inactivity.

Diabetes: A chronic energy-related disorder marked by high blood sugar levels due to either insufficient insulin production (Type 1) or insulin resistance (Type 2).

Dietary Supplement Health and Education Act of 1994: DSHEA is a U.S. law that defines and regulates dietary supplements, allowing them to be marketed without FDA approval for effectiveness.

DNA methylation: A process in which chemicals called methyl groups are added to DNA, affecting how genes work. It's essential for controlling gene activity and plays a role in cancer development and other biological processes.

Epigallocatechin gallate: EGCG is a powerful antioxidant found in green tea, known for its ability to prevent cancer by stopping cancer cells from growing and multiplying.

Epithelial-Mesenchymal Transition: EMT is a cellular process whereby epithelial cells lose their characteristics and transform into mesenchymal cells, often associated with increased migration and invasion.

Extra Virgin Olive Oil: EVOO is an olive oil rich in health-promoting antioxidants, beneficial for heart health, reducing inflammation, and potentially attacking cancer stem cells.

321

Fast Food Culture: The widespread habit of consuming quickly prepared, highly processed foods, often high in calories, fats, and sugars.

Fasting-Mimicking Diet (FMD): A diet that imitates the effects of fasting by restricting calorie intake and adjusting nutrient composition to trigger helpful health responses. Invented by Prof. Valter Longo of the University of Southern California (USC).

Fermented Wheat Germ Extract (FWGE): A supplement made from wheat germ, fermented with yeast, that's believed to help control cancer cell growth and support the immune system.

Food and Drug Administration: The FDA is a U.S. government agency responsible for regulating foods, dietary supplements, drugs, cosmetics, and medical devices.

Forest Bathing: A Japanese practice of being in nature to improve one's health.

Free radicals: Unstable molecules that can damage cells, potentially leading to health issues like aging and disease. Also called singlet oxygen.

Generally Recognized as Safe: "GRAS" is a U.S. Food and Drug Administration (FDA) designation that a substance added to food is considered safe by experts and so is exempted from the usual federal food additive tolerance requirements. The process must be started by the manufacturer of the product in question and, hence, is not all-inclusive.

Genome instability and changes: The genetic material of cancer cells is prone to frequent errors, which drive the disease's growth and diversity.

Glucosinolates: Natural compounds found in certain vegetables like broccoli and kale that contribute to their distinct taste and may have potential health benefits.

Glycolysis: A process in which cells break down sugar (glucose) for energy, which cancer cells use more than normal cells. This produces lactate (similar to lactic acid) as a waste material.

Gut microbiome: A complex community of microbes living in the digestive tracts of humans, which plays a crucial role in health and disease. The gut microbiome, technically, refers to all the genetic material in the intestines, whereas the *gut microbiota* refers to the organisms themselves.

Hallmarks of Cancer: Key traits delineated by Professors. Hanahan and Weinberg distinguishing cancer cells from normal cells include sustained growth signals, evasion of growth suppressors, and resistance to cell death. The number currently stands at ten.

Hemoglobin A1C: A blood test that measures the average blood sugar (glucose) level over the past two to three months, often used to monitor diabetes control. Also called HbA1C or just A1C.

Heterocyclic amines (HCAs): Chemical compounds formed when cooking meat at high temperatures, associated with cancer risk.

Imatinib (Gleevec): A targeted cancer drug used primarily to treat certain types of leukemia and other cancers by explicitly stopping a protein that promotes cancer cell growth.

Immune Checkpoint Blockers: A class of drugs used in cancer therapy that help the immune system recognize and attack cancer cells by stopping specific proteins that control immune responses. They fight cancer by boosting the body's immune response against cancer cells.

Immune surveillance: Immune surveillance is an old theory that posits that lymphocytes, a group of white blood cells, continuously monitor and eliminate transformed cells before they can evolve into tumors. This theory contributed to the rise of immune checkpoint blockers.

Immunotherapy: Treatments that use the body's immune system to fight disease, particularly cancer.

Inflammation: A natural process by which the body responds to injury or infection, which can become very difficult to treat if chronic.

Informed decision-making: Making healthcare decisions based on a thorough understanding of the available options, possible risks, and benefits.

Insulin-like growth factor 1: IGF-1, or Insulin-like Growth Factor 1: A hormone similar in molecular structure to insulin that normally plays an important role in childhood growth and promotes the building of muscle and other tissues in adults.

Insulin resistance: A condition where the body's cells don't respond effectively to insulin, leading to elevated blood sugar levels, often a precursor to type 2 diabetes.

Insulin sensitivity: The body's ability to effectively use insulin is important for adjusting blood sugar levels and can influence cancer risk.

Integrative medicine: A healthcare approach that combines traditional Western medicine with alternative or complementary treatments, like herbal medicine, acupuncture, and massage.

Intermittent fasting: An eating pattern that cycles between periods of fasting and eating, used for various health benefits.

Ketogenic (or keto) diet: A high-fat, low-carbohydrate diet that changes the body's metabolism to burn fats instead of carbohydrates, producing ketone bodies as a by-product.

Lentinan: A natural compound found in Shiitake mushrooms, known for boosting the immune system and stopping tumor growth.

Liver toxicity: This is liver damage, which can happen if someone consumes too much of a substance, like EGCG, that the liver struggles to process.

Lumpectomy: A less invasive surgical procedure for breast cancer that involves removing only the tumor and a small margin of surrounding tissue.

Luteolin: A plant compound found in foods like celery and green peppers, known for its allergy-relieving, heart-protecting, and possible anticancer qualities.

Median survival: The length of time from the start of treatment or diagnosis until half of the study participants have died, used as a measure to judge treatment effectiveness; for instance, a median survival of 24 months indicates that half of the patients lived longer than 24 months, while the other half lived less.

Mediterranean Diet: Also called the Med Diet, a dietary pattern typical of countries and territories in the Mediterranean region, marked by high intake of fruits, vegetables, whole grains, olive oil, and fish.

Meta-analysis: A study of studies utilizing a statistical analysis that combines the results of multiple clinical trials. It provides a broader understanding of a research topic than any single randomized controlled trial.

Metabolic syndrome: A cluster of disorders including high blood pressure, high blood sugar, excess body fat around the waist, and abnormal cholesterol levels, increasing the risk of heart disease, stroke, and diabetes.

Metastasis: The process by which cancer cells spread from the original tumor site to other parts of the body, forming new tumors. Cancerous spread.

Microbiome: A comprehensive term for the microorganisms in a specific environment, their genomes, and the environmental conditions, reflecting both the microbial community and its functional potential.

Microbiota: The collection of microorganisms, including bacteria, viruses, fungi, and archaea, that inhabit a specific environment, such as the human gut or skin.

Milk Thistle/Silymarin: This plant extract is known for its liver-protecting qualities and possible anticancer benefits, particularly good for liver health and managing cell damage from oxygen.

Mindful eating: Paying close attention to the eating experience, going beyond simply consuming food, and becoming conscious of all the sensations involved.

Myoglobin: A red protein containing heme, which carries and stores oxygen in muscle cells. It is structurally similar to a subunit of hemoglobin.

National Center for Complementary and Integrative Health (NCCIH): A center within the National Institutes of Health focusing on research and providing information on complementary and integrative health approaches. Formerly known as the Office of Alternative Medicine (OAM).

National Comprehensive Cancer Network: The NCCN is a not-for-profit alliance of top American cancer centers dedicated to improving the quality and effectiveness of cancer care.

National Institutes of Health (NIH): The primary agency of the United States government responsible for biomedical and public health research.

Natural killer (NK) Cells: A type of white blood cell that plays a crucial role in the body's immune system by attacking and destroying harmful cells, including cancer cells.

Natural selection: An evolutionary process where organisms better adapted to their environment tend to survive and produce more offspring.

Net carbs: Net carbs refer to the total carbohydrates in a food minus its fiber and sugar alcohols, representing the carbs that affect blood sugar levels.

Non-communicable diseases: Chronic diseases not passed from person to person, such as heart disease, stroke, and diabetes, are often associated with lifestyle factors.

Nutraceuticals: Foods that potentially positively affect health beyond essential nutrition, often containing specific nutrients or compounds that can improve health. This is a broad umbrella term that can be used to describe any product derived from food sources with extra health benefits in addition to the basic nutritional value found in foods. Also sometimes referred to as "functional food".

Obesity: A medical condition marked by excess body fat, which can increase the risk of various health issues like heart disease and type 2 diabetes.

Office of Alternative Medicine (OAM): An office established within the National Institutes of Health to explore and fund research in alternative medicine practices. It morphed into the National Center for Complementary and Integrative Health (NCCIH).

Oleacein: A compound found in extra virgin olive oil, known for its antioxidant properties and potential health benefits.

Oleocanthal (OC): A compound found in extra virgin olive oil known for its anti-inflammatory, antioxidant, and nerve-protective qualities. Oleocanthal is recognized for its ability to stop the COX enzymes, similar to ibuprofen.

Omega-3 Fatty Acids: Essential fats found in fish, flaxseeds, and walnuts are essential for heart and brain health and are known for their anti-inflammatory qualities.

ONCOblot: An experimental blood test used for early detection of various types of cancer, including prostate cancer. Not presently available.

Overall survival (OS): This is simply how long patients live after starting treatment, regardless of whether their cancer improves or worsens.

Oxidative phosphorylation: OxPhos is a complex process in cell mitochondria that uses oxygen to produce energy, typically efficient in normal cells but altered in cancer cells. Contrasts with aerobic glycolysis, a.k.a. the Warburg effect.

Oxidative stress: Cell damage from oxygen. A condition where there is an imbalance between dangerous free radicals and antioxidants in the body.

Patient-centered care: Medical care that is respectful of and responsive to individual patient preferences, needs, and values.

Piperine: A natural alkaloid found in peppercorns (*Piper nigrum*) and other plants, known for its ability to improve the availability of other nutrients, including curcumin from turmeric.

Polyphenol: A substance that is found in many plants and gives some flowers, fruits, and vegetables their color. Polyphenols have antioxidant activity. Also called polyphenolic compounds, they are key ingredients in *The Moss Method*.

Polysaccharides: A polysaccharide is a complex carbohydrate molecule composed of multiple sugar units bonded together in long chains, serving various structural and storage functions in living organisms. Found in mushrooms that can help adjust the immune system and may have anti-tumor qualities.

Positron emission tomography scan: Particularly in the context of cancer, a PET scan is a diagnostic imaging technique that uses a radioactive glucose analog called FDG to detect and measure the energy-related activity of tumors, as cancerous cells typically consume more glucose than normal cells.

Precision Medicine Initiative: A research endeavor, introduced by President Obama in his 2015 State of the Union address, that aims to tailor medical treatment to the individual traits of each patient, including their genetic makeup, environment, and lifestyle, to improve health outcomes.

Prediabetes: An energy-related condition where blood sugar levels are higher than usual but not high enough to be classified as diabetes, often a precursor to type 2 diabetes.

Programmed cell death: A regulated process by which cells are systematically dismantled and removed from an organism.

Programmed Death-Ligand 1: PD-L1 is a protein expressed on cancer cells that helps cancer cells evade immune system detection and destruction when binding to its receptor.

Progression-Free Survival: PFS is a term used in cancer research to describe the length of time during and after treatment that a patient lives with the disease, but it does not get worse.

Pulmonary embolism: This occurs when a blood clot dislodges from its site of origin, travels through the bloodstream, and lodges in the arteries of the lungs, potentially causing blockage and impaired blood flow.

Quercetin: A flavonoid found in fruits and vegetables that can improve the absorption and effectiveness of vitamin C, essential for immune function and skin health.

Randomized Controlled Trial (RCT): A scientific study where people are assigned by a computerized 'flip of a coin' to different groups to test a specific drug, treatment, or other intervention. This allows for fair and unbiased comparisons. Sometimes (less accurately) called randomized clinical trials.

Resveratrol: Found in red wine and berries, it influences how cells process energy and provides antioxidant protection, helping to stabilize DNA.

Roseto Effect: A phenomenon first observed in Roseto, Pennsylvania, where a close-knit community experienced low rates of heart disease, attributable to social cohesion and supportive relationships.

Self-help sphere: Activities and practices that people can undertake on their own to improve health and prevent disease.

Shingles: A disease caused by a Herpes Zoster infection. A painful skin rash caused by the reactivation of the chickenpox virus, typically occurring in older adults or those with weakened immune systems.

Signal networks: A series of interactions between molecules within a cell, which control its activities and can influence cancer growth and survival.

Stemness: The quality of a cell that allows it to behave like a stem cell, including self-renewal and the possibility of morphing into multiple cell types.

Sulforaphane: A naturally occurring compound found in cruciferous vegetables like broccoli, which is widely researched for its possible ability to promote health and protect against certain diseases by supporting the body's process of removing toxic compounds and reducing inflammation.

Surface markers: Specific proteins located on the surface of cells that identify and classify different types of cells, including cancer stem cells.

Sustaining proliferative signaling: The continuous self-triggered growth and division of cancer cells, much like a car stuck with the accelerator pedal always pressed.

Synbiotics: A combination of probiotic bacteria and prebiotics (usually from inulin) that enhances gut health by improving the survival and effectiveness of good gut bacteria.

Targeted therapies: Cancer treatments designed to specifically attack and interfere with molecules involved in tumor growth, such as proteins on the surface of cancer cells.

Time-restricted eating (TRE): A dietary approach where eating is limited to a certain number of contiguous hours each day, typically within an 8 to 12-hour window.

Toxicology: The scientific study of the harmful effects of chemicals, drugs, and substances on living organisms, as well as the method of toxicity.

Traditional, Complementary, and Integrative Medicine (TCI): A term the World Health Organization uses to describe a range of medical therapies that are not part of conventional Western medicine but may be integrated into it.

Tumor microenvironment: The environment around a tumor, including various cell types and molecules, can influence cancer growth and spread.

Tumor-promoting inflammation: Chronic inflammation in the body can unintentionally create conditions that help tumors to grow and spread.

Type 2 diabetes (T2D): A chronic condition where the body either doesn't produce enough insulin or doesn't use it effectively, leading to high blood sugar levels.

Venous thromboembolism (VTE): A condition marked by the formation of blood clots in the deep veins (deep vein thrombosis) that can travel to the lungs, causing a potentially life-threatening pulmonary embolism.

Vitamin C: A vital nutrient that supports the immune system, acts as an antioxidant, plays a role in skin and heart health, and may impact cancer stem cells. Also known as ascorbic acid.

Vitamin D3: A vitamin crucial for bone health, immune function, and overall well-being, with possible roles in cancer prevention and adjustment of cancer stem cells. Often referred to as the 'sunshine vitamin'.

Warburg effect: An energy-related feature of cancer cells where they preferentially use glycolysis (the breakdown of sugar) to generate energy, even in the presence of oxygen. Contrast with oxidative phosphorylation, or OxPhos.

A GLOSSARY OF ABBREVIATIONS

A1C: Also known as the hemoglobin A1C or HbA1c test, A1C is a blood test used primarily to diagnose and manage diabetes. Levels below 5.7% are considered normal, 5.7% to 6.4% indicating prediabetes, and 6.5% or higher signifying diabetes.

BMI: Body Mass Index, a numerical calculation using height and weight to estimate a person's body fat, categorizing them as underweight, normal weight, overweight, or obese.

CAM: Complementary and Alternative Medicine, a group of various medical practices and products not considered part of standard medical care.

CAPCAM: the former Cancer Advisory Panel on Complementary and Alternative Medicine of the National Institutes of Health. (RWM was a founding member.)

CDC: Centers for Disease Control and Prevention, the leading national public health institute of the United States.

CFU: Colony forming unit. A measure used in microbiology to estimate the number of viable microorganisms in a sample, with each unit potentially growing into a visible colony.

CSC: Cancer Stem Cell. A cell within a tumor is capable of self-renewal and driving tumor formation and spread.

CUFOX: A chemo regimen combining curcumin with the standard FOLFOX regimen of folinic acid, fluorouracil, and oxaliplatin, used in cancer treatment.

DNA: Deoxyribonucleic Acid, the molecule carrying genetic instructions for the development, functioning, growth, and reproduction of all known living organisms.

ECG: Epicatechin Gallate, a type of catechin found in green tea, known for its antioxidant properties and potential role in cardiovascular health.

ECGC: Epigallocatechin Gallate, the most abundant and potent catechin in green tea, celebrated for its antioxidant activity and researched for its potential to combat cancer and heart disease.

EFSA: The European Food Safety Authority, an agency of the European Union that provides independent scientific advice and communication on risks associated with the food chain.

EMT: Epithelial-Mesenchymal Transition is a process in which cells change from a stationary form to a mobile form, allowing them to move to different parts of the body. This is important for wound healing but can also contribute to the spread of cancer.

ENOX2: A class of proteins that are expressed only on the surface of cancer cells. Compounds or treatments that can attack ENOX2 include EGCG in green tea. Discovered by James and Dorothy Morré, Ph.D., of Purdue University.

EPIC: The European Prospective Investigation into Cancer and Nutrition. A massive research effort exploring the relationship between diet, nutritional status, lifestyle, environmental factors, cancer incidence, and other chronic diseases

EVOO: Extra Virgin Olive Oil, the highest-quality unrefined olive oil, marked by its superior taste and health benefits.

FDA: Food and Drug Administration, the U.S. government agency responsible for regulating food, drugs, medical devices, and other health-related products.

FDG: Fluorodeoxyglucose-18, a radioactive glucose analog used in PET scans to reveal areas of high glucose metabolism, such as actively growing tumors.

FOLFOX: A chemotherapy regimen combining folinic acid (leucovorin), fluorouracil, and oxaliplatin, commonly used to treat colorectal cancer.

FWGE: Fermented Wheat Germ Extract. A dietary supplement with possible anticancer qualities.

GRAS: Generally Recognized As Safe. A U.S. FDA designation for substances deemed safe in food.

I.e.: An abbreviation of the Latin phrase, *id est,* which translates to "that is" or "in other words." It is used to introduce a clarification, a specific list, or a restatement of something previously mentioned.

I3C: Indole-3-carbinol, a compound derived from the breakdown of glucosinolate glucobrassicin, found in cruciferous vegetables, known for its possible anti-cancer qualities and hormone balance control.

IARC: International Agency for Research on Cancer, a branch of the World Health Organization and therefore of the United Nations.

ICB: Immune checkpoint blockade: A cancer immunotherapy that involves inhibiting regulatory pathways to unleash the body's immune system against tumors.

JAMA: Journal of the American Medical Association. A widely circulated peer-reviewed medical journal.

MSKCC: Memorial Sloan Kettering Cancer Center, a world-renowned cancer treatment and research institution in New York City.

NCD: Non-Communicable Diseases. Chronic diseases not passed from person to person, such as heart disease, stroke, and diabetes.

NCI: National Cancer Institute. The U.S. federal government's principal agency for cancer research and training.

NDSR: Nutrition Data System for Research. A software tool used for dietary analysis and nutritional research.

NEJM: New England Journal of Medicine. A leading medical journal in the United States.

NF-κB: Nuclear Factor Kappa-light-chain-enhancer of activated B cells. A protein complex is involved in cell responses to stimuli like stress, harmful free radicals, and bacterial or viral antigens.

NLM: National Library of Medicine. A U.S. institution maintaining PubMed, a vast database of millions of journal articles and other forms of medical information.

OXPHOS: Oxidative phosphorylation is the energy-related pathway that generates energy in cells. It is a complex process in the body of the cell that uses oxygen to produce energy. This is typically present in normal cells but usually deficient in cancer cells. OxPhos contrasts with aerobic glycolysis, a.k.a. the Warburg effect.

PD-1: A protein in our immune system that can be exploited by cancer cells to evade detection and destruction.

PD-L1: A protein on cancer cells that can block our immune system from attacking them.

PET: Positron emission tomography. In its most common form, a diagnostic imaging technique that uses a radioactive glucose analog called FDG to detect and measure the energy-related activity of tumors.

PIN: Prostatic intraepithelial neoplasia. A condition characterized by abnormal cells in the prostate lining, considered a precursor to prostate cancer.

PMI: Precision Medicine Initiative, a U.S. government program.

PREDIMED: PREvención con Dieta MEDiterránea was a major clinical trial investigating the health benefits of the Mediterranean Diet, particularly in preventing heart diseases and diabetes. A subgroup analysis revealed a positive impact of olive oil on cancer.

T2D: Type 2 Diabetes, a chronic condition affecting the way the body processes blood sugar (glucose), marked by insulin resistance.

TCM: Traditional Chinese Medicine (TCM) is a holistic medical system that has been developed over thousands of years, incorporating practices such as herbal medicine, acupuncture, dietary therapy, and exercises like tai chi and qigong to prevent, diagnose, and treat diseases by restoring balance and harmony within the body.

TRE: Time-Restricted Eating. TRE is a dietary strategy that limits food intake to certain hours of the day, typically within an 8 to 12-hour window, to align with the body's natural circadian rhythms and potentially improve health outcomes.

UNESCO: United Nations Educational, Scientific and Cultural Organization, a specialized agency of the United Nations aimed at promoting world peace and security through international cooperation in education, the arts, the sciences, and culture.

VTE: Venous thromboembolism. A condition marked by the formation of blood clots in the deep veins (deep vein thrombosis) that can travel to the lungs, causing a potentially life-threatening pulmonary embolism.

WHO: The World Health Organization, a specialized agency of the United Nations responsible for international public health.

A Glossary of Names

Allison, James P., Ph.D.: An immunologist whose research on T-cell response methods led to the development of cancer immunotherapy, specifically CTLA-4 checkpoint blocking, earning him the Nobel Prize in Physiology or Medicine in 2018.

Atkins, Robert C., MD (1930-2003): American cardiologist, best known for the Atkins Diet, which requires close control of carbohydrate (carb) use and emphasizes protein and fat as the primary sources of dietary calories.

Aune, Dagfinn, Ph.D.: A renowned epidemiologist and researcher at Imperial College, London, known for his extensive work on the associations between diet, nutrition, lifestyle factors, and chronic diseases, including cancer.

Block, Keith I., MD: An integrative cancer treatment specialist, known for his work in optimizing chemo effectiveness through nutritional and lifestyle interventions, and for founding the Block Center for Integrative Cancer Treatment in Skokie, Illinois.

Dean Burk, Ph.D. (1904-1988): Co-founder of the National Cancer Institute and a biochemist known for his work on photosynthesis, fluoridation, and cancer metabolism.

Burnet, Sir MacFarlane (1899-1985): Nobel Laureate in Physiology or Medicine (1960). He suggested the "immune surveillance theory" of cancer, implying that the immune system continuously monitors and eliminates emerging tumor cells to prevent cancer development.

Duke, James. (1929-2017): Plant specialist at the United States Department of Agriculture (USDA) and an advisor to our "Cancer Chronicles" newsletter, known for his work in botany and plant chemicals.

Einstein, Albert (1879-1955): Theoretical physicist and Nobel laureate renowned for developing the theory of relativity, which revolutionized the understanding of space, time, and energy.

Epstein, Samuel S. (1926-2018): A prominent public health advocate and cancer researcher who was known for his work on environmental carcinogens and his criticism of industries and regulatory practices that he believed failed to protect public health.

Folkman, Judah, MD (1933-2008): Surgeon at Boston Children's Hospital and a pioneer in the field of blood vessel formation, his research laid the groundwork for developing targeted therapies that stop blood vessel growth to tumors.

Good, Robert A., MD, Ph.D. (1922-2003): Immunologist and the president of Memorial Sloan-Kettering Cancer Center, celebrated for his landmark contributions to the field of clinical immunology and bone marrow transplantation.

Hanahan, Douglas, Ph.D.: Professor at EPFL in Lausanne, Switzerland, known for co-authoring the seminal "Hallmarks of Cancer" papers which delineate the essential traits and behaviors of cancer cells.

Henning, Susanne, Ph.D., RD: Adjunct Professor, Department of Medicine, Center for Human Nutrition, Director of Nutritional Biomarker Laboratory, Center for Human Nutrition, University of California, Los Angeles (UCLA).

Hippocrates: A 5th-century BCE Greek physician often regarded as the "Father of Medicine," known for his lasting contributions to medical ethics and practice. Revised versions of his "Hippocratic oath" are recited upon graduation at many medical schools worldwide.

Honjo, Tasuku, MD, Ph.D.: Japanese immunologist awarded the Nobel Prize in Physiology or Medicine in 2018 for his discovery of the protein PD-1, which led to the development of PD-1 blockers, a new class of cancer immunotherapy drugs.

Katz, David L., MD: Director of the Yale-Griffin Prevention Research Center in New Haven, Connecticut, specializing in preventive medicine and lifestyle interventions to reduce chronic disease risks.

James Lind, MD (1716-1794): Scottish physician who conducted pioneering clinical trials in 1747 that demonstrated the effectiveness of citrus fruits in preventing and treating scurvy among sailors. Author of *A Treatise on the Scurvy.*

Livingstone, Stanley, MD (1813-1873): Scottish medical missionary and explorer renowned for his expeditions through Africa, mapping much of the continent previously unknown to Europeans.

Longo, Valter Ph.D.: Professor at the University of Southern California, Los Angeles, known for his research on fasting and lifespan, particularly how periodic fasting can reduce markers for aging and cancer.

Metchnikoff, Elie, Ph.D. (1845-1916). The discoverer of the macrophage cell, pioneer of gerontology (he coined the term), and sub-director of the Pasteur Institute in Paris, Metchnikoff is best remembered for his work on the importance of the microbiome in human health. He championed the ingestion of Bulgarian *Lactobacilli* in kefir and yogurt.

Morré, D. James, Ph.D. (1935-2016): Founding director of the Purdue Cancer Center, West Lafayette, Indiana from 1976 to 1986 and a Distinguished Professor there from 1986 to 2009 (AACR 2016).

Morré, Dorothy, Ph.D. (1935-2018): Researchers noted for her contributions to cancer research, including the co-discovery with her husband, James, of the ENOX2 protein which is specific to cancer cells and has implications in cancer diagnostics and treatment.

O'Brien, Catherine A., MD: Assistant Professor in the Department of Surgery at University Health Network and a Scientist at the Ontario Cancer Institute, she co-discovered cancer stem cells in colorectal cancer.

Old, Lloyd K., MD (1933-2011): Immunologist and vice president of Memorial Sloan-Kettering Cancer Center, recognized for his numerous contributions to the field of oncology, including cancer immunotherapy and vaccine development.

Pauling, Linus, Ph.D. (1901-1994): Chemist and a double Nobel laureate, receiving the Nobel Prize in Chemistry and the Nobel Peace Prize for his work in quantum chemistry and nuclear disarmament, respectively.

Peter Pedersen, Ph.D.: Professor of Biological Chemistry at Johns Hopkins University, recognized for his research on cellular metabolism and cancer, particularly the Warburg effect.

Quintana, Elsa, D.Pharm, Ph.D.: Vice President and Head of Cancer Immunology at REVOLUTION Medicines. While at the University of Michigan in 2012 she first discovered cancer stem cells in melanoma.

Ricci-Vitiani, Lucia, MD: Department of Hematology, Oncology and Molecular Medicine, Istituto Superiore di Sanità, Rome, Italy. Co-discoverer of cancer stem cells in colorectal cancer.

Rush, Benjamin, MD (1746–1813): A very influential early American physician, who was also a signer of the Declaration of Independence, an advocate for public health and education reforms, and for a time the Surgeon General of the Continental Army. He was also the first professor of chemistry at the University of Pennsylvania.

Schweitzer, Albert, MD (1875-1965): Nobel Peace Prize-winning medical missionary and philosopher known for his humanitarian work at his hospital in Lambaréné, now in *Gabon.*

Seyfried, Thomas N., Ph.D.: Professor of Biology at Boston College, known for his advocacy of metabolic therapy for cancer, including the use of ketogenic diets as a treatment to target cancer cell metabolism.

Sierra, Felipe, Ph.D.: Director Emeritus of the Division of Aging Biology at the National Institute on Aging, NIH, known for his research in the biology of aging and its implications on lifespan and health.

Silverstone, Herbert, Ph.D. (1913-1956): Former Manhattan Project researcher, at Michael Reese Hospital in Chicago focused on dietary factors and their impact on cancer, particularly how caloric intake influences cancer's growth.

Sheila K. Singh MD, Ph.D., FRCSC: A chief pediatric neurosurgeon at McMaster Children's Hospital in Ontario, Canada. She identified CSCs in brain tumors.

Spiegelman, Sol, Ph.D. (1914-1983): Pioneering molecular biologist and the director of the cancer institute at Columbia University, recognized for his innovations in genetic research and virology.

Spinoza, Baruch (1632-1677): Dutch philosopher who laid foundational ideas that advanced the Enlightenment and modern biblical criticism, focusing on rationalism and ethics.

Sugiura, Kanematsu, D.Sc.(1890-1979): Japanese-American scientist acclaimed for his pivotal contributions to cancer research, particularly in the development of chemo treatments.

Talalay, Paul, MD (1923-2019): German-American biochemist renowned for his research on the chemopreventive qualities of broccoli and other substances, advancing cancer prevention studies.

Tannenbaum, Albert, MD. (1901-1980): President of the American Association for Cancer Research (1956-1957), Manhattan Project researcher, at Michael Reese Hospital in Chicago studied the relationships between diet, energy-related rates, and cancer risks, proposing that calorie restriction could reduce tumor growth.

Thomas, Lewis, MD (1913-1993): Physician, poet, and essayist, celebrated for his reflective writings on biology and the human condition; he also served as president of Memorial Sloan-Kettering Cancer Center.

Trichopoulou, Antonia, Ph.D.: Professor at the University of Athens who has been instrumental in researching and promoting the Mediterranean Diet, linking dietary patterns to health outcomes and lifespan.

Warburg, Otto, MD, Ph.D. (1883-1970): Nobel Prize-winning biochemist known for his discovery of the nature and mode of action of the respiratory enzyme and his hypothesis on the altered metabolism of cancer cells (the Warburg effect).

Weinberg, Robert A. Ph.D.: Professor at the Massachusetts Institute of Technology (MIT) and a pioneering cancer biologist who discovered the first human oncogene and the first tumor suppressor gene, advancing the understanding of cancer biology.

Willett, Walter, Ph.D.: Professor at the Harvard T.H. Chan School of Public Health and a leading figure in public health and nutrition, particularly known for his research in dietary factors and their effects on health, including cancer epidemiology.

Zuniga, Krystle Ph.D.: Nutrition science educator and clinician, the University of Texas at Austin.

ANNOTATED BIBLIOGRAPHY

The great majority of the following references are indexed in PubMed, the U.S. National Library of Medicine's database of 37 million medical references. The citations are given in standard PubMed format, with some minor adjustments. Underscored titles provide live links in the eBook or pdf version, in many cases to free full texts.

[My personal annotations are included in bold and in brackets.]

Cited Works

AACR [American Association for Cancer Research]. In memoriam: D. James Morré. June 2016. Accessed May 2, 2024.

Abdul Ghani MA, Ugusman A, Latip J, et al. Role of terpenophenolics in modulating inflammation and apoptosis in cardiovascular diseases. Int J Mol Sci. 2023 Mar 10;24(6):5339. Doi: 10.3390/ijms24065339. PMID: 36982410; PMCID: PMC10049039.

Abdul Satar N, Ismail MN, Yahaya BH. Synergistic roles of curcumin in sensitizing the cisplatin effect on a cancer stem cell-like population derived from non-small cell lung cancer cell lines. Molecules. 2021 Feb 18;26(4):1056. Doi: 10.3390/molecules26041056. PMID: 33670440; PMCID: PMC7922800.

Abel U. Chemotherapy of advanced epithelial cancer–a critical review. Biomed Pharmacother. 1992;46(10):439-52. Doi: 10.1016/0753-3322(92)90002-o. PMID: 1339108. [Abel's writings inspired my book, *Questioning Chemotherapy*.]

Abugomaa A, Elbadawy M, Ishihara Y, et al. Anti-cancer activity of chaga mushroom (Inonotus obliquus) against dog bladder cancer organoids. Front Pharmacol. 2023 Apr 19;14:1159516. Doi: 10.3389/fphar.2023.1159516. PMID: 37153767; PMCID: PMC10154587.

Adams J. The proteasome: a suitable antineoplastic target. Nat Rev Cancer. 2004 May;4(5):349-60. Doi: 10.1038/nrc1361. PMID: 15122206.

Adams M. Information and education across the phases of cancer care. Semin Oncol Nurs. 1991 May;7(2):105-11. Doi: 10.1016/0749-2081(91)90088-7. PMID: 1882149.

Adamsson V, Reumark A, Fredriksson IB, et al. Effects of a healthy Nordic diet on cardiovascular risk factors in hypercholesterolaemic subjects: a randomized controlled trial (NORDIET). J Intern Med. 2011 Feb;269(2):150-9. Doi: 10.1111/j.1365-2796.2010.02290.x. Epub 2010 Oct 22. PMID: 20964740.

Adorno-Cruz V, Kibria G, Liu X, et al. Cancer stem cells: targeting the roots of cancer, seeds of metastasis, and sources of therapy resistance. Cancer Res. 2015 Mar 15;75(6):924-9. Doi:

10.1158/0008-5472.CAN-14-3225. Epub 2015 Jan 20. PMID: 25604264; PMCID: PMC4359955.

Afshari AR, Sanati M, Kesharwani P, et al. Recent advances in curcumin-based combination nanomedicines for cancer therapy. J Funct Biomater. 2023 Aug 2;14(8):408. doi: 10.3390/jfb14080408. PMID: 37623653; PMCID: PMC10455605.

Agarwal A, Ioannidis JPA. PREDIMED trial of Mediterranean diet: retracted, republished, still trusted? BMJ. 2019 Feb 7;364:l341. Doi: 10.1136/bmj.l341. PMID: 30733217.

Aggarwal BB, Shishodia S. Molecular targets of dietary agents for prevention and therapy of cancer. Biochem Pharmacol. 2006 May 14;71(10):1397-421. Doi: 10.1016/j.bcp.2006.02.009. Epub 2006 Feb 23. PMID: 16563357.

Aggarwal BB, Sundaram C, Malani N, et al. Curcumin: the Indian solid gold. Adv Exp Med Biol. 2007;595:1-75. Doi: 10.1007/978-0-387-46401-5_1. PMID: 17569205.

Aggarwal BB, Sung B. Pharmacological basis for the role of curcumin in chronic diseases: an age-old spice with modern targets. Trends Pharmacol Sci. 2009 Feb;30(2):85-94. Doi: 10.1016/j.tips.2008.11.002. Epub 2008 Dec 26. PMID: 19110321. [**Aggarwal was the leader of curcumin studies at M.D. Anderson Cancer Center, Houston for many years. I visited him in his lab in 2007.**]

Aggarwal BB, Yuan W, Li S, et al. Curcumin-free turmeric exhibits anti-inflammatory and anticancer activities: Identification of novel components of turmeric. Mol Nutr Food Res. 2013 Sep;57(9):1529-42. Doi: 10.1002/mnfr.201200838. Epub 2013 Jul 12. PMID: 23847105.

Aggarwal BB. Nuclear factor-kappaB: the enemy within. Cancer Cell. 2004 Sep;6(3):203-8. Doi: 10.1016/j.ccr.2004.09.003. PMID: 15380510.

Agnoli C, Grioni S, Sieri S, et al. Italian Mediterranean Index and risk of colorectal cancer in the Italian section of the EPIC cohort. Int J Cancer. 2013 Mar 15;132(6):1404-11. Doi: 10.1002/ijc.27740. Epub 2012 Aug 7. PMID: 22821300.

Ahn WS, Kim DJ, Chae GT, et al. Natural killer cell activity and quality of life were improved by consumption of a mushroom extract, Agaricus blazei Murill Kyowa, in gynecological cancer patients undergoing chemotherapy. Int J Gynecol Cancer. 2004 Jul-Aug;14(4):589-94. Doi: 10.1111/j.1048-891X.2004.14403.x. PMID: 15304151.

Alexander MS, Wilkes JG, Schroeder SR, et al. Pharmacologic ascorbate reduces radiation-induced normal tissue toxicity and enhances tumor radiosensitization in pancreatic cancer. Cancer Res. 2018 Dec 15;78(24):6838-6851. Doi: 10.1158/0008-5472.CAN-18-1680. Epub 2018 Sep 25. PMID: 30254147; PMCID: PMC6295907.

Al-Hajj M, Wicha MS, Benito-Hernandez A, et al. Prospective identification of tumorigenic breast cancer cells. Proc Natl Acad Sci U S A. 2003 Apr 1;100(7):3983-8. Doi: 10.1073/pnas.0530291100. Epub 2003 Mar 10. Erratum in: Proc Natl Acad Sci U S A. 2003

May 27;100(11):6890. PMID: 12629218; PMCID: PMC153034. [**This paper first established the existence of cancer stem cells in a solid tumor of the breast.**]

Al-Ishaq RK, Overy AJ, Büsselberg D. Phytochemicals and gastrointestinal cancer: cellular mechanisms and effects to change cancer progression. Biomolecules. 2020 Jan 8;10(1):105. Doi: 10.3390/biom10010105. PMID: 31936288; PMCID: PMC7022462.

Alsubhi NH, Al-Quwaie DA, Alrefaei GI, et al. Pomegranate pomace extract with antioxidant, anticancer, antimicrobial, and antiviral activity enhances the quality of strawberry-yogurt smoothie. Bioengineering (Basel). 2022 Nov 28;9(12):735. Doi: 10.3390/bioengineering9120735. PMID: 36550941; PMCID: PMC9774345.

American Association for Cancer Research [AACR]. Landmarks in cancer research, 2007-2017. Accessed January 23, 2024.

American Cancer Society [ACS]. *Cancer Facts & Figures 2024*, p. 1. Accessed February 16, 2024.

American Museum of Natural History (AMNH). The power of poison: poison as medicine. Exhibit Posts, November 13, 2013. [A version of this article first appeared in the AMNH member magazine *Rotunda*, Fall 2013.] Accessed June 11, 2024.

Ammon HPT. Boswellic extracts and 11-keto-ß-boswellic acids prevent type 1 and type 2 diabetes mellitus by suppressing the expression of proinflammatory cytokines. Phytomedicine. 2019 Oct;63:153002. Doi: 10.1016/j.phymed.2019.153002. Epub 2019 Jun 28. PMID: 31301539.

Anand P, Kunnumakkara AB, Newman RA, et al. Bioavailability of curcumin: problems and promises. Mol Pharm. 2007 Nov-Dec;4(6):807-18. Doi: 10.1021/mp700113r. Epub 2007 Nov 14. PMID: 17999464.

Anand P, Sundaram C, Jhurani S, et al. Curcumin and cancer: an "old-age" disease with an "age-old" solution. Cancer Lett. 2008 Aug 18;267(1):133-64. Doi: 10.1016/j.canlet.2008.03.025. Epub 2008 May 6. PMID: 18462866.

Andayani YD, Saleh MI, Sudoyo AW, et al. Effect of extra-virgin olive oil on hand foot syndrome and hs-CRP in patients receiving capecitabine: a randomized trial. Acta Med Indones. 2023 Oct;55(4):396-402. PMID: 38213043.

Anderson JW, Baird P, Davis RH Jr, et al. Health benefits of dietary fiber. Nutr Rev. 2009 Apr;67(4):188-205. Doi: 10.1111/j.1753-4887.2009.00189.x. PMID: 19335713.

Andreazzoli F, Levy Yurkovski I, Ben-Arye E, et al. Conceptualizing an integrative multiple myeloma care: the role of nutrition, supplements, and complementary modalities. Nutrients. 2024 Jan 11;16(2):237. Doi: 10.3390/nu16020237. PMID: 38257130; PMCID: PMC10818534. [**An important article from my colleagues Massimo Bonucci, Eran Ben-Arye, et al. that independently confirms many aspects of The Moss Method.**]

341

Andújar I, Recio MC, Giner RM, et al. Cocoa polyphenols and their potential benefits for human health. Oxid Med Cell Longev. 2012;2012:906252. Doi: 10.1155/2012/906252. Epub 2012 Oct 24. PMID: 23150750; PMCID: PMC3488419.

Anonymous. The relations of cancer to chronic inflammation. Hospital (Lond 1886). 1909 Jul 3;46(1195):349-350. PMID: 29815590; PMCID: PMC5200230.

Anonymous. Inching towards a cure for cancer. Washington Post, October 2, 1979.

Anonymous. Kefir. Halls J Health. 1884 Aug;31(8):151. PMID: 36491407; PMCID: PMC9231884.

Anonymous. Review of *Cancer: How it is Caused, How it can be Prevented*, by Barker, J. Ellis. Nature. 1924; No. 2866, vol. 114, p. 496. Accessed on December 1, 2023 from Google Books.

Anonymous. The burger that conquered the country. *Time,* Sept. 17, 1973. Accessed February 10, 2024.

Anonymous. What are phytochemicals? (And why should you eat more of them?) UCLA health website, May 10, 2023. Accessed on December 7, 2023.

Anonymous [Research and Markets]. Global fast food market worth $931 billion by 2027 – Industry assessment featuring Auntie Anne's, Domino's Pizza, Dunkin' Brands Group, McDonald's, Yum! Brands and More. CISION PR Newswire. July 20, 2020. Accessed on November 14, 2023.

Antonia SJ, Villegas A, Daniel D, et al. Overall survival with durvalumab after chemoradiotherapy in stage III NSCLC. N Engl J Med. 2018 Dec 13;379(24):2342-2350. Doi: 10.1056/NEJMoa1809697. Epub 2018 Sep 25. PMID: 30280658.

Apple, Sam. *Ravenous: Otto Warburg, the Nazis, and the Search for the Cancer-Diet Connection.* ISBN-13: 978-1631493157. New York: Liveright, 2021. **[A very interesting popular account of the founder of metabolic therapy.]**

Arora S, Singh S, Piazza GA, et al. Honokiol: a novel natural agent for cancer prevention and therapy. Curr Mol Med. 2012 Dec;12(10):1244-52. Doi: 10.2174/156652412803833508. PMID: 22834827; PMCID: PMC3663139.

Aune D, Chan DS, Lau R, et al. Dietary fibre, whole grains, and risk of colorectal cancer: systematic review and dose-response meta-analysis of prospective studies. BMJ. 2011 Nov 10;343:d6617. Doi: 10.1136/bmj.d6617. PMID: 22074852; PMCID: PMC3213242

Aune D, Keum N, Giovannucci E, et al. Nut consumption and risk of cardiovascular disease, total cancer, all-cause and cause-specific mortality: a systematic review and dose-response meta-analysis of prospective studies. BMC Med. 2016 Dec 5;14(1):207. Doi: 10.1186/s12916-016-0730-3. PMID: 27916000; PMCID: PMC5137221.

Aune D, Keum N, Giovannucci E, et al. Whole grain consumption and risk of cardiovascular disease, cancer, and all cause and cause specific mortality: systematic review and dose-response meta-analysis of prospective studies. BMJ. 2016 Jun 14;353:i2716. Doi: 10.1136/bmj.i2716. PMID: 27301975; PMCID: PMC4908315.

Autrup H, Barile FA, Berry SC, et al. Human exposure to synthetic endocrine disrupting chemicals (S-EDCs) is generally negligible as compared to natural compounds with higher or comparable endocrine activity: how to evaluate the risk of the S-EDCs? Arch Toxicol. 2020 Jul;94(7):2549-2557. Doi: 10.1007/s00204-020-02800-8. Epub 2020 Jun 8. PMID: 32514609; PMCID: PMC7367909.

Bach-Faig A, Berry EM, Lairon D, et al. Mediterranean diet pyramid today. Science and cultural updates. Public Health Nutr. 2011 Dec;14(12A):2274-84. Doi: 10.1017/S1368980011002515. PMID: 22166184.

Bae KH, Tan S, Yamashita A, et al. Hyaluronic acid-green tea catechin micellar nanocomplexes: fail-safe cisplatin nanomedicine for the treatment of ovarian cancer without off-target toxicity. Biomaterials. 2017 Dec;148:41-53. Doi: 10.1016/j.biomaterials.2017.09.027. Epub 2017 Sep 22. PMID: 28961534.

Bahari H, Ashtary-Larky D, Goudarzi K, et al. The effects of pomegranate consumption on glycemic indices in adults: a systematic review and meta-analysis. Diabetes Metab Syndr. 2024 Jan;18(1):102940. Doi: 10.1016/j.dsx.2024.102940. Epub 2024 Jan 3. PMID: 38194826 [cited as Bahari 2024a]

Bahari H, Omidian K, Goudarzi K, et al. The effects of pomegranate consumption on blood pressure in adults: a systematic review and meta-analysis. Phytother Res. 2024 Feb 27. Doi: 10.1002/ptr.8170. Epub ahead of print. PMID: 38410857. [Cited as Bahari 2024b]

Baharuddin P, Satar N, Fakiruddin KS, et al. Curcumin improves the efficacy of cisplatin by targeting cancer stem-like cells through p21 and cyclin D1-mediated tumor cell inhibition in non-small cell lung cancer cell lines. Oncol Rep. 2016 Jan;35(1):13-25. Doi: 10.3892/or.2015.4371. Epub 2015 Nov 2. PMID: 26531053; PMCID: PMC4699625.

Bashford A, Tracy SW. Introduction: modern airs, waters, and places. Bull Hist Med. 2012 Winter;86(4):495-514. Doi: 10.1353/bhm.2012.0084. PMID: 23263344.

Baur JA, Pearson KJ, Price NL, et al. Resveratrol improves health and survival of mice on a high-calorie diet. Nature. 2006 Nov 16;444(7117):337-42. Doi: 10.1038/nature05354. Epub 2006 Nov 1. PMID: 17086191; PMCID: PMC4990206. [Cited as Baur 2006a.]

Baur JA, Sinclair DA. Therapeutic potential of resveratrol: the in vivo evidence. Nat Rev Drug Discov. 2006 Jun;5(6):493-506. Doi: 10.1038/nrd2060. Epub 2006 May 26. PMID: 16732220.[Cited as Baur 2006b.]

Beard, James. *Beard On Food.* First published in 1974. Reprinted with a new preface by Mark Bittman. New York: Bloomsbury USA, 2007.

Beauchamp GK. Sensory and receptor responses to umami: an overview of pioneering work. Am J Clin Nutr. 2009 Sep;90(3):723S-727S. doi: 10.3945/ajcn.2009.27462E. Epub 2009 Jul 1. PMID: 19571221.

Beer TM, Ryan CW, Venner PM, et al. Double-blinded randomized study of high-dose calcitriol plus docetaxel compared with placebo plus docetaxel in androgen-independent prostate cancer: a report from the ASCENT Investigators. J Clin Oncol. 2007 Feb 20;25(6):669-74. Doi: 10.1200/JCO.2006.06.8197. PMID: 17308271.

Bell RB. The fourth modality: immunotherapy for head and neck cancer hits pay dirt. Oral Surg Oral Med Oral Pathol Oral Radiol. 2016 Jun;121(6):575-7. Doi: 10.1016/j.oooo.2016.03.019. Epub 2016 Apr 7. PMID: 27181440.

Bencze G, Bencze S, Rivera KD, et al. Mito-oncology agent: fermented extract suppresses the Warburg effect, restores oxidative mitochondrial activity, and inhibits in vivo tumor growth. Sci Rep. 2020 Aug 25;10(1):14174. Doi: 10.1038/s41598-020-71118-3. Erratum in: Sci Rep. 2021 Jan 29;11(1):3036. PMID: 32843660; PMCID: PMC7447799. [**This paper was the fruit of almost a decade of work at Cold Spring Harbor Laboratory on the science behind fermented wheat germ extract. James D. Watson was a co-author.**]

Bendix, Aria. Intermittent fasting linked to higher risk of cardiovascular death, research suggests. NBC News. March 18, 2024.

Benetou V, Orfanos P, Pettersson-Kymmer U, et al. Mediterranean diet and incidence of hip fractures in a European cohort. Osteoporos Int. 2013 May;24(5):1587-98. Doi: 10.1007/s00198-012-2187-3. Epub 2012 Oct 20. PMID: 23085859.

Benetou V, Trichopoulou A, Orfanos P, et al. Conformity to traditional Mediterranean diet and cancer incidence: the Greek EPIC cohort. Br J Cancer. 2008;99(1):191-195.

Berglas, A. *Cancer: Nature, Cause, and Cure.* Foreword by Dr. Albert Schweitzer, MD. Paris: Institut Pasteur, 1957: 27-58.

Bergman, Sylvia A. Letter and submission from Kemin Industries to Dr. Paulette Gaynor of the Food and Drug Administration (FDA), dated March 19, 2018.

Berrino F, Villarini A, Gargano G, et al. The effect of diet on breast cancer recurrence: the DIANA-5 randomized trial. Clin Cancer Res. 2024 Mar 1;30(5):965-974. Doi: 10.1158/1078-0432.CCR-23-1615. PMID: 37847493; PMCID: PMC10905522.

Bersanelli M, Cortellini A, Leonetti A, et al. Systematic vitamin D supplementation is associated with improved outcomes and reduced thyroid adverse events in patients with cancer treated with immune checkpoint inhibitors: results from the prospective PROVIDENCE study. Cancer Immunol Immunother. 2023 Nov;72(11):3707-3716. Doi: 10.1007/s00262-023-03522-3. Epub 2023 Aug 28. PMID: 37638980; PMCID: PMC10576732.

Berta J, Rózsás A, Megyesfalvi Z, et al. Thoracic irradiation as consolidation therapy in patients with extensive-stage small cell lung cancer. Curr Opin Oncol. 2023 Jan 1;35(1):54-60. Doi: 10.1097/CCO.0000000000000911. Epub 2022 Nov 16. PMID: 36420570.

Besasie BD, Saha A, DiGiovanni J, et al. Effects of curcumin and ursolic acid in prostate cancer: A systematic review. Urologia. 2024 Feb;91(1):90-106. Doi: 10.1177/03915603231202304. Epub 2023 Sep 30. PMID: 37776274; PMCID: PMC10976464.

Betts G, Twohig J, Van den Broek M, et al. The impact of regulatory T cells on carcinogen-induced sarcogenesis. Br J Cancer. 2007 Jun 18;96(12):1849-54. Doi: 10.1038/sj.bjc.6603824. Epub 2007 Jun 12. PMID: 17565340; PMCID: PMC2359957.

Bettuzzi S, Brausi M, Rizzi F, et al. Chemoprevention of human prostate cancer by oral administration of green tea catechins in volunteers with high-grade prostate intraepithelial neoplasia: a preliminary report from a one-year proof-of-principle study. Cancer Res. 2006 Jan 15;66(2):1234-40. Doi: 10.1158/0008-5472.CAN-05-1145. PMID: 16424063. [**Pioneering study of the effect of green tea in prostate cancer patients.**]

Bhaskara VK, Mittal B, Mysorekar VV, et al. Resveratrol, cancer and cancer stem cells from past to future. Curr Res Food Sci. 2020 Nov 24;3:284-295. Doi: 10.1016/j.crfs.2020.10.004. PMID: 33305295; PMCID: PMC7718213.

Bhattacharjee B, Chatterjee J. Identification of proapoptotic, anti-inflammatory, anti-proliferative, anti-invasive and anti-angiogenic targets of essential oils in cardamom by dual reverse virtual screening and binding pose analysis. Asian Pac J Cancer Prev. 2013;14(6):3735-42. Doi: 10.7314/apjcp.2013.14.6.3735. PMID: 23886174.

Bijangi-Vishehsaraei K, Reza Saadatzadeh M, Wang H, et al. Sulforaphane suppresses the growth of glioblastoma cells, glioblastoma stem cell-like spheroids, and tumor xenografts through multiple cell signaling pathways. J Neurosurg. 2017 Dec;127(6):1219-1230. Doi: 10.3171/2016.8.JNS161197. Epub 2017 Jan 6. PMID: 28059653; PMCID: PMC6086125.

Bilal I, Chowdhury A, Davidson J, et al. Phytoestrogens and prevention of breast cancer: the contentious debate. World J Clin Oncol. 2014 Oct 10;5(4):705-12. Doi: 10.5306/wjco.v5.i4.705. PMID: 25302172; PMCID: PMC4129534.

Biswas P, Dey D, Biswas PK, et al. A comprehensive analysis and anti-cancer activities of quercetin in ROS-mediated cancer and cancer stem cells. Int J Mol Sci. 2022 Oct 4;23(19):11746. Doi: 10.3390/ijms231911746. PMID: 36233051; PMCID: PMC9569933.

Block, Keith. The Paleo diet: what is it anyway? Life Over Cancer Blog, May 16, 2012. Accessed March 16, 2024.

Block KI, Gyllenhaal C, Lowe L, et al. A broad-spectrum integrative design for cancer prevention and therapy. Semin Cancer Biol. 2015 Dec;35 Suppl(Suppl):S276-S304. Doi: 10.1016/j.semcancer.2015.09.007. PMID: 26590477; PMCID: PMC4819002. [**This paper,** with 180 distinguished authors, has many points in common with The Moss Method.]

Bloomfield HE, Kane R, Koeller E, et al. Benefits and harms of the Mediterranean diet compared to other diets. Washington (DC): Department of Veterans Affairs (US); 2015 Nov. PMID: 27559560.

Bonandi E, Mori M, Infante P, et al. Design and synthesis of new Withaferin A inspired hedgehog pathway inhibitors. Chemistry. 2021 Jun 4;27(32):8350-8357. Doi: 10.1002/chem.202100315. Epub 2021 May 4. PMID: 33811701; PMCID: PMC8251939.

Boutas I, Kontogeorgi A, Dimitrakakis C, et al. Soy isoflavones and breast cancer risk: a meta-analysis. In Vivo. 2022 Mar-Apr;36(2):556-562. doi: 10.21873/invivo.12737. PMID: 35241506; PMCID: PMC8931889.

Brahmbhatt M, Gundala SR, Asif G, et al. Ginger phytochemicals exhibit synergy to inhibit prostate cancer cell proliferation. Nutr Cancer. 2013;65(2):263-72. Doi: 10.1080/01635581.2013.749925. PMID: 23441614; PMCID: PMC3925258.

Brandhorst, S, Choi IY., Wei M, et al. A periodic diet that mimics fasting promotes multi-system regeneration, enhanced cognitive performance, and healthspan. Cell Metab. 2015 Jul 7;22(1):86-99. Doi: 10.1016/j.cmet.2015.05.012.

Brincat, Clarissa. Intermittent fasting is linked to higher risk of heart disease death. New Scientist, March 23, 2024. Accessed April 6, 2024.

Brown JC, Crane TE, Meyerhardt JA, et al. LifeStyle factors, chapter 3. DeVita, Jr. VT, Rosenberg S, Lawrence T. DeVita, Hellman, and Rosenberg's Cancer. 12ᵗʰ Edition. Philadelphia: Wolters Kluwer Health, 2022 (online update 2024). Accessed April 8, 2024. [Subscription required.]

Brown K, Theofanous D, Britton RG, et al. Resveratrol for the management of human health: how far have we come? A systematic review of resveratrol clinical trials to highlight gaps and opportunities. Int J Mol Sci. 2024 Jan 6;25(2):747. Doi: 10.3390/ijms25020747. PMID: 38255828; PMCID: PMC10815776.

Brownstein, Maya. Red meat consumption is associated with increased type 2 diabetes risk. Harvard T.H. Chan School of Public Health press release. October 19, 2023. Accessed March 16, 2024.

Callahan, Alice. Is intermittent fasting bad for your heart? Here's what we know. New York Times, March 20, 2024. Accessed April 7, 2024. [Subscription required.]

Calle EE, Rodriguez C, Walker-Thurmond K, et al. Overweight, obesity, and mortality from cancer in a prospectively studied cohort of U.S. adults. N Engl J Med. 2003 Apr 24;348(17):1625-38. Doi: 10.1056/NEJMoa021423. PMID: 12711737.

Cameron E, Pauling L. Supplemental ascorbate in the supportive treatment of cancer: reevaluation of prolongation of survival times in terminal human cancer. Proc Natl Acad Sci U

S A. 1978 Sep;75(9):4538-42. Doi: 10.1073/pnas.75.9.4538. PMID: 279931; PMCID: PMC336151. [One of the scientific papers in support of the idea that high-dose intravenous vitamin C (IV-C) is of help to people with advanced stage cancer.]

Cao C, Sun L, Mo W, et al. Quercetin mediates β-catenin in pancreatic cancer stem-like cells. Pancreas. 2015 Nov;44(8):1334-9. Doi: 10.1097/MPA.0000000000000400. PMID: 26284537.

Cao Y, Cao R. Angiogenesis inhibited by drinking tea. Nature. 1999 Apr 1;398(6726):381. PMID: 10201366.

Carey TE, Prince ME, Brenner JC. Chapter 44: The molecular biology of head and neck cancers. In: DeVita, Jr VT, Rosenberg SA, Lawrence TS. DeVita, Hellman, and Rosenberg's Cancer. (11ᵗʰ Edition). Philadelphia: Wolters Kluwer Health; 2019 [Subscription required.] Accessed February 17, 2024 [Subscription required].

Carlson, Susan. GRAS Notice GRN 830 Agency Response Letter – Chicory flour. FDA letter to Blue Prairie Brands accepting their claim that chicory root powder is GRAS, through scientific procedures and common use. May 22, 2019.

Carluccio MA, Siculella L, Ancora MA, et al. Olive oil and red wine antioxidant polyphenols inhibit endothelial activation: anti-atherogenic properties of Mediterranean diet phytochemicals. Arterioscler Thromb Vasc Biol. 2003 Apr 1;23(4):622-9. Doi: 10.1161/01.ATV.0000062884.69432.A0. Epub 2003 Feb 20. PMID: 12615669.

Carnevale R, Silvestri R, Loffredo L, et al. Oleuropein, a component of extra virgin olive oil, lowers postprandial glycaemia in healthy subjects. Br J Clin Pharmacol. 2018 Jul;84(7):1566-1574. Doi: 10.1111/bcp.13589. Epub 2018 May 2. PMID: 29577365; PMCID: PMC6005585.

Casas AI, Hassan AA, Larsen SJ, et al. From single drug targets to synergistic network pharmacology in ischemic stroke. Proc Natl Acad Sci U S A. 2019 Apr 2;116(14):7129-7136. Doi: 10.1073/pnas.1820799116. Epub 2019 Mar 20. PMID: 30894481; PMCID: PMC6452748.

Castelvetro, Giacomo. The Fruit, Herbs & Vegetables of Italy. Translated with an introduction by Gillian Riley, Foreword by Jan Grigson. British Museum, Natural History. London: Viking, 1989. [Originally published in 1614.]

Castino R, Pucer A, Veneroni R, et al. Resveratrol reduces the invasive growth and promotes the acquisition of a long-lasting differentiated phenotype in human glioblastoma cells. J Agric Food Chem. 2011 Apr 27;59(8):4264-72. Doi: 10.1021/jf104917q. Epub 2011 Mar 11. PMID: 21395220.

Casto BC, Kresty LA, Kraly CL, et al. Chemoprevention of oral cancer by black raspberries. Anticancer Res. 2002 Nov-Dec;22(6C):4005-15. PMID: 12553025.

Center for Responsible Nutrition [CRN]. 2023 CRN Consumer Survey on Dietary Supplements. Accessed April 20, 2024.

Centers for Disease Control and Prevention [CDC]. Carb counting. Accessed November 9, 2023 [CDC 2023b]

Centers for Disease Control and Prevention [CDC]. National Center for Health Statistics. National Health Interview Survey, 1992–2021. Accessed November 8, 2023 from Cancer Survivors and Weight [CDC 2023a]

Centers for Disease Control and Prevention [CDC]. National Diabetes Statistics Report website. Table 1a: Estimated crude prevalence of diagnosed diabetes, undiagnosed diabetes, and total diabetes among adults aged 18 years or older, United States, 2017–2020. Accessed June 22, 2024. **[Crucial information on the prevalence of diabetes and prediabetes in the U.S.]**

Centers for Disease Control and Prevention [CDC]. Prediabetes. Accessed November 9, 2023 [CDC 2023c]

Chandler PD, Buring JE, Manson JE, et al. Circulating vitamin D levels and risk of colorectal cancer in women. Cancer Prev Res (Phila). 2015 Aug;8(8):675-82. Doi: 10.1158/1940-6207.CAPR-14-0470. Epub 2015 Mar 26. PMID: 25813525; PMCID: PMC4526335.

Chang CF, Islam A, Liu PF, Zhan JH, Chueh PJ. Capsaicin acts through tNOX (ENOX2) to induce autophagic apoptosis in p53-mutated HSC-3 cells but autophagy in p53-functional SAS oral cancer cells. Am J Cancer Res. 2020 Oct 1;10(10):3230-3247. PMID: 33163267; PMCID: PMC7642647.

Chan MM, Chen R, Fong D. Targeting cancer stem cells with dietary phytochemical—repositioned drug combinations. Cancer Lett. 2018 Oct 1;433:53-64. Doi: 10.1016/j.canlet.2018.06.034. Epub 2018 Jun 28. PMID: 29960048; PMCID: PMC7117025.

Charlesworth CJ, Smit E, Lee DS, et al. Polypharmacy among adults aged 65 years and older in the United States: 1988-2010. J Gerontol A Biol Sci Med Sci. 2015 Aug;70(8):989-95. Doi: 10.1093/348iochi/glv013. Epub 2015 Mar 1. PMID: 25733718; PMCID: PMC4573668.

Chao B, Llukani E, Lepor H. Two-year outcomes following focal laser ablation of localized prostate cancer. Eur Urol Oncol. 2018 Jun;1(2):129-133. Doi: 10.1016/j.euo.2018.03.011. Epub 2018 May 15. PMID: 31100236.

Cheng CS, Tan HY, Zhang C, et al. Berberine suppresses metastasis and recurrence of hepatocellular carcinoma by targeting circulating tumor cells: abridged secondary publication. Hong Kong Med J. 2022 Dec;28 Suppl 6(6):10-11. PMID: 36535791.

Cheng CW, Adams GB, Perin L, et al. Prolonged fasting reduces IGF-1/PKA to promote hematopoietic-stem-cell-based regeneration and reverse immunosuppression. Cell Stem Cell. 2014 June 5;14(6):810-23. Doi: 10.1016/j.stem.2014.04.014. Erratum in: Cell Stem Cell. 2016 Feb 4;18(2):291-2. PMID: 24905167; PMCID: PMC4102383.

Cheng JH, Tsai CL, Lien YY, et al. High molecular weight of polysaccharides from Hericium erinaceus against amyloid beta-induced neurotoxicity. BMC Complement Altern Med. 2016 Jun 7;16:170. Doi: 10.1186/s12906-016-1154-5. PMID: 27266872; PMCID: PMC4895996.

Cheng YM, Tsai CC, Hsu YC. Sulforaphane, a dietary isothiocyanate, induces G₂/M arrest in cervical cancer cells through cyclinb1 downregulation and GADD45β/CDC2 association. Int J Mol Sci. 2016 Sep 12;17(9):1530. Doi: 10.3390/ijms17091530. PMID: 27626412; PMCID: PMC5037805.

Chen KM, Sun YW, Kawasawa YI, et al. Black raspberry inhibits oral tumors in mice treated with the tobacco smoke constituent dibenzo(def,p)chrysene via genetic and epigenetic alterations. Cancer Prev Res (Phila). 2020 Apr;13(4):357-366. doi: 10.1158/1940-6207.CAPR-19-0496. Epub 2020 Jan 22. PMID: 31969344; PMCID: PMC7127947.

Chen L, Li WF, Wang HX, et al. Curcumin cytotoxicity is enhanced by PTEN disruption in colorectal cancer cells. World J Gastroenterol. 2013 Oct 28;19(40):6814-24. Doi: 10.3748/wjg.v19.i40.6814. PMID: 24187456; PMCID: PMC3812480.

Chen M, Zhong VW. Association between time-restricted eating and all-cause and cause-specific mortality. AHA EPI 2024, Session P01.11-Nutrition and Diet 1. [Abstract]. Published March 18, 2024. Accessed April 7, 2024.

Chen Q, Luo J, Wu C, et al. The miRNA-149-5p/MyD88 axis is responsible for ursolic acid-mediated attenuation of the stemness and chemoresistance of non-small cell lung cancer cells. Environ Toxicol. 2020 May;35(5):561-569. Doi: 10.1002/tox.22891. Epub 2019 Dec 19. PMID: 31855318.

Chen SS, Michael A, Butler-Manuel SA. Advances in the treatment of ovarian cancer: a potential role of antiinflammatory phytochemicals. Discov Med. 2012 Jan;13(68):7-17. PMID: 22284780.

Chen YX, Gao QY, Zou TH, et al. Berberine versus placebo for the prevention of recurrence of colorectal adenoma: a multicentre, double-blinded, randomized controlled study. Lancet Gastroenterol Hepatol. 2020 Mar;5(3):267-275. Doi: 10.1016/S2468-1253(19)30409-1. Epub 2020 Jan 8. PMID: 31926918.

Choi BY, Kim BW. Withaferin-A inhibits colon cancer cell growth by blocking stat3 transcriptional activity. J Cancer Prev. 2015 Sep;20(3):185-92. Doi: 10.15430/JCP.2015.20.3.185. PMID: 26473157; PMCID: PMC4597807.

Choi HY, Lim JE, Hong JH. Curcumin interrupts the interaction between the androgen receptor and Wnt/β-catenin signaling pathway in LNCaP prostate cancer cells. Prostate Cancer Prostatic Dis. 2010 Dec;13(4):343-9. Doi: 10.1038/pcan.2010.26. Epub 2010 Aug 3. PMID: 20680030.

Choudhury D, Ganguli A, Dastidar DG, et al. Apigenin shows synergistic anticancer activity with curcumin by binding at different sites of tubulin. Biochimie. 2013 June;95(6):1297-309. Doi: 10.1016/j.biochi.2013.02.010. Epub 2013 Feb 26. PMID: 23485682.

Chou TC, Talalay P. Quantitative analysis of dose-effect relationships: the combined effects of multiple drugs or enzyme inhibitors. Adv Enzyme Regul 22, 27–55 (1984).

Chou TC. Theoretical basis, experimental design, and computerized simulation of synergism and antagonism in drug combination studies. Pharmacol Rev. 2006 Sep;58(3):621-81. Doi: 10.1124/pr.58.3.10. Erratum in: Pharmacol Rev. 2007 Mar;59(1):124. PMID: 16968952.

Chu SC, Yu CC, Hsu LS, et al. Berberine reverses epithelial-to-mesenchymal transition and inhibits metastasis and tumor-induced angiogenesis in human cervical cancer cells. Mol Pharmacol. 2014 Dec;86(6):609-23. Doi: 10.1124/mol.114.094037. Epub 2014 Sep 12. Erratum in: Mol Pharmacol. 2017 Feb;91(2):158. PMID: 25217495.

Cifelli CJ, Agarwal S, Fulgoni VL 3rd. Association of yogurt consumption with nutrient intakes, nutrient adequacy, and diet quality in American children and adults. Nutrients. 2020 Nov 9;12(11):3435. doi: 10.3390/nu12113435. PMID: 33182430; PMCID: PMC7696083.

Clarke JD, Dashwood RH, Ho E. Multi-targeted prevention of cancer by sulforaphane. Cancer Lett. 2008 Oct 8;269(2):291-304. Doi: 10.1016/j.canlet.2008.04.018. Epub 2008 May 27. PMID: 18504070; PMCID: PMC2579766.

Clarke MF, Dick JE, Dirks PB, et al. Cancer stem cells—perspectives on current status and future directions: AACR Workshop on cancer stem cells. Cancer Res. 2006 Oct 1;66(19):9339-44. Doi: 10.1158/0008-5472.CAN-06-3126. Epub 2006 Sep 21. PMID: 16990346.

Clarke TC. The use of complementary health approaches among U.S. adults with a recent cancer diagnosis. J Altern Complement Med. 2018 Feb;24(2):139-145. Doi: 10.1089/acm.2016.0182. Epub 2017 Sep 20. PMID: 28930475; PMCID: PMC5820530.

Clifton KK, Ma CX, Fontana L, et al. Intermittent fasting in the prevention and treatment of cancer. CA Cancer J Clin. 2021 Nov;71(6):527-546. Doi: 10.3322/caac.21694. Epub 2021 Aug 12. PMID: 34383300.

Cockbain AJ, Volpato M, Race AD, et al. Anti-colorectal cancer activity of the omega-3 polyunsaturated fatty acid eicosapentaenoic acid. Gut. 2014 Nov;63(11):1760-8. Doi: 10.1136/gutjnl-2013-306445. Epub 2014 Jan 27. PMID: 24470281.

Cohen CW, Fontaine KR, Arend RC, et al. A ketogenic diet reduces central obesity and serum insulin in women with ovarian or endometrial cancer. J Nutr. 2018 Aug 1;148(8):1253-1260. Doi: 10.1093/jn/nxy119. PMID: 30137481; PMCID: PMC8496516.

Cohen SH, Gerding DN, Johnson S, et al. Clinical practice guidelines for Clostridium difficile infection in adults: 2010 update by the society for healthcare epidemiology of America (SHEA) and the infectious diseases society of America (IDSA). Infect Control Hosp Epidemiol. 2010 May;31(5):431-55. doi: 10.1086/651706. PMID: 20307191.

Colao A, Vetrani C, Muscogiuri G, et al. Towards a 'Planeterranean' diet. Italian scientists propose a global research programme for a model based on local adaptations of the Mediterranean Diet. Nature Italy. 10 May 2022. Accessed March 26, 2024.

Collins FS, Varmus H. A new initiative on Precision Medicine. N Engl J Med. 2015 Feb 26;372(9):793-5. Doi: 10.1056/NEJMp1500523. Epub 2015 Jan 30. PMID: 25635347; PMCID: PMC5101938. [A statement on "precision medicine" by two influential proponents of the somatic mutation theory.]

Colunga Biancatelli RML, Berrill M, Catravas JD, et al. Quercetin and vitamin C: an experimental, synergistic therapy for the prevention and treatment of SARS-CoV-2 related disease (COVID-19). Front Immunol. 2020 June 19;11:1451. Doi: 10.3389/fimmu.2020.01451. PMID: 32636851; PMCID: PMC7318306.

Congressional Budget Office [CBO]. *Research and Development in the Pharmaceutical Industry.* April 2021. Accessed January 7, 2024.

Coombs MRP, Harrison ME, Hoskin DW. Apigenin inhibits the inducible expression of programmed death ligand 1 by human and mouse mammary carcinoma cells. Cancer Lett. 2016 Oct 1;380(2):424-433. Doi: 10.1016/j.canlet.2016.06.023. Epub 2016 Jul 1. PMID: 27378243.

Cooperman, Tod, MD [Medical Editor and Reviewer]. Extra virgin olive oil and green tea reviews. Consumerlab.com, 2023. Accessed February 24, 2024. [Subscription required.]

Corominas-Faja B, Oliveras-Ferraros C, Cuyàs E, et al. Stem cell-like ALDH (bright) cellular states in EGFR-mutant non-small cell lung cancer: a novel mechanism of acquired resistance to erlotinib targetable with the natural polyphenol silibinin. Cell Cycle. 2013 Nov 1;12(21):3390-404. Doi: 10.4161/cc.26417. Epub 2013 Sep 17. PMID: 24047698; PMCID: PMC3895428.

Coussens LM, Werb Z. Inflammation and cancer. Nature. 2002 Dec 19-26;420(6917):860-7. Doi: 10.1038/nature01322. PMID: 12490959; PMCID: PMC2803035.

Crane C, Panner A, Pieper RO, et al. Honokiol-mediated inhibition of PI3K/mTOR pathway: a potential strategy to overcome immunoresistance in glioma, breast, and prostate carcinoma without impacting T cell function. J Immunother. 2009 Jul-Aug;32(6):585-92. Doi: 10.1097/CJI.0b013e3181a8efe6. PMID: 19483651; PMCID: PMC3795513.

Creagan ET, Moertel CG, O'Fallon JR, et al. Failure of high-dose vitamin C (ascorbic acid) therapy to benefit patients with advanced cancer. A controlled trial. N Engl J Med. 1979 Sep 27;301(13):687-90. Doi: 10.1056/NEJM197909273011303. PMID: 384241. [Because of its failure to distinguish the oral from intravenous routes of administration, this study set back vitamin C studies for decades.]

Crew KD, Brown P, Greenlee H, et al. Phase IB randomized, double-blinded, placebo-controlled, dose escalation study of Polyphenon E in women with hormone receptor-negative breast cancer. Cancer Prev Res (Phila). 2012 Sep;5(9):1144-54. Doi: 10.1158/1940-6207.CAPR-12-0117. Epub 2012 Jul 24. PMID: 22827973; PMCID: PMC3816771.

Crew KD, Ho KA, Brown P, et al. Effects of a green tea extract, Polyphenon E, on systemic biomarkers of growth factor signaling in women with hormone receptor-negative breast cancer. J Hum Nutr Diet. 2015 Jun;28(3):272-82. Doi: 10.1111/jhn.12229. Epub 2014 Mar 19. PMID: 24646362; PMCID: PMC4205214.

Cruz-Lozano M, González-González A, Marchal JA, et al. Hydroxytyrosol inhibits cancer stem cells and the metastatic capacity of triple-negative breast cancer cell lines by the simultaneous targeting of epithelial-to-mesenchymal transition, Wnt/β-catenin and TGFβ signaling pathways. Eur J Nutr. 2019 Dec;58(8):3207-3219. Doi: 10.1007/s00394-018-1864-1. Epub 2018 Nov 21. PMID: 30460610.

Culpepper T. The effects of kefir and kefir components on immune and metabolic physiology in pre-clinical studies: a narrative review. Cureus. 2022 Aug 8;14(8):e27768. Doi: 10.7759/cureus.27768. PMID: 36106262; PMCID: PMC9450431.

Dai F, Chen WF, Zhou B. Antioxidant synergism of green tea polyphenols with alpha-tocopherol and L-ascorbic acid in SDS micelles. Biochimie. 2008 Oct;90(10):1499-505. Doi: 10.1016/j.biochi.2008.05.007. Epub 2008 May 23. Erratum in: Biochimie. 2009 Nov-Dec;91(11-12):1535. PMID: 18554517.

Dai Q, He Y, Ho CT, et al. Effect of interaction of epigallocatechin gallate and flavonols on color alteration of simulative green tea infusion after thermal treatment. J Food Sci Technol. 2017 Aug;54(9):2919-2928. Doi: 10.1007/s13197-017-2730-5. Epub 2017 June 9. PMID: 28928532; PMCID: PMC5583122.

Dai X, Stanilka JM, Rowe CA, et al. Consuming Lentinula edodes (shiitake) mushrooms daily improves human immunity: a randomized dietary intervention in healthy young adults. J Am Coll Nutr. 2015;34(6):478-87. Doi: 10.1080/07315724.2014.950391. Epub 2015 Apr 11. PMID: 25866155.

Dai Z, Nair V, Khan M, et al. Pomegranate extract inhibits the proliferation and viability of MMTV-Wnt-1 mouse mammary cancer stem cells in vitro. Oncol Rep. 2010 Oct;24(4):1087-91. PMID: 20811693.

Dandawate PR, Subramaniam D, Jensen RA, et al. Targeting cancer stem cells and signaling pathways by phytochemicals: Novel approach for breast cancer therapy. Semin Cancer Biol. 2016 Oct;40-41:192-208. Doi: 10.1016/j.semcancer.2016.09.001. Epub 2016 Sep 5. PMID: 27609747; PMCID: PMC5565737.

Dang, Shirley. Science Communications Manager, Parker Institute for Cancer Immunotherapy (PICI). Probiotics are linked to poorer response to cancer immunotherapy in skin cancer patients. Press release, April 2, 2019. Accessed May 1, 2024.

De Gramont A, Tournigand C, Louvet C, et al. Oxaliplatine, acide folinique et 5-fluorouracile (folfox) en seconde ligne thérapeutique du cancer colorectal métastasé. Le GERCOD

[Oxaliplatin, folinic acid and 5-fluorouracil (folfox) in pretreated patients with metastatic advanced cancer. The GERCOD]. Rev Med Interne. 1997;18(10):769-75. French. Doi: 10.1016/s0248-8663(97)89966-3. PMID: 9500010.

De Groot S, Lugtenberg RT, Cohen D, et al. Fasting mimicking diet as an adjunct to neoadjuvant chemotherapy for breast cancer in the multicentre randomized phase 2 DIRECT trial. Nat Commun. 2020 June 23;11(1):3083. Doi: 10.1038/s41467-020-16138-3. PMID: 32576828; PMCID: PMC7311547.

Deloitte Center for Health Solutions. Seize the digital momentum: measuring the return from pharmaceutical innovation. January 2023. Accessed April 19, 2024.

De Lorgeril M, Salen P, Martin JL, et al. Mediterranean diet, traditional risk factors, and the rate of cardiovascular complications after myocardial infarction: final report of the Lyon Diet Heart Study. Circulation. 1999;99:779-785.

De Lorgeril M, Salen P, Martin JL, et al. Mediterranean dietary pattern in a randomized trial: prolonged survival and possible reduced cancer rate. Arch Intern Med. 1998 Jun 8;158(11):1181-7. Doi: 10.1001/archinte.158.11.1181. PMID: 9625397.

Del Saz-Lara A, López de Las Hazas MC, Visioli F, et al. Nutri-epigenetic effects of phenolic compounds from extra virgin olive oil: a systematic review. Adv Nutr. 2022 Oct 2;13(5):2039-2060. Doi: 10.1093/advances/nmac067. PMID: 35679085; PMCID: PMC9526845.

Deng G, Lin H, Seidman A, et al. A phase I/II trial of a polysaccharide extract from Grifola frondosa (maitake mushroom) in breast cancer patients: immunological effects. J Cancer Res Clin Oncol. 2009 Sep;135(9):1215-21. Doi: 10.1007/s00432-009-0562-z. Epub 2009 Mar 1. PMID: 19253021; PMCID: PMC3751581. **[An unusual paper from MSKCC substantiating the use of a popular complementary treatment.]**

Derrien M, Vaughan EE, Plugge CM, et al. Akkermansia muciniphila gen. nov., sp. Nov., a human intestinal mucin-degrading bacterium. Int J Syst Evol Microbiol. 2004 Sep;54(Pt 5):1469-1476. Doi: 10.1099/ijs.0.02873-0. PMID: 15388697.

De Sousa Almeida-Filho B, De Luca Vespoli H, Pessoa EC, et al. Vitamin D deficiency is associated with poor breast cancer prognostic features in postmenopausal women. J Steroid Biochem Mol Biol. 2017 Nov;174:284-289. Doi: 10.1016/j.jsbmb.2017.10.009. Epub 2017 Oct 12. PMID: 29031688.

Dhermain F. Radiotherapy of high-grade gliomas: current standards and new concepts, innovations in imaging and radiotherapy, and new therapeutic approaches. Chin J Cancer. 2014;33(1):16-24.

Dhillon N, Aggarwal BB, Newman RA, et al. Phase II trial of curcumin in patients with advanced pancreatic cancer. Clin Cancer Res. 2008 Jul 15;14(14):4491-9. doi: 10.1158/1078-0432.CCR-08-0024. PMID: 18628464.

353

Diaz M, Rosado JL, Allen LH, et al. The efficacy of a local ascorbic acid-rich food in improving iron absorption from Mexican diets: a field study using stable isotopes. Am J Clin Nutr. 2003 Sep;78(3):436-40. Doi: 10.1093/ajcn/78.3.436. PMID: 12936926.

Dickinson SE, Rusche JJ, Bec SL, et al. The effect of sulforaphane on histone deacetylase activity in keratinocytes: differences between in vitro and in vivo analyses. Mol Carcinog. 2015 Nov;54(11):1513-20. Doi: 10.1002/mc.22224. Epub 2014 Oct 12. Erratum in: Mol Carcinog. 2016 Jul;55(7):1210. PMID: 25307283; PMCID: PMC4394046.

Diehl A, Yarchoan M, Hopkins A, et al. Relationships between lymphocyte counts and treatment-related toxicities and clinical responses in patients with solid tumors treated with PD-1 checkpoint inhibitors. Oncotarget. 2017 Dec 14;8(69):114268-114280. Doi: 10.18632/oncotarget.23217. PMID: 29371985; PMCID: PMC5768402.

Dow LE, O'Rourke KP, Simon J, et al. APC restoration promotes cellular differentiation and reestablishes crypt homeostasis in colorectal cancer. Cell. 2015;161(7):1539-52.

Drenkhahn SK, Jackson GA, Slusarz A, et al. Inhibition of Hedgehog/Gli signaling by botanicals: a review of compounds with potential hedgehog pathway inhibitory activities. Curr Cancer Drug Targets. 2013 June;13(5):580-95. Doi: 10.2174/15680096113139990003. PMID: 23675897.

Dresen E, Lee ZY, Hill A, et al. History of scurvy and use of vitamin C in critical illness: a narrative review. Nutr Clin Pract. 2023 Feb;38(1):46-54. Doi: 10.1002/ncp.10914. Epub 2022 Sep 25. PMID: 36156315.

Drewnowski A. Why do we like fat? J Am Diet Assoc. 1997 Jul;97(7 Suppl):S58-62. Doi: 10.1016/s0002-8223(97)00732-3. PMID: 9216570.

Du FY, Zhou QF, Sun WJ, et al. Targeting cancer stem cells in drug discovery: Current state and future perspectives. World J Stem Cells. 2019 Jul 26;11(7):398-420. doi: 10.4252/wjsc.v11.i7.398. PMID: 31396368; PMCID: PMC6682504.

Duke, James. *The Green Pharmacy: New Discoveries in Herbal Remedies for Common Diseases.* New York: St. Martins, 1998. **[A lifetime of wisdom from the USDA scientist who also served as my mentor and advisor on all things herbal.]**

Dunbar RIM. Breaking bread: the functions of social eating. Adapt Human Behav Physiol. 2017;3(3):198-211. Doi: 10.1007/s40750-017-0061-4. Epub 2017 Mar 11. PMID: 32025474; PMCID: PMC6979515.

Durgo K, Koncar M, Komes D, et al. Cytotoxicity of blended versus single medicinal mushroom extracts on human cancer cell lines: contribution of polyphenol and polysaccharide content. Int J Med Mushrooms. 2013;15(5):435-48. Doi: 10.1615/intjmedmushr.v15.i5.20. PMID: 24266369.

Dutta A, Chakraborty A. Cinnamon in anticancer armamentarium–a molecular approach. J Toxicol. 2018 Mar 29;2018:8978731. Doi: 10.1155/2018/8978731. PMID: 29796019; PMCID: PMC5896244.

Earls, Ellis. Clinical trial delays: America's patient recruitment dilemma. Clinicaltrialsarena.com, July 18, 2012. Clinical Trials Arena. Accessed January 10, 2024.

EFSA Panel on Food Additives and Nutrient Sources added to Food (ANS); Younes M, Aggett P, et al. Scientific opinion on the safety of green tea catechins. EFSA J. 2018 Apr 18;16(4):e05239. Doi: 10.2903/j.efsa.2018.5239. PMID: 32625874; PMCID: PMC7009618.

Egolf B, Lasker J, Wolf S, et al. The Roseto effect: 50-year comparison of mortality rates. Am J Public Health. 1992 Aug;82(8):1089-92. Doi: 10.2105/ajph.82.8.1089. PMID: 1636828; PMCID: PMC1695733.

El-Benhawy SA, Morsi MI, Fahmy EI, et al. Role of resveratrol as radiosensitizer by targeting cancer stem cells in radioresistant prostate cancer cells (PC-3). Asian Pac J Cancer Prev. 2021 Dec 1;22(12):3823-3837. Doi: 10.31557/APJCP.2021.22.12.3823. PMID: 34967561; PMCID: PMC9080384.

Epstein, Samuel S. The Politics of Cancer. ISBN-13: 978-08715619. New York: Random House, 1982.

Epstein SS, Moss RW. Have we lost the war on cancer? [Op-ed]. Chicago Tribune, December 12, 1991. [Prof. Epstein and I wrote a number of op-eds on the occasion of the 20th anniversary of the war on cancer.]

Ericsson CI, Pacheco LS, Romanos-Nanclares A, et al. Prospective study of avocado consumption and cancer risk in U.S. men and women. Cancer Prev Res (Phila). 2023 Apr 3;16(4):211-218. Doi: 10.1158/1940-6207.CAPR-22-0298. PMID: 36490225; PMCID: PMC10073249.

Eroglu Z, Erdem C, Oktem G, et al. Effect of SIRT1 activators and inhibitors on CD44+/CD133+-enriched non-small cell lung cancer cells. Mol Med Rep. 2020 Jul;22(1):575-581. Doi: 10.3892/mmr.2020.11113. Epub 2020 May 4. PMID: 32377734.

Ervin RB. Prevalence of metabolic syndrome among adults 20 years of age and over, by sex, age, race and ethnicity, and body mass index: United States, 2003-2006. Natl Health Stat Report. 2009 May 5;(13):1-7. PMID: 19634296.

Estruch R, Ros E, Salas-Salvadó J, et al. Primary prevention of cardiovascular disease with a Mediterranean diet supplemented with extra-virgin olive oil or nuts. N Engl J Med. 2018 June 21;378(25):e34. Doi: 10.1056/NEJMoa1800389. Epub 2018 Jun 13. PMID: 29897866. [Key paper concerning the PREDIMED clinical trial.]

Fahey JW, Zhang Y, Talalay P. Broccoli sprouts: an exceptionally rich source of inducers of enzymes that protect against chemical carcinogens. Proc Natl Acad Sci U S A. 1997 Sep 16;94(19):10367-72. Doi: 10.1073/pnas.94.19.10367. PMID: 9294217; PMCID: PMC23369.

[The paper that introduced broccoli sprouts as an anticancer detoxification mechanism.]

Falcon, Andrea. Aristotle on causality. *The Stanford Encyclopedia of Philosophy*. Edward N. Zalta & Uri Nodelman, editors. Spring 2023 edition.

Faqar-Uz-Zaman WF, Schmidt KG, Thomas D, et al. S1P Lyase siRNA dampens malignancy of DLD-1 colorectal cancer cells. Lipids. 2021 Mar;56(2):155-166. Doi: 10.1002/lipd.12282. Epub 2020 Sep 24. PMID: 32971566.

Farkas E. Szupportív kezelés fermentált búzacsíra-kivonattal colorectalis carcinomában [Fermented wheat germ extract in the supportive therapy of colorectal cancer]. Orv Hetil. 2005 Sep 11;146(37):1925-31. Hungarian. PMID: 16255377.

Fearon, Henry. An improved method of amputating a cancerous breast; with an account of two cases in which it was performed with success. Lond Med J. 1783 Oct-Dec;4(4):406-412. PMID: 29139873; PMCID: PMC5545505. [The first references to the surgical treatment of cancer in the PubMed database.]

Feng W, Yang CX, Zhang L, et al. Curcumin promotes the apoptosis of human endometrial carcinoma cells by downregulating the expression of androgen receptor through Wnt signal pathway. Eur J Gynaecol Oncol. 2014;35(6):718-23. PMID: 25556280.

Feres M, Feres MFN. Absence of evidence is not evidence of absence. J Appl Oral Sci. 2023 Mar 27;31:ed001. Doi: 10.1590/1678-7757-2023-ed001. PMID: 36995884; PMCID: PMC10065758.

Fernandes G, Yunis EJ, Good RA. Influence of diet on survival of mice. Proc Natl Acad Sci U S A. 1976 Apr;73(4):1279-83. Doi: 10.1073/pnas.73.4.1279. PMID: 1063408; PMCID: PMC430247.

Fernández-Elías VE, Ortega JF, Nelson RK, et al. Relationship between muscle water and glycogen recovery after prolonged exercise in the heat in humans. Eur J Appl Physiol. 2015 Sep;115(9):1919-26. Doi: 10.1007/s00421-015-3175-z. Epub 2015 Apr 25. PMID: 25911631.

Ferrara LA, Raimondi AS, d'Episcopo L, et al. Olive oil and reduced need for antihypertensive medications. Arch Intern Med. 2000 Mar 27;160(6):837-42. Doi: 10.1001/archinte.160.6.837. PMID: 10737284.

Finkelstein EA, Trogdon JG, Cohen JW, et al. Annual medical spending attributable to obesity: payer-and service-specific estimates. Health Aff (Millwood). 2009 Sep-Oct;28(5):w822-31. Doi: 10.1377/hlthaff.28.5.w822. Epub 2009 Jul 27. PMID: 19635784.

Fisher, Sir Ronald Aylmer. *Statistical Methods for Research Workers*. Edinburgh and London: Oliver & Boyd, 1925.

Fischler, C. Food, self and identity. Social Science Information, 1988;27(2), 275-292.

Fleming, John, MD. Surgeon on the Bengal Establishment. *A Catalog of Indian Medicinal Plants and Drugs: With Their Names in the Hindustani and Sanskrit Languages.* Calcutta: The Hindstani Press, 1810.

Flood PM, Qian L, Peterson LJ, et al. Transcriptional factor NF-κB as a target for therapy in Parkinson's disease. Parkinsons Dis. 2011;2011:216298. Doi: 10.4061/2011/216298. Epub 2011 Mar 30. PMID: 21603248; PMCID: PMC3095232.

Florio R, De Filippis B, Veschi S, et al. Resveratrol derivative exhibits marked antiproliferative actions, affecting stemness in pancreatic cancer cells. Int J Mol Sci. 2023 Jan 19;24(3):1977. Doi: 10.3390/ijms24031977. PMID: 36768301; PMCID: PMC9916441.

Fogacci F, Grassi D, Rizzo M, et al. Metabolic effect of berberine-silymarin association: a meta-analysis of randomized, double-blind, placebo-controlled clinical trials. Phytother Res. 2019 Apr;33(4):862-870. Doi: 10.1002/ptr.6282. Epub 2019 Jan 10. PMID: 30632209; PMCID: PMC6590227.

Folkman J, Shing Y. Angiogenesis. J Biol Chem. 1992 Jun 5;267(16):10931-4. PMID: 1375931. [**Judah Folkman introduced the idea of controlling cancer by blocking new blood vessel formation.**]

Food and Drug Administration [FDA]. Food labeling: health claims; soy protein and coronary heart disease. Final rule. Fed Regist. 1999 Oct 26;64(206):57700-33. Accessed January 28, 2024.

Fortune Business Insights. Olive oil market size, share & industry analysis.... June 3, 2024. Accessed June 20, 2024.

Freedland SJ, Carducci M, Kroeger N, et al. A double-blind, randomized, neoadjuvant study of the tissue effects of POMx pills in men with prostate cancer before radical prostatectomy. Cancer Prev Res (Phila). 2013 Oct;6(10):1120-7. Doi: 10.1158/1940-6207.CAPR-12-0423. Epub 2013 Aug 28. PMID: 23985577; PMCID: PMC3806642. [**A randomized trial of a combination of four food extracts on cancer.**]

Friedenreich CM, Neilson HK, Farris MS, et al. Physical activity and cancer outcomes: a precision medicine approach. Clin Cancer Res. 2016 Oct 1;22(19):4766-4775. Doi: 10.1158/1078-0432.CCR-16-0067. Epub 2016 Jul 12. PMID: 27407093.

Fryar CD, Hughes JP, Herrick KA, et al. Fast food consumption among adults in the United States, 2013-2016. NCHS Data Brief. 2018 Oct;(322):1-8. PMID: 30312154.

Fuhrman J. The hidden dangers of fast and processed food. Am J Lifestyle Med. 2018 Apr 3;12(5):375-381. Doi: 10.1177/1559827618766483. PMID: 30283262; PMCID: PMC6146358.

Fujiki H, Suganuma M, Imai K, et al. Green tea: cancer preventive beverage and/or drug. Cancer Lett. 2002 Dec 15;188(1-2):9-13. Doi: 10.1016/s0304-3835(02)00379-8. PMID: 12406542.

Fujiki H, Watanabe T, Sueoka E, et al. Cancer prevention with green tea and its principal constituent, EGCG: from early investigations to current focus on human cancer stem cells. Mol Cells. 2018 Feb 28;41(2):73-82. Doi: 10.14348/molcells.2018.2227. Epub 2018 Jan 31. PMID: 29429153; PMCID: PMC5824026.

Fu Y, Chang H, Peng X, et al. Resveratrol inhibits breast cancer stem-like cells and induces autophagy via suppressing Wnt/β-catenin signaling pathway. PloS One. 2014 Jul 28;9(7):e102535. Doi: 10.1371/journal.pone.0102535. PMID: 25068516; PMCID: PMC4113212.

Fu Z, Cao X, Liu L, et al. Soy isoflavones inhibits lung cancer cell stem-like characteristics by modulating MnSOD and FoxM1 expression. Oncol Lett. 2020 Sep;20(3):2506-2515. Doi: 10.3892/ol.2020.11802. Epub 2020 Jul 1. PMID: 32782570; PMCID: PMC7400602.

Gabon. Countries and their cultures. Everyculture.com. Website accessed January 19, 2024.

Gano CA, Fatima S, Failes TW, et al. Anti-cancer potential of synergistic phytochemical combinations is influenced by the genetic profile of prostate cancer cell lines. Front Nutr. 2023 Mar 7;10:1119274. Doi: 10.3389/fnut.2023.1119274. PMID: 36960209; PMCID: PMC10029761.

Gao J, Wei W, Wang G, et al. Circulating vitamin D concentration and risk of prostate cancer: a dose-response meta-analysis of prospective studies. Ther Clin Risk Manag. 2018 Jan 9;14:95-104. Doi: 10.2147/TCRM.S149325. PMID: 29386901; PMCID: PMC5767091.

Gao J, Zhao H, Hylands PJ, et al. Secondary metabolite mapping identifies Scutellaria inhibitors of human lung cancer cells. J Pharm Biomed Anal. 2010 Nov 2;53(3):723-8. Doi: 10.1016/j.jpba.2010.04.019. Epub 2010 Apr 20. PMID: 20457505.

García-Martínez BI, Ruiz-Ramos M, Pedraza-Chaverri J, et al. Effect of resveratrol on markers of oxidative stress and sirtuin 1 in elderly adults with type 2 diabetes. Int J Mol Sci. 2023 Apr 18;24(8):7422. Doi: 10.3390/ijms24087422. PMID: 37108584; PMCID: PMC10138491.

Geng W, Guo X, Zhang L, et al. Resveratrol inhibits proliferation, migration and invasion of multiple myeloma cells via NEAT1-mediated Wnt/β-catenin signaling pathway. Biomed Pharmacother. 2018 Nov;107:484-494. Doi: 10.1016/j.biopha.2018.08.003. Epub 2018 Aug 11. PMID: 30107344.

Gersey ZC, Rodriguez GA, Barbarite E, et al. Curcumin decreases malignant characteristics of glioblastoma stem cells via induction of reactive oxygen species. BMC Cancer. 2017 Feb 4;17(1):99. Doi: 10.1186/s12885-017-3058-2. PMID: 28160777; PMCID: PMC5292151.

Ghadirian P, Ekoé JM, Thouez JP. Food habits and esophageal cancer: an overview. Cancer Detect Prev. 1992;16(3):163-8. PMID: 1458505.

Ghadirian P. Food habits of the people of the Caspian Littoral of Iran in relation to esophageal cancer. Nutr Cancer. 1987;9(2-3):147-57. Doi: 10.1080/01635588709513922. PMID: 3562293.

Ghanbari-Movahed M, Shafiee S, Burcher JT, et al. Anticancer potential of apigenin and isovitexin with focus on oncogenic metabolism in cancer stem cells. Metabolites. 2023 Mar 9;13(3):404. Doi: 10.3390/metabo13030404. PMID: 36984844; PMCID: PMC10051376.

Ghannam Y, Laville A, Kirova Y, et al. Radiotherapy of the primary disease for synchronous metastatic cancer: a systematic review. Cancers (Basel). 2022 Nov 30;14(23):5929. Doi: 10.3390/cancers14235929. PMID: 36497410; PMCID: PMC9736289.

Ghosh J, Myers CE. Inhibition of arachidonate 5-lipoxygenase triggers massive apoptosis in human prostate cancer cells. Proc Natl Acad Sci U S A. 1998 Oct 27;95(22):13182-7.

Giacosa A, Barale R, Bavaresco L, et al. Cancer prevention in Europe: the Mediterranean diet as a protective choice. Eur J Cancer Prev. 2013 Jan;22(1):90-5. Doi: 10.1097/CEJ.0b013e328354d2d7. PMID: 22644232.

Gibbs, David, CEO. Yum! Brands 2023 Annual Report. Accessed April 24, 2024.

Giovannucci E, Harlan DM, Archer MC, et al. Diabetes and cancer: a consensus report. Diabetes Care. 2010 Jul;33(7):1674-85. Doi: 10.2337/dc10-0666. PMID: 20587728; PMCID: PMC2890380.

Giovannucci E. Metabolic syndrome, hyperinsulinemia, and colon cancer. Am J Clin Nutr. 2007 Sep;86(3):s836-42. Doi: 10.1093/ajcn/86.3.836S. PMID: 18265477.

Giovannucci E. Tomatoes, tomato-based products, lycopene, and cancer: review of the epidemiologic literature. J Natl Cancer Inst. 1999 Feb 17;91(4):317-31. Doi: 10.1093/jnci/91.4.317. PMID: 10050865. [**Report from Edward Giovannucci of Harvard that boosted use of lycopene vs. prostate cancer risk.**]

Gioxari A, Tzanos D, Kostara C, et al. Mediterranean diet implementation to protect against advanced lung cancer index (ALI) rise: study design and preliminary results of a Randomised Controlled Trial. Int J Environ Res Public Health. 2021 Apr 1;18(7):3700. Doi: 10.3390/ijerph18073700. PMID: 33916252; PMCID: PMC8036451.

Goel A, Kunnumakkara AB, Aggarwal BB. Curcumin as "Curecumin": from kitchen to clinic. Biochem Pharmacol. 2008 Feb 15;75(4):787-809. Doi: 10.1016/j.bcp.2007.08.016. Epub 2007 Aug 19. PMID: 17900536.

Golden EB, Lam PY, Kardosh A, et al. Green tea polyphenols block the anticancer effects of bortezomib and other boronic acid-based proteasome inhibitors. Blood. 2009 Jun 4;113(23):5927-37. Doi: 10.1182/blood-2008-07-171389. Epub 2009 Feb 3. PMID: 19190249.

Gollier C, Treich N, Precautionary Principle – an overview | ScienceDirect Topics. In: *Encyclopedia of Energy, Natural Resource, and Environmental Economics,* Elsevier Science, 2011. Accessed January 31, 2024.

Golombick T, Diamond TH, Manoharan A, et al. Monoclonal gammopathy of undetermined significance, smoldering multiple myeloma, and curcumin: a randomized, double-blind placebo-controlled crossover 4g study and an open-label 8g extension study. Am J Hematol. 2012 May;87(5):455-60. Doi: 10.1002/ajh.23159. Epub 2012 Apr 4. PMID: 22473809.

Gong X, Jiang L, Li W, et al. Curcumin induces apoptosis and autophagy inhuman renal cell carcinoma cells via Akt/mTOR suppression. Bioengineered. 2021 Dec;12(1):5017-5027. Doi: 10.1080/21655979.2021.1960765. PMID: 34402718; PMCID: PMC8806675.

González-Rodríguez M, Ait Edjoudi D, Cordero-Barreal A, et al. Oleocanthal, an antioxidant phenolic compound in extra virgin olive oil (EVOO): a comprehensive systematic review of its potential in inflammation and cancer. Antioxidants (Basel). 2023 Dec 14;12(12):2112. Doi: 10.3390/antiox12122112. PMID: 38136231; PMCID: PMC10741130.

González-Vallinas M, Molina S, Vicente G, et al. Expression of microRNA-15b and the glycosyltransferase GCNT3 correlates with antitumor efficacy of Rosemary diterpenes in colon and pancreatic cancer. PloS One. 2014 Jun 3;9(6):e98556. Doi: 10.1371/journal.pone.0098556. PMID: 24892299; PMCID: PMC4043684.

Graham JG, Quinn ML, Fabricant DS, et al. Plants used against cancer – an extension of the work of Jonathan Hartwell. J Ethnopharmacol. 2000 Dec;73(3):347-77. Doi: 10.1016/s0378-8741(00)00341-x. PMID: 11090989. [**Hartwell began the scientific study of anticancer plant constituents at the NIH.**]

Green S. Oxygenation therapy: unproven treatments for cancer and AIDS. QuackWatch, June 17, 2001. Accessed February 29, 2024.

Gregory K, Zhao L, Felder TM, et al. Prevalence of health behaviors among cancer survivors in the United States. J Cancer Surviv. 2023 Mar 18:1–9. Doi: 10.1007/s11764-023-01347-8. Epub ahead of print. PMID: 36933085; PMCID: PMC10024006.

Guasch-Ferré M, Bulló M, Martínez-González MÁ, et al. Frequency of nut consumption and mortality risk in the PREDIMED nutrition intervention trial. BMC Med. 2013 Jul 16;11:164. Doi: 10.1186/1741-7015-11-164. PMID: 23866098; PMCID: PMC3738153.

Guasch-Ferré M, Li Y, Willett WC, et al. Consumption of olive oil and risk of total and cause-specific mortality among U.S. adults. J Am Coll Cardiol. 2022 Jan 18;79(2):101-112. Doi: 10.1016/j.jacc.2021.10.041. PMID: 35027106; PMCID: PMC8851878.

Gussow JD. Mediterranean diets: are they environmentally responsible? Am J Clin Nutr. 1995 Jun;61(6 Suppl):1383S-1389S. doi: 10.1093/ajcn/61.6.1383S. PMID: 7754992.

Gutierrez RMP, Velazquez EG, Carrera SPP. Spinacia oleracea Linn considered as one of the most perfect foods: a pharmacological and phytochemical review. Mini Rev Med Chem. 2019;19(20):1666-1680. Doi: 10.2174/1389557519666190603090347. PMID: 31161986.

Habib M, Saif MW. Pancreatic cancer stem cells: their role in pancreatic cancer patient outcomes and what is the future? JOP. 2013 Jul 10;14(4):401-4. Doi: 10.6092/1590-8577/1658. PMID: 23846937.

Hanahan D, Coussens LM. Accessories to the crime: functions of cells recruited to the tumor microenvironment. Cancer Cell. 2012 Mar 20;21(3):309-22. Doi: 10.1016/j.ccr.2012.02.022. PMID: 22439926. [A paper in which Hanahan writes favorably about the cancer stem cell concept.]

Hanahan D, Weinberg RA. Hallmarks of cancer: the next generation. Cell. 2011 Mar 4;144(5):646-74. Doi: 10.1016/j.cell.2011.02.013. PMID: 21376230. [H&W's most influential paper.]

Hanahan D, Weinberg RA. The hallmarks of cancer. Cell. 2000 Jan 7;100(1):57-70. Doi: 10.1016/s0092-8674(00)81683-9. PMID: 10647931. [Classic statement of the hallmarks of cancer.]

Hanahan D. Hallmarks of cancer: new dimensions. Cancer Discov. 2022 Jan;12(1):31-46. Doi: 10.1158/2159-8290.CD-21-1059. PMID: 35022204. [Hanahan's solo summation.]

Hanau C, Morré DJ, Morré DM. Cancer prevention trial of a synergistic mixture of green tea concentrate plus Capsicum (CAPSOL-T) in a random population of subjects ages 40-84. Clin Proteomics. 2014 Jan 6;11(1):2. Doi: 10.1186/1559-0275-11-2. PMID: 24393573; PMCID: PMC3901999. [The Morrés' last paper with vital information on the synergy between EGCG and capsaicin.]

Han H, Lim JW, Kim H. Lycopene inhibits activation of epidermal growth factor receptor and expression of cyclooxygenase-2 in gastric cancer cells. Nutrients. 2019 Sep 5;11(9):2113. Doi: 10.3390/nu11092113. PMID: 31491956; PMCID: PMC6770769.

Han M, Lu Y, Tao Y, et al. Luteolin protects pancreatic β cells against apoptosis through regulation of autophagy and ros clearance. Pharmaceuticals (Basel). 2023 July 7;16(7):975. Doi: 10.3390/ph16070975. PMID: 37513887; PMCID: PMC10385282.

Han MA, Zeraatkar D, Guyatt GH, et al. Reduction of red and processed meat intake and cancer mortality and incidence: a systematic review and meta-analysis of cohort studies. Ann Intern Med. 2019 Nov 19;171(10):711-720. Doi: 10.7326/M19-0699. Epub 2019 Oct 1. PMID: 31569214.

Harris HR, Orsini N, Wolk A. Vitamin C and survival among women with breast cancer: a meta-analysis. Eur J Cancer. 2014 May;50(7):1223-31. Doi: 10.1016/j.ejca.2014.02.013. Epub 2014 Mar 7. PMID: 24613622.

Hassan ZK, Elamin MH, Omer SA, et al. Oleuropein induces apoptosis via the p53 pathway in breast cancer cells. Asian Pac J Cancer Prev. 2014 Jan;14(11):6739-42. Doi: 10.7314/apjcp.2013.14.11.6739. PMID: 24377598.

Hayflick L. The limited in vitro lifetime of human diploid cell strains. Exp Cell Res. 1965 Mar;37:614-36. Doi: 10.1016/0014-4827(65)90211-9. PMID: 14315085. [A classic of biology, cited over 4,500 times in other journal articles.]

361

Heidari H, Bagherniya M, Majeed M, et al. Curcumin-piperine co-supplementation and human health: a comprehensive review of preclinical and clinical studies. Phytother Res. 2023 Apr;37(4):1462-1487. Doi: 10.1002/ptr.7737. Epub 2023 Jan 31. PMID: 36720711.

Helmus DS, Thompson CL, Zelenskiy S, et al. Red meat-derived heterocyclic amines increase risk of colon cancer: a population-based case-control study. Nutr Cancer. 2013;65(8):1141-50. Doi: 10.1080/01635581.2013.834945. Epub 2013 Oct 29. PMID: 24168237; PMCID: PMC4045458.

Henning SM, Wang P, Said JW, et al. Randomized clinical trial of brewed green and black tea in men with prostate cancer prior to prostatectomy. Prostate. 2015 Apr 1;75(5):550-9. Doi: 10.1002/pros.22943. Epub 2014 Dec 24. PMID: 25545744; PMCID: PMC4334734.

Hermann PC, Huber SL, Herrler T, et al. Distinct populations of cancer stem cells determine tumor growth and metastatic activity in human pancreatic cancer. Cell Stem Cell. 2007 Sep 13;1(3):313-23. Doi: 10.1016/j.stem.2007.06.002. PMID: 18371365.

He X, Shu J, Xu L, et al. Inhibitory effect of Astragalus polysaccharides on lipopolysaccharide-induced TNF-a and IL-1β production in THP-1 cells. Molecules. 2012 Mar 12;17(3):3155-64. Doi: 10.3390/molecules17033155. PMID: 22410422; PMCID: PMC6268450.

He Z, Subramaniam D, Zhang Z, et al. Honokiol as a radiosensitizing agent for colorectal cancers. Curr Colorectal Cancer Rep. 2013 Dec;9(4):10.1007/s11888-013-0191-4. Doi: 10.1007/s11888-013-0191-4. PMID: 24307888; PMCID: PMC3844429.

Hilakivi-Clarke L, Verma V, McDermott M, et al. Foods may modify responsiveness to cancer immune checkpoint blockers by altering both the gut microbiota and activation of estrogen receptors in immune cells. Front Microbiomes 2022;1: 12 December 2022.

Hinzey, Elaine and Chien, Shanley. Mediterranean diet do's & don'ts. U.S. News & World Report, April 2, 2024. Accessed April 12, 2024.

Hitchcock J, Hughes K, Pensa S, et al. The immune environment of the mammary gland fluctuates during post-lactational regression and correlates with tumor growth rate. Development. 2022 Apr 15;149(8):dev200162. Doi: 10.1242/dev.200162. Epub 2022 Apr 29. PMID: 35420674; PMCID: PMC9124574.

Holloszy JO, Fontana L. Caloric restriction in humans. Exp Gerontol. 2007 Aug;42(8):709-12. Doi: 10.1016/j.exger.2007.03.009. Epub 2007 Mar 31. PMID: 17482403; PMCID: PMC2020845.

Holt-Lunstad J, Smith TB, Layton JB. Social relationships and mortality risk: a meta-analytic review. PLoS Med. 2010 Jul 27;7(7):e1000316. Doi: 10.1371/journal.pmed.1000316. PMID: 20668659; PMCID: PMC2910600.

Holzapfel NP, Shokoohmand A, Wagner F, et al. Lycopene reduces ovarian tumor growth and intraperitoneal metastatic load. Am J Cancer Res. 2017 June 1;7(6):1322-1336. PMID: 28670494; PMCID: PMC5489781.

362

Hong HR, Jeong JO, Kong JY, et al. Effect of walking exercise on abdominal fat, insulin resistance and serum cytokines in obese women. J Exerc Nutrition Biochem. 2014 Sep;18(3):277-85. Doi: 10.5717/jenb.2014.18.3.277. Epub 2014 Sep 10. PMID: 25566464; PMCID: PMC4241903.

Hopkins BD, Goncalves MD, Cantley LC. Obesity and cancer mechanisms: cancer metabolism. J Clin Oncol. 2016 Dec 10;34(35):4277-4283. Doi: 10.1200/JCO.2016.67.9712. Epub 2016 Nov 7. PMID: 27903152; PMCID: PMC5562429.

Howells LM, Iwuji COO, Irving GRB, et al. Curcumin combined with FOLFOX chemotherapy is safe and tolerable in patients with metastatic colorectal cancer in a randomized Phase Iia trial. J Nutr. 2019 July 1;149(7):1133-1139. Doi: 10.1093/jn/nxz029. PMID: 31132111; PMCID: PMC6602900. [Extremely important clinical trial establishing the value of adding curcumin supplements to chemo in advanced colorectal cancer.]

Hrelia S, Di Renzo L, Bavaresco L, et al. Moderate wine consumption and health: a narrative review. Nutrients. 2022 Dec 30;15(1):175. Doi: 10.3390/nu15010175. PMID: 36615832; PMCID: PMC9824172.

Hsieh TC, Wu JM. Suppression of cell proliferation and gene expression by combinatorial synergy of EGCG, resveratrol and gamma-tocotrienol in estrogen receptor-positive MCF-7 breast cancer cells. Int J Oncol. 2008 Oct;33(4):851-9. PMID: 18813800.

Hsieh TC, Wu JM. Targeting CWR22Rv1 prostate cancer cell proliferation and gene expression by combinations of the phytochemicals EGCG, genistein, and quercetin. Anticancer Res. 2009 Oct;29(10):4025-32. PMID: 19846946; PMCID: PMC3641843.

Hsing AW, Chokkalingam AP, Gao YT, et al. Allium vegetables and risk of prostate cancer: a population-based study. J Natl Cancer Inst. 2002 Nov 6;94(21):1648-51. Doi: 10.1093/jnci/94.21.1648. PMID: 12419792.

Hsu HS, Lin JH, Huang WC, et al. Chemoresistance of lung cancer stem like cells depends on activation of Hsp27. Cancer. 2011 Apr 1;117(7):1516-28. Doi: 10.1002/cncr.25599. Epub 2010 Nov 8. PMID: 21425153.

Huang KJ, Kuo CH, Chen SH, et al. Honokiol inhibits in vitro and in vivo growth of oral squamous cell carcinoma through induction of apoptosis, cell cycle arrest and autophagy. J Cell Mol Med. 2018 Mar;22(3):1894-1908. Doi: 10.1111/jcmm.13474. Epub 2018 Jan 24. PMID: 29363886; PMCID: PMC5824386.

Huang X, Chen S, Xu L, et al. Genistein inhibits p38 map kinase activation, matrix metalloproteinase type 2, and cell invasion in human prostate epithelial cells. Cancer Res. 2005 Apr 15;65(8):3470-8. Doi: 10.1158/0008-5472.CAN-04-2807. PMID: 15833883.

Huang X, Dai S, Dai J, et al. Luteolin decreases invasiveness, deactivates STAT3 signaling, and reverses interleukin-6 induced epithelial-mesenchymal transition and matrix metalloproteinase secretion of pancreatic cancer cells. Onco Targets Ther. 2015 Oct 19;8:2989-3001. Doi: 10.2147/OTT.S91511. PMID: 26527884; PMCID: PMC4621199.

Hu FB, Li TY, Colditz GA, et al. Television watching and other sedentary behaviors in relation to risk of obesity and type 2 diabetes mellitus in women. JAMA. 2003 Apr 9;289(14):1785-91. Doi: 10.1001/jama.289.14.1785. PMID: 12684356.

Hu HY, Li KP, Wang XJ, et al. Set9, NF-κB, and microRNA-21 mediate berberine-induced apoptosis of human multiple myeloma cells. Acta Pharmacol Sin. 2013 Jan;34(1):157-66. Doi: 10.1038/aps.2012.161. Epub 2012 Dec 17. PMID: 23247593; PMCID: PMC4086496.

Hu J, Webster D, Cao J, Shao A. The safety of green tea and green tea extract consumption in adults – Results of a systematic review. Regul Toxicol Pharmacol. 2018 Jun;95:412-433. Doi: 10.1016/j.yrtph.2018.03.019. Epub 2018 Mar 24. PMID: 29580974.

Huntly BJ, Gilliland DG. Leukemia stem cells and the evolution of cancer-stem-cell research. Nat Rev Cancer. 2005 Apr;5(4):311-21. Doi: 10.1038/nrc1592. PMID: 15803157.

Hu Q, Xie B. Effect of maitake D-fraction in advanced laryngeal and pharyngeal cancers during concurrent chemoradiotherapy: a randomized clinical trial. Acta Biochim Pol. 2022 Sep 7;69(3):625-632. Doi: 10.18388/abp.2020_5996. PMID: 36070433.

Hu Y, Teng C, Yu S, et al. Inonotus obliquus polysaccharide regulates gut microbiota of chronic pancreatitis in mice. AMB Express. 2017 Dec;7(1):39. Doi: 10.1186/s13568-017-0341-1. Epub 2017 Feb 14. PMID: 28197985; PMCID: PMC5309192.

IARC Working Group on the Evaluation of Carcinogenic Risks to Humans. *IARC Monographs on the Evaluation of Carcinogenic Risks to Humans*, No. 114. Lyon (FR): International Agency for Research on Cancer; 2018. Accessed February 11, 2024.

IATP [Institute for Agriculture & Trade Policy]. Broccoli sprout patent invalid, November 6, 2001. Accessed April 19, 2024.

Imran M, Rauf A, Abu-Izneid T, et al. Luteolin, a flavonoid, as an anticancer agent: a review. Biomed Pharmacother. 2019 Apr;112:108612. Doi: 10.1016/j.biopha.2019.108612. Epub 2019 Feb 21. Erratum in: Biomed Pharmacother. 2019 Aug;116:109084. PMID: 30798142.

Ina K, Furuta R, Kataoka T, et al. Lentinan prolonged survival in patients with gastric cancer receiving S-1-based chemotherapy. World J Clin Oncol. 2011 Oct 10;2(10):339-43. Doi: 10.5306/wjco.v2.i10.339. PMID: 21994907; PMCID: PMC3191325.

Institute of Medicine (U.S.) [IOM], Committee on Quality of HealthCare in America. *Crossing the Quality Chasm: a New Health System for the 21st Century.* Washington (DC): National Academies Press (U.S.); 2001. PMID: 25057539. **[IOM is now the National Academy of Medicine, or NAM]**

Islami F, Boffetta P, Ren JS, et al. High-temperature beverages and foods and esophageal cancer risk–a systematic review. Int J Cancer. 2009 Aug 1;125(3):491-524. Doi: 10.1002/ijc.24445. PMID: 19415743; PMCID: PMC2773211.

Jacobs DR Jr, Gross MD, Tapsell LC. Food synergy: an operational concept for understanding nutrition. Am J Clin Nutr. 2009 May;89(5):1543S-1548S. doi: 10.3945/ajcn.2009.26736B. Epub 2009 Mar 11. PMID: 19279083; PMCID: PMC2731586.

Jacobs DR Jr, Steffen LM. Nutrients, foods, and dietary patterns as exposures in research: a framework for food synergy. Am J Clin Nutr. 2003 Sep;78(3 Suppl):508S-513S. doi: 10.1093/ajcn/78.3.508S. PMID: 12936941.

Jiang L, Wang J, Xiong K, et al. Intake of fish and marine n-3 polyunsaturated fatty acids and risk of cardiovascular Disease mortality: a meta-analysis of prospective cohort studies. Nutrients. 2021 Jul 9;13(7):2342. Doi: 10.3390/nu13072342. PMID: 34371852; PMCID: PMC8308510.

Jakab F, Mayer A, Hoffmann A, Hidvégi M. First clinical data of a natural immunomodulator in colorectal cancer. Hepatogastroenterology. 2000 Mar-Apr;47(32):393-5. PMID: 10791198. **[Early report on fermented wheat germ extract by Maté Hidvegi, of Budapest.]**

Jakobušić Brala C, Karković Marković A, Kugić A, et al. Combination chemotherapy with selected polyphenols in preclinical and clinical studies-an update overview. Molecules. 2023 Apr 26;28(9):3746. Doi: 10.3390/molecules28093746. PMID: 37175156; PMCID: PMC10180288.

Jakubikova J, Cervi D, Ooi M, et al. Anti-tumor activity and signaling events triggered by the isothiocyanates, sulforaphane and phenethyl isothiocyanate, in multiple myeloma. Haematologica. 2011 Aug;96(8):1170-9. Doi: 10.3324/haematol.2010.029363. Epub 2011 Jun 28. PMID: 21712538; PMCID: PMC3148911.

Jang JY, Im E, Kim ND. Mechanism of resveratrol-induced programmed cell death and new drug discovery against cancer: a review. Int J Mol Sci. 2022 Nov 8;23(22):13689. Doi: 10.3390/ijms232213689. PMID: 36430164; PMCID: PMC9697740.

Jeandet P, Hébrard C, Deville MA, et al. Deciphering the role of phytoalexins in plant-microorganism interactions and human health. Molecules. 2014 Nov 5;19(11):18033-56. Doi: 10.3390/molecules191118033. PMID: 25379642; PMCID: PMC6271817.

Jiang X, Wu H, Zhao W, et al. Lycopene improves the efficiency of anti-PD-1 therapy via activating IFN signaling of lung cancer cells. Cancer Cell Int. 2019 Mar 21;19:68. Doi: 10.1186/s12935-019-0789-y. PMID: 30948928; PMCID: PMC6429703.

Jiang ZB, Wang WJ, Xu C, et al. Luteolin and its derivative apigenin suppress the inducible PD-L1 expression to improve anti-tumor immunity in KRAS-mutant lung cancer. Cancer Lett. 2021 Sep 1;515:36-48. Doi: 10.1016/j.canlet.2021.05.019. Epub 2021 May 28. PMID: 34052328.

Jiao J, Moudon AV, Kim SY, et al. Health implications of adults' eating at and living near fast food or quick service restaurants. Nutr Diabetes. 2015 Jul 20;5(7):e171. Doi: 10.1038/nutd.2015.18. PMID: 26192449; PMCID: PMC4521173.

Jin P, Zhang C, Li N. Berberine exhibits antitumor effects in human ovarian cancer cells. Anticancer Agents Med Chem. 2015;15(4):511-6. Doi: 10.2174/1871520614666141226124110. PMID: 25544381.

Joehrer K, Çiçek SS. Multiple myeloma inhibitory activity of plant natural products. Cancers (Basel). 2021 May 29;13(11):2678. Doi: 10.3390/cancers13112678. PMID: 34072312; PMCID: PMC8198565.

Johnson, Steven Ross. Food insecurity is tied to shorter life, early death. U.S. News. January 9, 2024. Accessed April 6, 2024.

Kabat-Zinn, John. *Full Catastrophe Living: Using the Wisdom of Your Body and Mind to Face Stress, Pain, and Illness,* 1990; revised edition. New York: Bantam, 2013. Accessed January 17, 2024.

Kakarala M, Brenner DE, Korkaya H, et al. Targeting breast stem cells with the cancer preventive compounds curcumin and piperine. Breast Cancer Res Treat. 2010 Aug;122(3):777-85. Doi: 10.1007/s10549-009-0612-x. Epub 2009 Nov 7. PMID: 19898931; PMCID: PMC3039120.

Kalam F, James DL, Li YR, et al. Intermittent fasting interventions to leverage metabolic and circadian mechanisms for cancer treatment and supportive care outcomes. JNCI Monographs, Volume 2023, Issue 61, June 2023, Pages 84–103.

Kalluru H, Kondaveeti SS, Telapolu S, et al. Turmeric supplementation improves the quality of life and hematological parameters in breast cancer patients on paclitaxel chemotherapy: A case series. Complement Ther Clin Pract. 2020 Nov;41:101247. doi: 10.1016/j.ctcp.2020.101247. Epub 2020 Oct 13. PMID: 33099272.

Kanai M, Yoshimura K, Asada M, et al. A phase I/II study of gemcitabine-based chemotherapy plus curcumin for patients with gemcitabine-resistant pancreatic cancer. Cancer Chemother Pharmacol. 2011 Jul;68(1):157-64. doi: 10.1007/s00280-010-1470-2. Epub 2010 Sep 22. PMID: 20859741.

Kang DY, Sp N, Jang KJ, et al. Antitumor effects of natural bioactive ursolic acid in embryonic cancer stem cells. J Oncol. 2022 Feb 16;2022:6737248. Doi: 10.1155/2022/6737248. PMID: 35222644; PMCID: PMC8866021.

Kang HJ, Youn YK, Hong MK, et al. Antiproliferation and redifferentiation in thyroid cancer cell lines by polyphenol phytochemicals. J Korean Med Sci. 2011 Jul;26(7):893-9. Doi: 10.3346/jkms.2011.26.7.893. Epub 2011 June 20. PMID: 21738342; PMCID: PMC3124719.

Kapała A, Szlendak M, Motacka E. The anti-cancer activity of lycopene: a systematic review of human and animal studies. Nutrients. 2022 Dec 3;14(23):5152. Doi: 10.3390/nu14235152. PMID: 36501182; PMCID: PMC9741066.

Katz DL, Meller S. Can we say what diet is best for health? Annu Rev Public Health. 2014;35:83-103. Doi: 10.1146/annurev-publhealth-032013-182351. PMID: 24641555.

Kaufman, Francine R. *Diabesity.* New York: Bantam, 2005. Accessed February 3, 2024 from Google Books.

Kawasaki BT, Hurt EM, Mistree T, et al. Targeting cancer stem cells with phytochemicals. Mol Interv. 2008 Aug;8(4):174-84. Doi: 10.1124/mi.8.4.9. PMID: 18829843. [**The first report from the NIH on a core focus of The Moss Method, the use of plant chemicals to target CSCs.**]

Kaya M, Abuaisha A, Suer I, et al. Turmeric inhibits MDA-MB-231 cancer cell proliferation, altering miR-638-5p and its potential targets. Eur J Breast Health. 2024 Apr 1;20(2):102-109. Doi: 10.4274/ejbh.galenos.2024.2023-12-2. PMID: 38571691; PMCID: PMC10985573.

Kciuk M, Alam M, Ali N, et al. Epigallocatechin-3-gallate therapeutic potential in cancer: mechanism of action and clinical implications. Molecules. 2023 July 6;28(13):5246. Doi: 10.3390/molecules28135246. PMID: 37446908; PMCID: PMC10343677.

Kelly SP, Gomez-Ramirez M, Montesi JL, et al. L-theanine and caffeine in combination affect human cognition as evidenced by oscillatory alpha-band activity and attention task performance. J Nutr. 2008 Aug;138(8):1572S-1577S. doi: 10.1093/jn/138.8.1572S. PMID: 18641209.

Kensler TW, Wakabayashi N, Biswal S. Cell survival responses to environmental stresses via the Keap1-Nrf2-ARE pathway. Annu Rev Pharmacol Toxicol. 2007;47:89-116. Doi: 10.1146/annurev.pharmtox.46.120604.141046. PMID: 16968214.

Key TJ, Appleby PN, Crowe FL, et al. Cancer in British vegetarians: updated analyses of 4998 incident cancers in a cohort of 32,491 meat eaters, 8612 fish eaters, 18,298 vegetarians, and 2246 vegans. Am J Clin Nutr. 2014 Jul;100 Suppl 1(1):378S-85S. doi: 10.3945/ajcn.113.071266. Epub 2014 Jun 4. Erratum in: Am J Clin Nutr. 2022 June 7;115(6):1658-1659. PMID: 24898235; PMCID: PMC4144109.

Khammissa RAG, Fourie J, Motswaledi MH, et al. The biological activities of vitamin D and its receptor in relation to calcium and bone homeostasis, cancer, immune and cardiovascular systems, skin biology, and oral health. Biomed Res Int. 2018 May 22;2018:9276380. Doi: 10.1155/2018/9276380. PMID: 29951549; PMCID: PMC5987305.

Khan SH, Alhumaydhi FA, Khan MA, et al. Therapeutic potential of polyphenols and their nanoformulations in the treatment of colorectal cancer. Anticancer Agents Med Chem. 2021 Oct 28;21(16):2117-2129. Doi: 10.2174/1871520621666201231144007. PMID: 33390126.

Kim ND, Mehta R, Yu W, et al. Chemopreventive and adjuvant therapeutic potential of pomegranate (Punica granatum) for human breast cancer. Breast Cancer Res Treat. 2002 Feb;71(3):203-17. Doi: 10.1023/a:1014405730585. PMID: 12002340.

Kim YS, Farrar W, Colburn NH, et al. Cancer stem cells: Potential target for bioactive food components. J Nutr Biochem. 2012 Jul;23(7):691-8. Doi: 10.1016/j.jnutbio.2012.03.002. PMID: 22704055; PMCID: PMC4518442.

Kiokias S, Oreopoulou V. A review of the health protective effects of phenolic acids against a range of severe pathologic conditions (including coronavirus-based infections). Molecules. 2021 Sep 6;26(17):5405. Doi: 10.3390/molecules26175405. PMID: 34500838; PMCID: PMC8433690.

Kiselev VI, Ashrafyan LA, Muyzhnek EL, et al. A new promising way of maintenance therapy in advanced ovarian cancer: a comparative clinical study. BMC Cancer. 2018 Sep 20;18(1):904. Doi: 10.1186/s12885-018-4792-9. PMID: 30236079; PMCID: PMC6148762.

Kleckner A, Reschke JE, Altman BJ, et al. A 10-hour time-restricted eating intervention to address cancer-related fatigue among cancer survivors. J Clin Oncol 39, 2021 (suppl 15; abstr 12109).

Klement RJ, Kämmerer U. Is there a role for carbohydrate restriction in the treatment and prevention of cancer? Nutr Metab (Lond). 2011 Oct 26;8:75. Doi: 10.1186/1743-7075-8-75. PMID: 22029671; PMCID: PMC3267662.

Kluge HHP. Shaking up the status quo that separates different approaches to medicine and health. World Health Organization–Europe. Statement. Accessed December 21, 2023.

Kobori M, Yoshida M, Ohnishi-Kameyama M, et al. Ergosterol peroxide from an edible mushroom suppresses inflammatory responses in RAW264.7 macrophages and growth of HT29 colon adenocarcinoma cells. Br J Pharmacol. 2007 Jan;150(2):209-19. Doi: 10.1038/sj.bjp.0706972. Epub 2006 Dec 11. PMID: 17160010; PMCID: PMC2042906.

Kodama N, Komuta K, Nanba H. Can maitake MD-fraction aid cancer patients? Altern Med Rev. 2002 Jun;7(3):236-9. PMID: 12126464.

Kodama N, Komuta K, Nanba H. Effect of maitake (Grifola frondosa) D-fraction on the activation of NK cells in cancer patients. J Med Food. 2003 Winter;6(4):371-7. Doi: 10.1089/109662003772519949. PMID: 14977447.

Kornel A, Nadile M, Retsidou MI, et al. Ursolic acid against prostate and urogenital cancers: a review of in vitro and in vivo studies. Int J Mol Sci. 2023 Apr 18;24(8):7414. Doi: 10.3390/ijms24087414. PMID: 37108576; PMCID: PMC10138876.

Kroon MA, Berbee JK, Majait S, et al. Non-therapeutic plasma levels in individuals utilizing curcumin supplements in daily life. Front Nutr. 2023 Nov 30;10:1267035. Doi: 10.3389/fnut.2023.1267035. PMID: 38099182; PMCID: PMC10720437.

Kubatka P, Kello M, Kajo K, et al. Oregano demonstrates distinct tumor-suppressive effects in the breast carcinoma model. Eur J Nutr. 2017 Apr;56(3):1303-1316. Doi: 10.1007/s00394-016-1181-5. Epub 2016 Feb 23. PMID: 26907089.

Kubatka P, Uramova S, Kello M, et al. Anticancer activities of thymus vulgaris L. in experimental breast carcinoma in vivo and in vitro. Int J Mol Sci. 2019 Apr 9;20(7):1749. Doi: 10.3390/ijms20071749. PMID: 30970626; PMCID: PMC6479806.

Kubo K, Aoki H, Nanba H. Anti-diabetic activity present in the fruit body of Grifola frondosa (maitake). I. Biol Pharm Bull. 1994 Aug;17(8):1106-10. Doi: 10.1248/bpb.17.1106. PMID: 7820117.

Kuć J. Phytoalexins and disease resistance mechanisms from a perspective of evolution and adaptation. Ciba Found Symp. 1984;102:100-18. Doi: 10.1002/9780470720837.ch7. PMID: 6559110.

Kyrø C, Skeie G, Loft S, et al. Adherence to a healthy Nordic food index is associated with a lower incidence of colorectal cancer in women: the Diet, Cancer and Health cohort study. Br J Nutr. 2013 Mar 14;109(5):920-7. Doi: 10.1017/S0007114512002085. Epub 2012 Jul 3. Erratum in: Br J Nutr. 2014 Feb;111(4):758-9. PMID: 22874538.

Lapidot T, Sirard C, Vormoor J, et al. A cell initiating human acute myeloid leukemia after transplantation into SCID mice. Nature. 1994 Feb 17;367(6464):645-8. Doi: 10.1038/367645a0. PMID: 7509044. [Paper from the Toronto lab that announced the isolation of cancer stem cells.]

Laplane, Lucie. Cancer Stem Cells: Philosophy and Therapies. Cambridge, MA: Harvard University Press, 2016. ISBN-13: 978-0674088740. [How a French philosopher interprets the discovery of cancer stem cells.]

Lasolle H, Schiavo A, Tourneur A, et al. Dual targeting of MAPK and PI3K pathways unlocks redifferentiation of Braf-mutated thyroid cancer organoids. Oncogene. 2024 Jan;43(3):155-170. Doi: 10.1038/s41388-023-02889-y. Epub 2023 Nov 20. PMID: 37985676; PMCID: PMC10786723.

Lauby-Secretan B, Scoccianti C, Loomis D, et al. Body fatness and cancer–Viewpoint of the IARC Working Group. N Engl J Med. 2016 Aug 25;375(8):794-8. Doi: 10.1056/NEJMsr1606602. PMID: 27557308; PMCID: PMC6754861.

Leach DR, Krummel MF, Allison JP. Enhancement of antitumor immunity by CTLA-4 blockade. Science. 1996 Mar 22;271(5256):1734-6. Doi: 10.1126/science.271.5256.1734. PMID: 8596936.

Leacock, Stephen. "The Second Voyage–Stadacona." The Mariner of St. Malo: A Chronicle of the Voyages of Jacques Cartier. Chronicles of Canada, vol. 2. Edited by George M. Wrong and H. H. Langton. Toronto, 1915. [Historically, the very first step in the discovery of vitamin C.]

Lee A, Thurnham DI, Chopra M. Consumption of tomato products with olive oil but not sunflower oil increases the antioxidant activity of plasma. Free Radic Biol Med. 2000 Nov 15;29(10):1051-5. Doi: 10.1016/s0891-5849(00)00440-8. PMID: 11084294.

Lee C, Longo V. Dietary restriction with and without caloric restriction for healthy aging. F1000Res. 2016 Jan 29;5:F1000 Faculty Rev-117. Doi: 10.12688/f1000research.7136.1. PMID: 26918181; PMCID: PMC4755412.

Lee J, Sehrawat A, Singh SV. Withaferin A causes activation of Notch2 and Notch4 in human breast cancer cells. Breast Cancer Res Treat. 2012 Nov;136(1):45-56. Doi: 10.1007/s10549-012-2239-6. Epub 2012 Sep 11. PMID: 22965833; PMCID: PMC3474857.

Lee JH, Khor TO, Shu L, et al. Dietary phytochemicals and cancer prevention: nrf2 signaling, epigenetics, and cell death mechanisms in blocking cancer initiation and progression. Pharmacol Ther. 2013 Feb;137(2):153-71. Doi: 10.1016/j.pharmthera.2012.09.008. Epub 2012 Oct 3. PMID: 23041058; PMCID: PMC3694988.

Lee KA, Luong MK, Shaw H, et al. The gut microbiome: what the oncologist ought to know. Br J Cancer. 2021 Oct;125(9):1197-1209. Doi: 10.1038/s41416-021-01467-x. Epub 2021 Jul 14. PMID: 34262150; PMCID: PMC8548300.

Lee KA, Thomas AM, Bolte LA, et al. Cross-cohort gut microbiome associations with immune checkpoint inhibitor response in advanced melanoma. Nat Med. 2022 Mar;28(3):535-544. Doi: 10.1038/s41591-022-01695-5. Epub 2022 Feb 28. PMID: 35228751; PMCID: PMC8938272.

Lee MJ, Maliakal P, Chen L, et al. Pharmacokinetics of tea catechins after ingestion of green tea and (-)-epigallocatechin-3-gallate by humans: formation of different metabolites and individual variability. Cancer Epidemiol Biomarkers Prev. 2002 Oct;11(10 Pt 1):1025-32. PMID: 12376503.

Lee SH, Cekanova M, Baek SJ. Multiple mechanisms are involved in 6-gingerol-induced cell growth arrest and apoptosis in human colorectal cancer cells. Mol Carcinog. 2008 Mar;47(3):197-208. Doi: 10.1002/mc.20374. PMID: 18058799; PMCID: PMC2430145.

Lee SH, Park S, Blanck HM. Consumption of added sugars by states and factors associated with added sugars intake among US adults in 50 states and the District of Columbia-2010 and 2015. Nutrients. 2023 Jan 11;15(2):357. Doi: 10.3390/nu15020357. PMID: 36678228; PMCID: PMC9863459.

Lee SO, Lee IS. Induction of quinone reductase, the phase 2 anticarcinogenic marker enzyme, in Hepa1c1c7 cells by radish sprouts, Raphanus sativus L. Journal of Food Science, 2006;71(2).S144-S148.

Leigh S. Cancer survivorship: a consumer movement. Semin Oncol. 1994 Dec;21(6):783-6. PMID: 7992094.

León-Muñoz LM, Guallar-Castillón P, Graciani A, et al. Adherence to the Mediterranean diet pattern has declined in Spanish adults. J Nutr. 2012 Oct;142(10):1843-50. Doi: 10.3945/jn.112.164616. Epub 2012 Aug 8. PMID: 22875552.

Levantesi G, Marfisi R, Mozaffarian D, et al. Wine consumption and risk of cardiovascular events after myocardial infarction: results from the GISSI-Prevenzione trial. Int J Cardiol. 2013 Mar 10;163(3):282-287. Doi: 10.1016/j.ijcard.2011.06.053. Epub 2011 Jul 6. PMID: 21737162.

Liang X, Or B, Tsoi MF, et al. Prevalence of metabolic syndrome in the United States National Health and Nutrition Examination Survey 2011-18. Postgrad Med J. 2023 Aug 22;99(1175):985-992. doi: 10.1093/postmj/qgad008. PMID: 36906842.

Liang Z, Lu L, Mao J, et al. Curcumin reversed chronic tobacco smoke exposure induced urocystis EMT and acquisition of cancer stem cells properties via Wnt/β-catenin. Cell Death Dis. 2017 Oct 5;8(10):e3066. Doi: 10.1038/cddis.2017.452. PMID: 28981096; PMCID: PMC5680574.

Liao W, Zhang L, Chen X, et al. Targeting cancer stem cells and signaling pathways through phytochemicals: a promising approach against colorectal cancer. Phytomedicine. 2023 Jan;108:154524. Doi: 10.1016/j.phymed.2022.154524. Epub 2022 Oct 31. PMID: 36375238.

Li C, Du Y, Yang Z, et al. GALNT1-mediated glycosylation and activation of Sonic Hedgehog Signaling maintains the self-renewal and tumor-initiating capacity of bladder cancer stem cells. Cancer Res. 2016 Mar 1;76(5):1273-83. Doi: 10.1158/0008-5472.CAN-15-2309. Epub 2015 Dec 16. PMID: 26676748.

Li C, Heidt DG, Dalerba P, et al. Identification of pancreatic cancer stem cells. Cancer Res. 2007 Feb 1;67(3):1030-7. Doi: 10.1158/0008-5472.CAN-06-2030. PMID: 17283135.

Li C, Wu JJ, Hynes M, et al. c-Met is a marker of pancreatic cancer stem cells and therapeutic target. Gastroenterology. 2011 Dec;141(6):2218-2227.e5. doi: 10.1053/j.gastro.2011.08.009. Epub 2011 Aug 22. PMID: 21864475.

Li E, Zhang T, Sun X, et al. Sonic hedgehog pathway mediates soy isoflavones inhibition of renal cancer stem cells. Oncol Lett. 2019 Sep;18(3):3081-3091. Doi: 10.3892/ol.2019.10657. Epub 2019 July 24. PMID: 31452785; PMCID: PMC6704282.

Liese AD, Krebs-Smith SM, Subar AF, et al. The Dietary Patterns Methods Project: synthesis of findings across cohorts and relevance to dietary guidance. J Nutr. 2015 Mar;145(3):393-402. Doi: 10.3945/jn.114.205336. Epub 2015 Jan 21. PMID: 25733454; PMCID: PMC4336525.

Li J, Liu F, Jiang S, et al. Berberine hydrochloride inhibits cell proliferation and promotes apoptosis of non-small cell lung cancer via the suppression of the MMP2 and Bcl-2/Bax signaling pathways. Oncol Lett. 2018 May;15(5):7409-7414. Doi: 10.3892/ol.2018.8249. Epub 2018 Mar 13. PMID: 29725453; PMCID: PMC5920480.

Li J, Qiu M, Chen L,et al. Resveratrol promotes regression of renal carcinoma cells via a renin-angiotensin system suppression-dependent mechanism. Oncol Lett. 2017 Feb;13(2):613-620. Doi: 10.3892/ol.2016.5519. Epub 2016 Dec 20. PMID: 28356937; PMCID: PMC5351218.

Lind, James. *A Treatise on the Scurvy, in Three Parts. Containing an Inquiry into the Nature, Causes, and Cure, of that Disease. Together with a Critical and Chronological View of What has Been Published on the Subject.* 3rd edition, enlarged and improved. London: S. Crowder, 1772.

Li LW, Na C, Tian SY, et al. Ellagic acid induces HeLa cell apoptosis via regulating signal transducer and activator of transcription 3 signaling. Exp Ther Med. 2018 Jul;16(1):29-36. Doi: 10.3892/etm.2018.6182. Epub 2018 May 17. PMID: 29896225; PMCID: PMC5995030.

Li N, Wu X, Zhuang W, et al. Tomato and lycopene and multiple health outcomes: an umbrella review. Food Chem. 2021 May 1;343:128396. Doi: 10.1016/j.foodchem.2020.128396. Epub 2020 Oct 15. PMID: 33131949.

Lin A, Giuliano CJ, Palladino A, et al. Off-target toxicity is a common mechanism of action of cancer drugs undergoing clinical trials. Sci Transl Med. 2019 Sep 11;11(509):eaaw8412. Doi: 10.1126/scitranslmed.aaw8412. PMID: 31511426; PMCID: PMC7717492. [Study showing that many drugs do not work the way scientists say they do.]

Lin H, de Stanchina E, Zhou XK, et al. Maitake beta-glucan promotes recovery of leukocytes and myeloid cell function in peripheral blood from paclitaxel hematotoxicity. Cancer Immunol Immunother. 2010 Jun;59(6):885-97. Doi: 10.1007/s00262-009-0815-3. Epub 2010 Feb 6. PMID: 20140432; PMCID: PMC3268513.

Lin J, Ding D. The prognostic role of the cancer stem cell marker CD44 in ovarian cancer: a meta-analysis. Cancer Cell Int. 2017 Jan 5;17:8. Doi: 10.1186/s12935-016-0376-4. PMID: 28070170; PMCID: PMC5216581.

Lin JY, Lin YJ, Chen CC, et al. Cardiotoxic protein from edible mushrooms. Nature. 1974 Nov 15;252(5480):235-7. Doi: 10.1038/252235a0. PMID: 4472852.

Lin MG, Liu LP, Li CY, et al. Scutellaria extract decreases the proportion of side population cells in a myeloma cell line by down-regulating the expression of ABCG2 protein. Asian Pac J Cancer Prev. 2013;14(12):7179-86. Doi: 10.7314/apjcp.2013.14.12.7179. PMID: 24460272.

Linnewiel-Hermoni K, Khanin M, Danilenko M, et al. The anti-cancer effects of carotenoids and other phytonutrients reside in their combined activity. Arch Biochem Biophys. 2015 Apr 15;572:28-35. Doi: 10.1016/j.abb.2015.02.018. Epub 2015 Feb 21. PMID: 25711533.

Li Q. Effects of forest environment (Shinrin-yoku/forest bathing) on health promotion and disease prevention -the establishment of "forest medicine." Environ Health Prev Med. 2022;27:43. Doi: 10.1265/ehpm.22-00160. PMID: 36328581; PMCID: PMC9665958.

Liskova A, Kubatka P, Samec M, et al. Dietary phytochemicals targeting cancer stem cells. Molecules. 2019 Mar 4;24(5):899. Doi: 10.3390/molecules24050899. PMID: 30836718; PMCID: PMC6429493.

Liu GH, Yao ZQ, Chen GQ, Li YL, Liang B. Potential benefits of green tea in prostate cancer prevention and treatment: a comprehensive review. Chin J Integr Med. 2024 Apr 2. Doi: 10.1007/s11655-024-4100-2. Epub ahead of print. PMID: 38561489.

Liu K, Sun Q, Liu Q, et al. Focus on immune checkpoint PD-1/PD-L1 pathway: new advances of polyphenol phytochemicals in tumor immunotherapy. Biomed Pharmacother.

2022 Oct;154:113618. Doi: 10.1016/j.biopha.2022.113618. Epub 2022 Aug 30. PMID: 36055113.

Liu L, Lim MA, Jung SN, et al. The effect of curcumin on multi-level immune checkpoint blockade and T cell dysfunction in head and neck cancer. Phytomedicine. 2021 Nov;92:153758. Doi: 10.1016/j.phymed.2021.153758. Epub 2021 Sep 16. PMID: 34592487.

Liu N, Zou S, Xie C, et al. Effect of the β-glucan from Lentinus edodes on colitis-associated colorectal cancer and gut microbiota. Carbohydr Polym. 2023 Sep 15;316:121069. Doi: 10.1016/j.carbpol.2023.121069. Epub 2023 May 26. PMID: 37321711.

Liu RH. Health benefits of fruit and vegetables are from additive and synergistic combinations of phytochemicals. Am J Clin Nutr. 2003 Sep;78(3 Suppl):517S-520S. doi: 10.1093/ajcn/78.3.517S. PMID: 12936943.

Liu RH. Health-promoting components of fruits and vegetables in the diet. Adv Nutr. 2013 May 1;4(3):384S-92S. doi: 10.3945/an.112.003517. PMID: 23674808; PMCID: PMC3650511.

Liu X, Qi M, Li X, et al. Curcumin: a natural organic component that plays a multi-faceted role in ovarian cancer. J Ovarian Res. 2023 Mar 1;16(1):47. Doi: 10.1186/s13048-023-01120-6. PMID: 36859398; PMCID: PMC9976389.

Liu Y, Liu X, Zhang N, et al. Berberine diminishes cancer cell PD-L1 expression and facilitates antitumor immunity via inhibiting the deubiquitination activity of CSN5. Acta Pharm Sin B. 2020 Dec;10(12):2299-2312. Doi: 10.1016/j.apsb.2020.06.014. Epub 2020 June 30. PMID: 33354502; PMCID: PMC7745128.

Liu Y, Yao Y, Zhang Y, et al. Identification of prognostic stemness-related genes in kidney renal papillary cell carcinoma. BMC Med Genomics. 2024 May 3;17(1):121. Doi: 10.1186/s12920-024-01870-2. PMID: 38702698.

Li WQ, Zhang JY, Ma JL, et al. Effects of Helicobacter pylori treatment and vitamin and garlic supplementation on gastric cancer incidence and mortality: follow-up of a randomized intervention trial. BMJ. 2019 Sep 11;366:l5016. Doi: 10.1136/bmj.l5016. PMID: 31511230; PMCID: PMC6737461.

Li X, Meng Y, Xie C, et al. Diallyl trisulfide inhibits breast cancer stem cells via suppression of Wnt/β-catenin pathway. J Cell Biochem. 2018 May;119(5):4134-4141. Doi: 10.1002/jcb.26613. Epub 2018 Jan 22. PMID: 29243835.

Li X, Zhou N, Wang J, et al. Quercetin suppresses breast cancer stem cells (CD44+/CD24-) by inhibiting the PI3K/Akt/mTOR-signaling pathway. Life Sci. 2018 Mar 1;196:56-62. Doi: 10.1016/j.lfs.2018.01.014. Epub 2018 Jan 21. PMID: 29355544.

Li XX, Liu C, Dong SL, et al Anticarcinogenic potentials of tea catechins. Front Nutr. 2022 Dec 5;9:1060783. Doi: 10.3389/fnut.2022.1060783. PMID: 36545470; PMCID: PMC9760998.

Li Y, Hu Y, Yang L, et al. Luteolin directly binds to KDM4C and attenuates ovarian cancer stemness via epigenetic suppression of PPP2CA/YAP axis. Biomed Pharmacother. 2023 Apr;160:114350. Doi: 10.1016/j.biopha.2023.114350. Epub 2023 Feb 16. PMID: 36804120.

Li Y, Wicha MS, Schwartz SJ, et al. Implications of cancer stem cell theory for cancer chemoprevention by natural dietary compounds. J Nutr Biochem. 2011 Sep;22(9):799-806. Doi: 10.1016/j.jnutbio.2010.11.001. Epub 2011 Feb 4. PMID: 21295962; PMCID: PMC3248810.

Li Y, Zhang T, Korkaya H, et al. Sulforaphane, a dietary component of broccoli/broccoli sprouts, inhibits breast cancer stem cells. Clin Cancer Res. 2010 May 1;16(9):2580-90. Doi: 10.1158/1078-0432.CCR-09-2937. Epub 2010 Apr 13. PMID: 20388854; PMCID: PMC2862133.

Li Y, Zhang T. Targeting cancer stem cells with sulforaphane, a dietary component from broccoli and broccoli sprouts. Future Oncol. 2013 Aug;9(8):1097-103. Doi: 10.2217/fon.13.108. PMID: 23902242.

Li Z, Wang H, Wang Y, et al. Luteolin inhibits the TGF-β signaling pathway to overcome bortezomib resistance in multiple myeloma. Cancer Lett. 2023 Feb 1;554:216019. Doi: 10.1016/j.canlet.2022.216019. Epub 2022 Nov 26. PMID: 36442773.

Lo-Coco F, Avvisati G, Vignetti M, et al. Retinoic acid and arsenic trioxide for acute promyelocytic leukemia. N Engl J Med. 2013 Jul 11;369(2):111-21. Doi: 10.1056/NEJMoa1300874. PMID: 23841729.

Long J, Ji Z, Yuan P, et al. Nut consumption and risk of cancer: a meta-analysis of prospective studies. Cancer Epidemiol Biomarkers Prev. 2020 Mar;29(3):565-573. Doi: 10.1158/1055-9965.EPI-19-1167. Epub 2020 Feb 10. PMID: 32041895.

Longo VD, Mattson MP. Fasting: molecular mechanisms and clinical applications. Cell Metab. 2014 Feb 4;19(2):181-92. Doi: 10.1016/j.cmet.2013.12.008. Epub 2014 Jan 16. PMID: 24440038; PMCID: PMC3946160.

Longo VD, Panda S. Fasting, circadian rhythms, and time-restricted feeding in healthy lifespan. Cell Metab. 2016 Jun 14;23(6):1048-1059. Doi: 10.1016/j.cmet.2016.06.001. PMID: 27304506; PMCID: PMC5388543.

Loomis D, Guyton KZ, International Agency for Research on Cancer Monograph Working Group, et al. Carcinogenicity of drinking coffee, mate, and very hot beverages. Lancet Oncol. 2016 Jul;17(7):877-878. Doi: 10.1016/S1470-2045(16)30239-X. Epub 2016 Jun 15. PMID: 27318851

Lopéz, Ana M. Fast-casual restaurants' revenue in Spain 2015-2022, August 15, 2023. Accessed February 10, 2024.

Lowe L, LaValley JW, Felsher DW. Tackling heterogeneity in treatment-resistant breast cancer using a broad-spectrum therapeutic approach. Cancer Drug Resist. 2022 Oct 12;5(4):917-925. Doi: 10.20517/cdr.2022.40. PMID: 36627896; PMCID: PMC9771755.

Low SA, Vogel S. Direct and intermediated marketing of local foods in the United States, ERR-128, U.S. Department of Agriculture, Economic Research Service, November 2011.

Luce, Henry R. A Letter from the publisher. Time, December 14, 1962. Retrieved January 22, 2024.

Luo J, Hendryx M, Manson JE, et al. Intentional weight loss and obesity-related cancer risk. JNCI Cancer Spectrum. 2019 Aug 9;3(4):pkz054. Doi: 10.1093/jncics/pkz054. PMID: 31737862; PMCID: PMC6795232.

Luo L, Lin C, Wang P, et al. Combined use of immune checkpoint inhibitors and phytochemicals as a novel therapeutic strategy against cancer. J Cancer. 2023 July 24;14(12):2315-2328. Doi: 10.7150/jca.85966. PMID: 37576404; PMCID: PMC10414047.

Luo Y, Shang P, Li D. Luteolin: a flavonoid that has multiple cardio-protective effects and its molecular mechanisms. Front Pharmacol. 2017 Oct 6;8:692. Doi: 10.3389/fphar.2017.00692. PMID: 29056912; PMCID: PMC5635727.

Lustig, Robert H. Sugar: The Bitter Truth. An official University of California (UCSF) video, Show ID: 16717, recorded on May 26, 2009. Accessed April 1, 2024. [Lustig is UCSF professor of pediatric endocrinology. This YouTube video has had over 24 million views.]

Lv Y, Liu Z, Jia H, et al. Properties of flavonoids in the treatment of bladder cancer (Review). Exp Ther Med. 2022 Sep 19;24(5):676. Doi: 10.3892/etm.2022.11612. PMID: 36185766; PMCID: PMC9522619.

Lyu C, Wang L, Stadlbauer B, et al. Identification of EZH2 as Cancer stem cell marker in clear cell renal cell carcinoma and the anti-tumor effect of epigallocatechin-3-gallate (EGCG). Cancers (Basel). 2022 Aug 30;14(17):4200. Doi: 10.3390/cancers14174200. PMID: 36077742; PMCID: PMC9454898.

Macrae F. Epidemiology and risk factors for colorectal cancer. UpToDate. Philadelphia: Wolters Kluwer, updated March 18, 2024. Accessed April 2, 2024. [Subscription required].

Maeda N, Matsubara K, Yoshida H, et al. Anti-cancer effect of spinach glycoglycerolipids as angiogenesis inhibitors based on the selective inhibition of DNA polymerase activity. Mini Rev Med Chem. 2011 Jan;11(1):32-8. Doi: 10.2174/138955711793564042. PMID: 21034405.

Ma H, Wang X, Li X, et al. Food insecurity and premature mortality and life expectancy in the US. JAMA Intern Med. 2024 Mar 1;184(3):301-310. Doi: 10.1001/jamainternmed.2023.7968. PMID: 38285593; PMCID: PMC10825785.

Mahn A, Pérez CE, Zambrano V, et al. Maximization of sulforaphane content in broccoli sprouts by blanching. Foods. 2022 Jun 27;11(13):1906. Doi: 10.3390/foods11131906. PMID: 35804720; PMCID: PMC9266238. [**Soaking broccoli sprouts in 60º-70º Celsius water for 3 minutes increases sulforaphane content.**]

Makhov P, Golovine K, Canter D, et al. Co-administration of piperine and docetaxel results in improved anti-tumor efficacy via inhibition of CYP3A4 activity. Prostate. 2012 May 1;72(6):661-7. Doi: 10.1002/pros.21469. Epub 2011 Jul 27. PMID: 21796656; PMCID: PMC3208085.

Mancebo-Campos V, Salvador MD, Fregapane G. EFSA Health Claims-Based Virgin Olive Oil Shelf-Life. Antioxidants (Basel). 2023 Aug 4;12(8):1563. Doi: 10.3390/antiox12081563. PMID: 37627558; PMCID: PMC10452016.

Manocha A, Brockton NT, Cook L, et al. Low serum vitamin D associated with increased tumor size and higher grade in premenopausal Canadian women with breast cancer. Clin Breast Cancer. 2023 Aug;23(6):e368-e376. Doi: 10.1016/j.clbc.2023.06.003. Epub 2023 Jun 14. PMID: 37357130.

Mantovani A, Allavena P, Sica A, et al. Cancer-related inflammation. Nature. 2008 Jul 24;454(7203):436-44. Doi: 10.1038/nature07205. PMID: 18650914.

Mao GX, Cao YB, Lan XG, et al. Therapeutic effect of forest bathing on human hypertension in the elderly. J Cardiol. 2012 Dec;60(6):495-502. Doi: 10.1016/j.jjcc.2012.08.003. Epub 2012 Sep 1. PMID: 22948092.

Marinac CR, Nelson SH, Breen CI, et al. Prolonged nightly fasting and breast cancer prognosis. JAMA Oncol. 2016 Aug 1;2(8):1049-55. Doi: 10.1001/jamaoncol.2016.0164. PMID: 27032109; PMCID: PMC4982776. [**Prolonging the nightly fast to at least 13 hours is associated with fewer breast cancer recurrences.**]

Markowiak P, Śliżewska K. Effects of probiotics, prebiotics, and synbiotics on human health. Nutrients. 2017 Sep 15;9(9):1021. Doi: 10.3390/nu9091021. PMID: 28914794; PMCID: PMC5622781.

Marshall, Michael. We're finally working out why the Mediterranean diet is so good for us. New Scientist, January 9, 2024. Accessed March 19, 2024.

Martínez-González MA, Gea A, Ruiz-Canela M. The Mediterranean diet and cardiovascular health. Circ Res. 2019 Mar;124(5):779-798. Doi: 10.1161/CIRCRESAHA.118.313348. PMID: 30817261.

Martínez-González MA, Salas-Salvadó J, Estruch R, et al. Benefits of the Mediterranean diet: insights from the PREDIMED study. Prog Cardiovasc Dis. 2015 Jul-Aug;58(1):50-60. Doi: 10.1016/j.pcad.2015.04.003. Epub 2015 May 1. PMID: 25940230.

Martin KR, Brophy SK. Commonly consumed and specialty dietary mushrooms reduce cellular proliferation in MCF-7 human breast cancer cells. Exp Biol Med (Maywood). 2010 Nov;235(11):1306-14. Doi: 10.1258/ebm.2010.010113. Epub 2010 Oct 4. PMID: 20921274.

Matson V, Fessler J, Bao R, et al. The commensal microbiome is associated with anti-PD-1 efficacy in metastatic melanoma patients. Science. 2018 Jan 5;359(6371):104-108. Doi: 10.1126/science.aao3290. PMID: 29302014; PMCID: PMC6707353.

Matthewman C, Krishnakumar IM, Swick AG. Review: bioavailability and efficacy of 'free' curcuminoids from curcumagalactomannoside (CGM) curcumin formulation. *Nutrition Research Reviews.* 2023:1-18. Doi:10.1017/S0954422423000033.

Matusheski NV, Jeffery EH. Comparison of the bioactivity of two glucoraphanin hydrolysis products found in broccoli, sulforaphane and sulforaphane nitrile. J Agric Food Chem. 2001 Dec;49(12):5743-9. Doi: 10.1021/jf010809a. PMID: 11743757.

Matusheski NV, Juvik JA, Jeffery EH. Heating decreases epithiospecifier protein activity and increases sulforaphane formation in broccoli. Phytochemistry. 2004 May;65(9):1273-81. Doi: 10.1016/j.phytochem.2004.04.013. PMID: 15184012.

Ma X, Zhou J, Zhang CX, et al. Modulation of drug-resistant membrane and apoptosis proteins of breast cancer stem cells by targeting berberine liposomes. Biomaterials. 2013 June;34(18):4452-65. Doi: 10.1016/j.biomaterials.2013.02.066. Epub 2013 Mar 18. PMID: 23518403.

Mayo Clinic. Cancer causes: Popular myths about the causes of cancer. Website, Accessed March 24, 2024.

McCulloch EA, Till JE. Regulatory mechanisms acting on hematopoietic stem cells: some clinical implications. Am J Pathol. 1971 Dec;65(3):601-19. PMID: 4941070; PMCID: PMC2047583.

Meerson A, Khatib S, Mahajna J. Natural products targeting cancer stem cells for augmenting cancer therapeutics. Int J Mol Sci. 2021 Dec 2;22(23):13044. Doi: 10.3390/ijms222313044. PMID: 34884848; PMCID: PMC8657727.

Mekkawy SA, Abdalla MS, Omran MM, et al. Cancer stem cells as a prognostic biomarker and therapeutic target using curcumin/ piperine extract for multiple myeloma. Asian Pac J Cancer Prev. 2022 Oct 1;23(10):3507-3515. Doi: 10.31557/APJCP.2022.23.10.3507. PMID: 36308377; PMCID: PMC9924316.

Méndez-del Villar M, González-Ortiz M, Martínez-Abundis E, et al. Effect of resveratrol administration on metabolic syndrome, insulin sensitivity, and insulin secretion. Metab Syndr Relat Disord. 2014 Dec;12(10):497-501. Doi: 10.1089/met.2014.0082. Epub 2014 Aug 19. PMID: 25137036.

Meng S, Zhu Y, Li JF, et al. Apigenin inhibits renal cell carcinoma cell proliferation. Oncotarget. 2017 Mar 21;8(12):19834-19842. Doi: 10.18632/oncotarget.15771. PMID: 28423637; PMCID: PMC5386726.

Messina M. Insights gained from 20 years of soy research. J Nutr. 2010 Dec;140(12):2289S-2295S. doi: 10.3945/jn.110.124107. Epub 2010 Oct 27. PMID: 20980639.

Messina M. Soy and health update: evaluation of the clinical and epidemiologic literature. Nutrients. 2016 Nov 24;8(12):754. Doi: 10.3390/nu8120754. PMID: 27886135; PMCID: PMC5188409.

Metchnikoff, Elie. *The Prolongation of Life: Optimistic Studies.* English translation by P. Chalmers Mitchell. New York: Putnam and Sons, 1908. **[A foundational work on the relationship of the gut microbiome to longevity and health.]**

Michie S, Abraham C, Whittington C, et al. Effective techniques in healthy eating and physical activity interventions: a meta-regression. Health Psychol. 2009 Nov;28(6):690-701. Doi: 10.1037/a0016136. PMID: 19916637.

Milner CE, Cote KA. Benefits of napping in healthy adults: impact of nap length, time of day, age, and experience with napping. J Sleep Res. 2009 Jun;18(2):272-81. Doi: 10.1111/j.1365-2869.2008.00718.x. PMID: 19645971.

Mogg, Katie. Why one particular diet is found to be the best year after year. NBC News website. January 28, 2024. Accessed March 31, 2024.

Mohos V, Fliszár-Nyúl E, Ungvári O, et al. Inhibitory effects of quercetin and its main methyl, sulfate, and glucuronic acid conjugates on cytochrome P450 enzymes, and on OATP, BCRP and MRP2 transporters. Nutrients. 2020 Jul 31;12(8):2306. doi: 10.3390/nu12082306. PMID: 32751996; PMCID: PMC7468908.

Moon DO. Curcumin in cancer and inflammation: an in-depth exploration of molecular interactions, therapeutic potentials, and the role in disease management. Int J Mol Sci. 2024 Mar 2;25(5):2911. Doi: 10.3390/ijms25052911. PMID: 38474160; PMCID: PMC10932100.

Moore J, Yousef M, Tsiani E. Anticancer effects of rosemary (Rosmarinus officinalis L.) extract and rosemary extract polyphenols. Nutrients. 2016 Nov 17;8(11):731. Doi: 10.3390/nu8110731. PMID: 27869665; PMCID: PMC5133115.

Morré DJ, Hostetler B, Taggart DJ, et al. ENOX2-based early detection (ONCOblot) of asbestos-induced malignant mesothelioma 4-10 years in advance of clinical symptoms. Clin Proteomics. 2016 Jan 22;13:2. Doi: 10.1186/s12014-016-9103-3. Erratum in: Clin Proteomics. 2016;13:3. PMID: 26807072; PMCID: PMC4724078.

Morré DM, Morré DJ. Catechin-vanilloid synergies with potential clinical applications in cancer. Rejuvenation Res. 2006 Spring;9(1):45-55. Doi: 10.1089/rej.2006.9.45. PMID: 16608395. **[How and why green tea and guajillo peppers have a synergistic effect.]**

Morris JN. Exercise in the prevention of coronary heart disease: today's best buy in public health. Med Sci Sports Exerc. 1994 Jul;26(7):807-14. PMID: 7934752.

Morze J, Danielewicz A, Hoffmann G, et al. Diet quality as assessed by the healthy eating index, alternate healthy eating index, dietary approaches to stop hypertension score, and health outcomes: a second update of a systematic review and meta-analysis of cohort studies. J Acad Nutr Diet. 2020 Dec;120(12):1998-2031.e15. doi: 10.1016/j.jand.2020.08.076. Epub 2020 Oct 14. PMID: 33067162.

Morze J, Danielewicz A, Przybyłowicz K, et al. An updated systematic review and meta-analysis on adherence to Mediterranean diet and risk of cancer. Eur J Nutr. 2021 Apr;60(3):1561-1586. Doi: 10.1007/s00394-020-02346-6. Epub 2020 Aug 8. PMID: 32770356; PMCID: PMC7987633.

Moselhy J, Srinivasan S, Ankem MK, Damodaran C. Natural products that target cancer stem cells. Anticancer Res. 2015 Nov;35(11):5773-88. PMID: 26503998; PMCID: PMC7523548.

Moss, Jacob (director). *Immunotherapy: The Battle Within*. Documentary film, 2020. Accessed November 7, 2023. **[This documentary, produced by *The Moss Report*, won a Colorado International Activism Film Festival award as an Official Selection in The Big Apple Film Festival.]**

Moss RW. Should patients undergoing chemotherapy and radiotherapy be prescribed antioxidants? Integr Cancer Ther. 2006 Mar;5(1):63-82. Doi: 10.1177/1534735405285882. PMID: 16484715. **[My contribution to the "concurrent usage debate" of antioxidants and conventional oncology.]**

Moustafa EM, Abdel Salam HS, Mansour SZ. Withania somnifera modulates radiation-induced generation of lung cancer stem cells via restraining the hedgehog signaling factors. Dose Response. 2022 Feb 24;20(1):15593258221076711. Doi: 10.1177/15593258221076711. PMID: 35250409; PMCID: PMC8891860.

Mozaffarian D. Dietary and policy priorities for cardiovascular disease, diabetes, and obesity: a comprehensive review. Circulation. 2016 Jan 12;133(2):187-225. Doi: 10.1161/CIRCULATIONAHA.115.018585. PMID: 26746178; PMCID: PMC4814348.

Mukherjee, Siddharta. *The Emperor of All Maladies*. New York: Charles Scribner's Sons, 2010. **[This history of the war on cancer by a prominent New York oncologist won a Pulitzer Prize.]**

Mukherjee, Siddhartha. The cancer sleeper cell [also titled The riddle of cancer relapse]. New York Times, Sunday, October 29, 2010, p. 40. [Subscription required.]

Mumtaz S, Ali S, Khan R, et al Therapeutic role of garlic and vitamins C and E against toxicity induced by lead on various organs. Environ Sci Pollut Res Int. 2020 Mar;27(9):8953-8964. Doi: 10.1007/s11356-020-07654-2. Epub 2020 Feb 8. PMID: 32036533.

Naasani I, Oh-Hashi F, Oh-Hara T, et al. Blocking telomerase by dietary polyphenols is a major mechanism for limiting the growth of human cancer cells in vitro and in vivo. Cancer Res. 2003 Feb 15;63(4):824-30. PMID: 12591733.

Nahin RL, Rhee A, Stussman B. Use of complementary health approaches overall and for pain management by US adults. JAMA. 2024 Jan 25:e2326775. Doi: 10.1001/jama.2023.26775. Epub ahead of print. PMID: 38270938; PMCID: PMC10811586.

Nair MP, Kandaswami C, Mahajan S, et al. The flavonoid, quercetin, differentially regulates Th-1 (IFNgamma) and Th-2 (IL4) cytokine gene expression by normal peripheral blood mononuclear cells. Biochim Biophys Acta. 2002 Dec 16;1593(1):29-36. Doi: 10.1016/s0167-4889(02)00328-2. PMID: 12431781.

Nakano H, Namatame K, Nemoto H, et al. A multi-institutional prospective study of lentinan in advanced gastric cancer patients with unresectable and recurrent diseases: effect on prolongation of survival and improvement of quality of life. Kanagawa Lentinan Research Group. Hepatogastroenterology. 1999 Jul-Aug;46(28):2662-8. PMID: 10522061.

National Cancer Institute [NCI]. Cell metabolism and cancer. Accessed November 30, 2023.

National Cancer Institute [NCI]. Common Terminology Criteria for Adverse Events (CTCAE) Version 5.0, published November 27, 2017. Accessed November 11, 2023.**[A classic ranking of cancer drug side effects.]**

National Cancer Institute [NCI]. Genetic Testing Fact Sheet – NCI Cancer.gov. Accessed September 23, 2023. [Designated NCI 2023b]

National Cancer Institute [NCI]. The Mediterranean eating plan: "The Program." Evidence Based Cancer Control Programs. March 29, 2023. Accessed March 14, 2024. [designated 2023a]

National Center for Complementary and Integrative Health [NCCIH]. NIH analysis reveals a significant rise in use of complementary health approaches, especially for pain management. News release, January 31, 2024. Accessed February 2, 2024. **[The NCCIH is the former Office of Alternative Medicine.]**

National Institutes of Health [NIH]. Cancer trends progress report 2022 update. Accessed November 8, 2023.

National Oceanic and Atmospheric Administration [NOAA]. Office of General Counsel: International Section. Cross cutting issues: Precautionary approach, updated March 22, 2024.

NatMED PRO. A TRC Healthcare brand. 1,400+ comprehensive monographs on natural medicine products. Accessed January 17, 2024. [Subscription required.]

Nature Medical. FAQs about POMI-T. 2016. Accessed March 9, 2024.

Naujokat C, McKee DL. The "Big Five" phytochemicals targeting cancer stem cells: curcumin, EGCG, sulforaphane, resveratrol and soy isoflavones. Curr Med Chem. 2021;28(22):4321-4342. Doi: 10.2174/0929867327666200228110738. PMID: 32107991. **[A** fine summary from two integrative oncologists of the relationship between five plant chemicals and CSCs.]

Nautiyal J, Kanwar SS, Yu Y, et al. Combination of dasatinib and curcumin eliminates chemo-resistant colon cancer cells. J Mol Signal. 2011 Jul 20;6:7. Doi: 10.1186/1750-2187-6-7. PMID: 21774804; PMCID: PMC3162943.

Naveen CR, Gaikwad S, Agrawal-Rajput R. Berberine induces neuronal differentiation through inhibition of cancer stemness and epithelial-mesenchymal transition in neuroblastoma cells. Phytomedicine. 2016 Jun 15;23(7):736-44. Doi: 10.1016/j.phymed.2016.03.013. Epub 2016 Apr 13. PMID: 27235712.

Nazemi A, Huang WC, Wysock J, et al. A prospective pilot study investigating performance of 18F-fluciclovine PET imaging for detection of prostate cancer 2 years following primary partial gland cryoablation. Nucl Med Mol Imaging. 2022 Aug;56(4):196-201. Doi: 10.1007/s13139-022-00755-5. Epub 2022 Jun 21. PMID: 35846414; PMCID: PMC9276896.

NCD Risk Factor Collaboration (NCD-RisC). Worldwide trends in underweight and obesity from 1990 to 2022: a pooled analysis of 3663 population-representative studies with 222 million children, adolescents, and adults. Lancet. 2024 Mar 16;403(10431):1027-1050. Doi: 10.1016/S0140-6736(23)02750-2. Epub 2024 Feb 29. PMID: 38432237; PMCID: PMC7615769.

Nechuta SJ, Caan BJ, Chen WY, et al. Soy food intake after diagnosis of breast cancer and survival: an in-depth analysis of combined evidence from cohort studies of U.S. and Chinese women. Am J Clin Nutr. 2012 Jul;96(1):123-32. Doi: 10.3945/ajcn.112.035972. Epub 2012 May 30. PMID: 22648714; PMCID: PMC3374736.

Neetha MC, Panchaksharappa MG, Pattabhiramasastry S, et al. Chemopreventive synergism between green tea extract and curcumin in patients with potentially malignant oral disorders: a double-blind, randomized preliminary study. J Contemp Dent Pract. 2020 May 1;21(5):521-531. PMID: 32690834.

Ng TB. A review of research on the protein-bound polysaccharide (polysaccharopeptide, PSP) from the mushroom Coriolus versicolor (Basidiomycetes: Polyporaceae). Gen Pharmacol. 1998 Jan;30(1):1-4. Doi: 10.1016/s0306-3623(97)00076-1. PMID: 9457474.

Nguyen MM, Karboune S. Combinatorial interactions of essential oils enriched with individual polyphenols, polyphenol mixes, and plant extracts: multi-antioxidant systems. Antioxidants (Basel). 2023 Feb 15;12(2):486. Doi: 10.3390/antiox12020486. PMID: 36830046; PMCID: PMC9952583.

Niedzwiecki A, Roomi MW, Kalinovsky T, et al. Anticancer efficacy of polyphenols and their combinations. Nutrients. 2016 Sep 9;8(9):552. Doi: 10.3390/nu8090552. PMID: 27618095; PMCID: PMC5037537.

Nijveldt RJ, van Nood E, van Hoorn DE, et al. Flavonoids: a review of probable mechanisms of action and potential applications. Am J Clin Nutr. 2001 Oct;74(4):418-25. Doi: 10.1093/ajcn/74.4.418. PMID: 11566638.

Nimee F, Gioxari A, Papandreou P, et al. The effect of melatonin supplementation on cancer-related fatigue during chemotherapy treatment of breast cancer patients: adouble-blind, randomized controlled study. Cancers (Basel). 2024 Feb 16;16(4):802. Doi: 10.3390/cancers16040802. PMID: 38398193; PMCID: PMC10887218.

Nobel Foundation. Nobel Lectures, Physiology or Medicine 1922-1941. Otto Warburg. Amsterdam: Elsevier Publishing Company, 1965. Accessed online on December 1, 2023.

Norouzkhani N, Karimi AG, Badami N, et al. From kitchen to clinic: pharmacotherapeutic potential of common spices in Indian cooking in age-related neurological disorders. Front Pharmacol. 2022 Nov 10;13:960037. Doi: 10.3389/fphar.2022.960037. PMID: 36438833; PMCID: PMC9685814.

NYAS [New York Academy of Sciences]. Cancer prevention: from the laboratory to the clinic: implications of genetic, molecular, and preventive research. Proceedings of an international conference. New York City, New York, USA. September 22-24, 1994. Ann N Y Acad Sci. 1995 Sep 30;768:1-342. PMID: 9729205.[**The conference at which Prof. Nanba introduced maitake D-Fraction to the U.S.**]

O'Brien CA, Pollett A, Gallinger S, et al. A human colon cancer cell capable of initiating tumor growth in immunodeficient mice. Nature. 2007 Jan 4;445(7123):106-10. Doi: 10.1038/nature05372. Epub 2006 Nov 19. PMID: 17122772. [**Discovery of CSCs in colorectal cancer.**]

O'Hare, TJ, Williams, DJ, Zhang B, et al. Radish sprouts versus broccoli sprouts: a comparison of anti-cancer potential based on glucosinolate breakdown products. Acta Hortic. 2009;841,187-192. DOI: 10.17660/ActaHortic.2009.841.21 [**A detailed explanation of how and why radish sprouts are superior to broccoli sprouts.**]

O'Hare TJ, Wong LS, Force LE, et al. Glucosinolate composition and anti-cancer potential of daikon and radish sprouts. Acta Hortic. 2008;765: 237-244. DOI: 10.17660/ActaHortic.2008.765.29.

Obolskiy D, Pischel I, Siriwatanametanon N, et al. Garcinia mangostana L.: a phytochemical and pharmacological review. Phytother Res. 2009 Aug;23(8):1047-65. Doi: 10.1002/ptr.2730. PMID: 19172667.

Olvera-Sandoval C, Fabela-Illescas HE, Fernández-Martínez E, et al. Potential mechanisms of the improvement of glucose homeostasis in Type 2 diabetes by pomegranate juice. Antioxidants (Basel). 2022 Mar 15;11(3):553. Doi: 10.3390/antiox11030553. PMID: 35326203; PMCID: PMC8945221.

Otto C, Kaemmerer U, Illert B, et al. Growth of human gastric cancer cells in nude mice is delayed by a ketogenic diet supplemented with omega-3 fatty acids and medium-chain triglycerides. BMC Cancer. 2008 Apr 30;8:122. Doi: 10.1186/1471-2407-8-122. PMID: 18447912; PMCID: PMC2408928.

O'Hare, TJ. Personal communications, April 18, 2024.

Padayatty SJ, Sun H, Wang Y, et al. Vitamin C pharmacokinetics: implications for oral and intravenous use. Ann Intern Med. 2004;140:533-537. [The NIH study that helped reverse the negative verdict on vitamin C.]

Paget S. The distribution of secondary growths in cancer of the breast [1889]. Reprinted in Cancer Metastasis Rev. 1989 Aug;8(2):98-101. PMID: 2673568.

Pallav K, Dowd SE, Villafuerte J, et al. Effects of polysaccharopeptide from Trametes versicolor and amoxicillin on the gut microbiome of healthy volunteers: a randomized clinical trial. Gut Microbes. 2014 Jul 1;5(4):458-67. Doi: 10.4161/gmic.29558. Epub 2014 Jul 9. PMID: 25006989.

Paller CJ, Pantuck A, Carducci MA. A review of pomegranate in prostate cancer. Prostate Cancer Prostatic Dis. 2017 Sep;20(3):265-270. Doi: 10.1038/pcan.2017.19. Epub 2017 Apr 25. PMID: 28440320; PMCID: PMC5555799.

Paller CJ, Ye X, Wozniak PJ, et al. A randomized phase II study of pomegranate extract for men with rising PSA following initial therapy for localized prostate cancer. Prostate Cancer Prostatic Dis. 2013 Mar;16(1):50-5. Doi: 10.1038/pcan.2012.20. Epub 2012 Jun 12. PMID: 22689129; PMCID: PMC3549301.

Palozza P, Colangelo M, Simone R, et al. Lycopene induces cell growth inhibition by altering mevalonate pathway and Ras signaling in cancer cell lines. Carcinogenesis. 2010 Oct;31(10):1813-21. Doi: 10.1093/carcin/bgq157. Epub 2010 Aug 10. PMID: 20699249.

Pandey KB, Rizvi SI. Plant polyphenols as dietary antioxidants in human health and disease. Oxid Med Cell Longev. 2009 Nov-Dec;2(5):270-8. Doi: 10.4161/oxim.2.5.9498. PMID: 20716914; PMCID: PMC2835915.

Pandey KR, Naik SR, Vakil BV. Probiotics, prebiotics and synbiotics- a review. J Food Sci Technol. 2015 Dec;52(12):7577-87. Doi: 10.1007/s13197-015-1921-1. Epub 2015 Jul 22. PMID: 26604335; PMCID: PMC4648921.

Pandey PR, Okuda H, Watabe M, et al. Resveratrol suppresses growth of cancer stem-like cells by inhibiting fatty acid synthase. Breast Cancer Res Treat. 2011 Nov;130(2):387-98. Doi: 10.1007/s10549-010-1300-6. Epub 2010 Dec 29. PMID: 21188630; PMCID: PMC3404809.

Pan H, Zhou W, He W, et al. Soy isoflavones inhibits MDA-MB-231 triple-negative breast cancer cell growth by inhibiting NF-κB activity via the Notch-1 pathway. Int J Mol Med. 2012 Aug;30(2):337-43. Doi: 10.3892/ijmm.2012.990. Epub 2012 May 9. PMID: 22580499.

Pan L, Sha J, Lin W, et al. Curcumin inhibits prostate cancer progression by regulating the miR-30a-5p/PCLAF axis. Exp Ther Med. 2021 Sep;22(3):969. Doi: 10.3892/etm.2021.10401. Epub 2021 Jul 7. PMID: 34335911; PMCID: PMC8290411.

Pan MH, Hsieh MC, Kuo JM, et al. 6-Shogaol induces apoptosis in human colorectal carcinoma cells via ROS production, caspase activation, and GADD 153 expression. Mol Nutr Food Res. 2008 May;52(5):527-37. Doi: 10.1002/mnfr.200700157. PMID: 18384088.

Pan MH, Lai CS, Ho CT. Anti-inflammatory activity of natural dietary flavonoids. Food Funct. 2010 Oct;1(1):15-31. Doi: 10.1039/c0fo00103a. Epub 2010 Sep 13. PMID: 21776454.

Pantuck AJ, Leppert JT, Zomorodian N, et al. Phase II study of pomegranate juice for men with rising prostate-specific antigen following surgery or radiation for prostate cancer. Clin Cancer Res. 2006 Jul 1;12(13):4018-26. Doi: 10.1158/1078-0432.CCR-05-2290. PMID: 16818701.

Parkinson L, Keast R. Oleocanthal, a phenolic derived from virgin olive oil: a review of the beneficial effects on inflammatory disease. Int J Mol Sci. 2014 Jul 11;15(7):12323-34. doi: 10.3390/ijms150712323. PMID: 25019344; PMCID: PMC4139846.

Park YK, Lee HB, Jeon EJ, et al. Chaga mushroom extract inhibits oxidative DNA damage in human lymphocytes as assessed by comet assay. Biofactors. 2004;21(1-4):109-12. Doi: 10.1002/biof.552210120. PMID: 15630179.

Patel S, Waghela B, Shah K, et al. Silibinin, a natural blend in polytherapy formulation for targeting cd44v6 expressing colon cancer stem cells. Sci Rep. 2018 Nov 19;8(1):16985. Doi: 10.1038/s41598-018-35069-0. Erratum in: Sci Rep. 2018 Dec 17;8(1):17992. PMID: 30451890; PMCID: PMC6242811.

Patridge E, Gareiss P, Kinch MS, et al. An analysis of FDA-approved drugs: natural products and their derivatives. Drug Discov Today. 2016 Feb;21(2):204-7. Doi: 10.1016/j.drudis.2015.01.009. Epub 2015 Jan 21. PMID: 25617672.

Patterson, James T. The Dread Disease: Cancer and Modern American Culture. ISBN-13: 978-0674216259. Cambridge, Mass.: Harvard University Press, 1987.

Paul B, Li Y, Tollefsbol TO. The effects of combinatorial soy isoflavones and sulforaphane in breast tumor inhibition: role in epigenetic regulation. Int J Mol Sci. 2018 Jun 13;19(6):1754. Doi: 10.3390/ijms19061754. PMID: 29899271; PMCID: PMC6032337.

PDQ Integrative, Alternative, and Complementary Therapies Editorial Board. Curcumin (Curcuma, Turmeric) and Cancer (PDQ®): Health Professional Version. 2024 Apr 5. In: PDQ Cancer Information Summaries [Internet]. Bethesda (MD): National Cancer Institute (US); 2002-. Accessed June 20, 2024.

Pepe G, Salviati E, Rapa SF, et al. Citrus sinensis and Vitis vinifera protect cardiomyocytes from doxorubicin-induced oxidative stress: evaluation of onco nutraceutical potential of vegetable smoothies. Antioxidants (Basel). 2020 May 2;9(5):378. doi: 10.3390/antiox9050378. PMID: 32370308; PMCID: PMC7278676.

Piana, Ronald. The Halifax Project: a new approach to combination therapy. The ASCO Post, September 25, 2016. [A rare recognition by the American Society of Clinical Oncology of a major effort towards a more integrative treatment.]

Piao L, Mukherjee S, Chang Q, et al. TriCurin, a novel formulation of curcumin, epicatechin gallate, and resveratrol, inhibits the tumorigenicity of human papillomavirus-positive head and neck squamous cell carcinoma. Oncotarget. 2016 Jul 16;8(36):60025-60035. doi: 10.18632/oncotarget.10620. PMID: 28947951; PMCID: PMC5601119.

Pintova S, Dharmupari S, Moshier E, et al. Genistein combined with FOLFOX or FOLFOX-Bevacizumab for the treatment of metastatic colorectal cancer: phase I/II pilot study. Cancer Chemother Pharmacol. 2019 Sep;84(3):591-598. doi: 10.1007/s00280-019-03886-3. Epub 2019 Jun 15. PMID: 31203390.

Poff AM, Ari C, Seyfried TN, et al. The ketogenic diet and hyperbaric oxygen therapy prolong survival in mice with systemic metastatic cancer. PLoS One. 2013 Jun 5;8(6):e65522. doi: 10.1371/journal.pone.0065522. PMID: 23755243; PMCID: PMC3673985.

Pollock W. Case of tænia in an infant, cured by decoction of pomegranate. Edinb Med Surg J. 1814 Oct 1;10(40):419-421. PMID: 30329372; PMCID: PMC5743259. [Very early reference to the healing effects of pomegranate.]

Polyak K, Weinberg RA. Transitions between epithelial and mesenchymal states: Acquisition of malignant and stem cell traits. Nat Rev Cancer. 2009;9(4):265-273.

Ponnurangam S, Mammen JM, Ramalingam S, et al. Honokiol in combination with radiation targets Notch signaling to inhibit colon cancer stem cells. Mol Cancer Ther. 2012 Apr;11(4):963-72. doi: 10.1158/1535-7163.MCT-11-0999. Epub 2012 Feb 8. PMID: 22319203; PMCID: PMC3324630.

Popkin BM. Does excessive fast-food consumption impair our health? Am J Clin Nutr. 2022 Jul 6;116(1):11-12. doi: 10.1093/ajcn/nqac110. PMID: 35679428.

Pradhan R, Paul S, Acharya SS, et al. Nano formulated resveratrol inhibits PD-L1 in oral cancer cells by deregulating the association between tumor associated macrophages and cancer associated fibroblasts through IL-6/JAK2/STAT3 signaling axis. J Nutr Biochem. 2024 Jan 5:109568. doi: 10.1016/j.jnutbio.2024.109568. Epub ahead of print. PMID: 38185347.

Prasher P, Sharma M, Singh SK, et al. Luteolin: a flavonoid with a multifaceted anticancer potential. Cancer Cell Int. 2022 Dec 8;22(1):386. doi: 10.1186/s12935-022-02808-3. PMID: 36482329; PMCID: PMC9730645.

Prud'homme GJ. Cancer stem cells and novel targets for antitumor strategies. Curr Pharm Des. 2012;18(19):2838-49. doi: 10.2174/138161212800626120. PMID: 22390767.

Psaltopoulou T, Sergentanis TN, Panagiotakos DB, et al. Mediterranean diet, stroke, cognitive impairment, and depression: a meta-analysis. Ann Neurol. 2013 Oct;74(4):580-91. doi: 10.1002/ana.23944. Epub 2013 Sep 16. PMID: 23720230.

Quintana E, Shackleton M, Sabel MS, et al. Efficient tumor formation by single human melanoma cells. Nature. 2008 Dec 4;456(7222):593-8. doi: 10.1038/nature07567. PMID: 19052619; PMCID: PMC2597380.

Rafter J, Bennett M, Caderni G, et al. Dietary synbiotics reduce cancer risk factors in polypectomized and colon cancer patients. Am J Clin Nutr. 2007 Feb;85(2):488-96. doi: 10.1093/ajcn/85.2.488. PMID: 17284748.

Rajaram N, Yap B, Eriksson M, et al. A randomized controlled trial of soy isoflavone intake on mammographic density among Malaysian women. Nutrients. 2023 Jan 6;15(2):299. doi: 10.3390/nu15020299. PMID: 36678170; PMCID: PMC9862880.

Ramasamy TS, Ayob AZ, Myint HH, et al. Targeting colorectal cancer stem cells using curcumin and curcumin analogues: insights into the mechanism of the therapeutic efficacy. Cancer Cell Int. 2015 Oct 9;15:96. doi: 10.1186/s12935-015-0241-x. PMID: 26457069; PMCID: PMC4599442.

Rao M, Afshin A, Singh G, et al. Do healthier foods and diet patterns cost more than less healthy options? A systematic review and meta-analysis. BMJ Open. 2013 Dec 5;3(12):e004277. doi: 10.1136/bmjopen-2013-004277. PMID: 24309174; PMCID: PMC3855594.

Rawangkan A, Wongsirisin P, Namiki K, et al. Green tea catechin is an alternative immune checkpoint inhibitor that inhibits PD-L1 expression and lung tumor growth. Molecules. 2018 Aug 18;23(8):2071. doi: 10.3390/molecules23082071. PMID: 30126206; PMCID: PMC6222340. [The paper that established that EGCG from green tea targeted PD-L1, thus opening up the field of natural immune checkpoint inhibitors.]

Rayalam S, Della-Fera MA, Baile CA. Synergism between resveratrol and other phytochemicals: implications for obesity and osteoporosis. Mol Nutr Food Res. 2011 Aug;55(8):1177-85. doi: 10.1002/mnfr.201000616. Epub 2011 May 2. PMID: 21538845.

Reuter S, Gupta SC, Chaturvedi MM, et al. Oxidative stress, inflammation, and cancer: how are they linked? Free Radic Biol Med. 2010 Dec 1;49(11):1603-16. doi: 10.1016/j.freeradbiomed.2010.09.006. Epub 2010 Sep 16. PMID: 20840865; PMCID: PMC2990475.

Reya T, Morrison SJ, Clarke MF, et al. Stem cells, cancer, and cancer stem cells. Nature. 2001 Nov 1;414(6859):105-11. doi: 10.1038/35102167. PMID: 11689955.

Ricci H, Gaeta M, Franchi C, et al. Fish intake in relation to fatal and non-fatal cardiovascular risk: a systematic review and meta-analysis of cohort studies. Nutrients. 2023 Oct 26;15(21):4539. doi: 10.3390/nu15214539. PMID: 37960192; PMCID: PMC10647504.

Ricci-Vitiani L, Lombardi DG, Pilozzi E, et al. Identification and expansion of human colon-cancer-initiating cells. Nature. 2007 Jan 4;445(7123):111-5. doi: 10.1038/nature05384. Epub 2006 Nov 19. PMID: 17122771.

Richards, Victor. _Cancer: The Wayward Cell, Its Origins, Nature, and Treatment._ ISBN-13 978-0520358829. Berkeley: University of California Press, 1972.

Rijpma, Sjoerd. _David Livingstone and the Myth of African Poverty and Disease (Afrika-Studiecentrum, 35)._ ISBN-13: 978-9004277831. Leiden: Brill, 2015. Accessed February 3, 2024.

Rinkenbaugh AL, Baldwin AS. The NF-κB pathway and cancer stem cells. Cells. 2016 Apr 6;5(2):16. doi: 10.3390/cells5020016. PMID: 27058560; PMCID: PMC4931665.

Roberts, Sam. Dr. Samuel Epstein, 91, Cassandra of cancer prevention, dies. New York Times, April 25, 2018, p. Section A, Page 24. Accessed December 16, 2023. [Subscription required.] **[Obituary of Sam Epstein, MD, an indefatigable fighter against environmental pollution.]**

Rodríguez-Cañamero S, Cobo-Cuenca AI, Carmona-Torres JM, et al. Impact of physical exercise in advanced-stage cancer patients: Systematic review and meta-analysis. Cancer Med. 2022 Oct;11(19):3714-3727. doi: 10.1002/cam4.4746. Epub 2022 Apr 11. PMID: 35411694; PMCID: PMC9554454.

Rojas Gil AP, Kodonis I, Ioannidis A, et al. The effect of dietary intervention with high-oleocanthal and oleacein olive oil in patients with early-stage chronic lymphocytic leukemia: a pilot randomized trial. Front Oncol. 2022 Jan 21;11:810249. doi: 10.3389/fonc.2021.810249. PMID: 35127522; PMCID: PMC8814521. **[The first clinical trials of high-polyphenol olive oil as a treatment for leukemia. Results were positive.]**

Roomi MW, Monterrey JC, Kalinovsky T, Rath M, Niedzwiecki A. Comparative effects of EGCG, green tea and a nutrient mixture on the patterns of MMP-2 and MMP-9 expression in cancer cell lines. Oncol Rep. 2010 Sep;24(3):747-57. doi: 10.3892/or_00000917. PMID: 20664983.

Rothenberg SM, McFadden DG, Palmer EL, et al. Redifferentiation of iodine-refractory BRAF V600E-mutant metastatic papillary thyroid cancer with dabrafenib. Clin Cancer Res 2015;21(5):1028–1035.

Roullier-Gall C, Boutegrabet L, Gougeon RD, et al. A grape and wine chemodiversity comparison of different appellations in Burgundy: vintage vs terroir effects. Food Chem. 2014;152:100-7. doi: 10.1016/j.foodchem.2013.11.056. Epub 2013 Nov 19. PMID: 24444912.

Roy S, Khanna S, Alessio HM, et al. Anti-angiogenic property of edible berries. Free Radic Res. 2002 Sep;36(9):1023-31. doi: 10.1080/1071576021000006662. PMID: 12448828.

Rush, Benjamin. An account of the late Dr. Hugh Martin's cancer powder; with brief observations on cancers. Transactions of the American Philosophical Society. 1786;2:212-217. Reprinted in the _London Medical Journal, 1787;8(Pt 1):89-96._ PMID: 29139908; PMCID: PMC5545550. **[One of the earliest articles on cancer in PubMed. A fascinating attempt by Rush to evaluate an "alternative" Native American-derived remedy for cancer.]**

Saha A, Kuzuhara T, Echigo N, et al. New role of (-)-epicatechin in enhancing the induction of growth inhibition and apoptosis in human lung cancer cells by curcumin. Cancer Prev Res (Phila). 2010 Aug;3(8):953-62. doi: 10.1158/1940-6207.CAPR-09-0247. Epub 2010 Jul 6. PMID: 20606042.

Sahin K, Yenice E, Tuzcu M, et al. Lycopene protects against spontaneous ovarian cancer formation in laying hens. J Cancer Prev. 2018 Mar;23(1):25-36. doi: 10.15430/JCP.2018.23.1.25. Epub 2018 Mar 30. PMID: 29629346; PMCID: PMC5886492.

Salas-Salvadó J, Bulló M, Babio N, et al. Reduction in the incidence of type 2 diabetes with the Mediterranean diet: results of the PREDIMED-Reus nutrition intervention randomized trial. Diabetes Care. 2011;34(1):14-19.

Salas-Salvadó J, Bulló M, Estruch R, et al. Prevention of diabetes with Mediterranean diets: a subgroup analysis of a randomized trial. Ann Intern Med. 2014 Jan 7;160(1):1-10. doi: 10.7326/M13-1725. Erratum in: Ann Intern Med. 2018 Aug 21;169(4):271-272. PMID: 24573661.

Salas-Salvadó J, Casas-Agustench P, Murphy MM, et al. The effect of nuts on inflammation. Asia Pac J Clin Nutr. 2008;17 Suppl 1:333-6. PMID: 18296371. [Cited as 2008b]

Salas-Salvadó J, Fernández-Ballart J, Ros E, et al. Effect of a Mediterranean diet supplemented with nuts on metabolic syndrome status. Arch Intern Med. 2008;168(22):2449-2458. [Cite as 2008a]

Salas-Salvadó J, Guasch-Ferré M, Lee CH, et al. Protective effects of the Mediterranean diet on type 2 diabetes and metabolic syndrome. J Nutr. 2015 Apr 1;146(4):920S-927S. doi: 10.3945/jn.115.218487. PMID: 26962178; PMCID: PMC4807638.

Samykutty A, Shetty AV, Dakshinamoorthy G, et al. Piperine, a bioactive component of pepper spice, exerts therapeutic effects on androgen dependent and androgen independent prostate cancer cells. PLoS One. 2013 Jun 18;8(6):e65889. doi: 10.1371/journal.pone.0065889. PMID: 23824300; PMCID: PMC3688824.

Sánchez-Villegas A, Delgado-Rodríguez M, Alonso A, et al. Association of the Mediterranean dietary pattern with the incidence of depression: the Seguimiento Universidad de Navarra/University of Navarra follow-up (SUN) cohort. Arch Gen Psychiatry. 2009 Oct;66(10):1090-8. doi: 10.1001/archgenpsychiatry.2009.129. PMID: 19805699.

Sánchez-Villegas A, Martínez-González MA, Estruch R, et al. Mediterranean dietary pattern and depression: the PREDIMED randomized trial. BMC Med. 2013 Sep 20;11:208. doi: 10.1186/1741-7015-11-208. PMID: 24229349; PMCID: PMC3848350.

Santo L, Liao LM, Andreotti G, et al. Alcohol consumption and risk of multiple myeloma in the NIH-AARP Diet and Health Study. Int J Cancer. 2019 Jan 1;144(1):43-48. doi: 10.1002/ijc.31648. Epub 2018 Oct 30. PMID: 29971781; PMCID: PMC10309010.

Santosa D, Suharti C, Riwanto I, et al. Curcumin as adjuvant therapy to improve remission in myeloma patients: A pilot randomized clinical trial. Caspian J Intern Med. 2022 Spring;13(2):375-384. doi: 10.22088/cjim.13.2.9. PMID: 35919637; PMCID: PMC9301229.

Sassano M, Seyyedsalehi MS, Collatuzzo G, et al. Dietary intake of vitamin C and gastric cancer: a pooled analysis within the Stomach cancer Pooling (StoP) Project. Gastric Cancer. 2024 May;27(3):461-472. doi: 10.1007/s10120-024-01476-8. Epub 2024 Mar 4. PMID: 38436761; PMCID: PMC11016516.

Scarmeas N, Stern Y, Mayeux R, et al. Mediterranean diet and mild cognitive impairment. Arch Neurol. 2009 Feb;66(2):216-25. doi: 10.1001/archneurol.2008.536. PMID: 19204158; PMCID: PMC2653223phytochemical

Scheiner G. Treating hypos: one-size does not fit all! diatribe learn: making sense of diabetes. Published: June 13, 2013. Updated October 8, 2021. Accessed February 14, 2024.

Schick B. A tea prepared from needles of pine trees against scurvy. Science. 1943 Sep 10;98(2541):241-2. doi: 10.1126/science.98.2541.241. PMID: 17752698.

Schmidt M, Pfetzer N, Schwab M, et al. Effects of a ketogenic diet on the quality of life in 16 patients with advanced cancer: a pilot trial. Nutr Metab (Lond). 2011 Jul 27;8(1):54. doi: 10.1186/1743-7075-8-54. PMID: 21794124; PMCID: PMC3157418.

Schmutzler C, Köhrle J. Retinoic acid redifferentiation therapy for thyroid cancer. Thyroid. 2000 May;10(5):393-406. doi: 10.1089/thy.2000.10.393. PMID: 10884186.

Schröder FH, Roobol MJ, Boevé ER, et al. Randomized, double-blind, placebo-controlled crossover study in men with prostate cancer and rising PSA: effectiveness of a dietary supplement. Eur Urol. 2005 Dec;48(6):922-30; discussion 930-1. doi: 10.1016/j.eururo.2005.08.005. Epub 2005 Oct 17. PMID: 16263208.

Schroeder K, Ratcliffe SJ, Perez A, et al. Dance for health: an intergenerational program to increase access to physical activity. J Pediatr Nurs. 2017 Nov-Dec;37:29-34. doi: 10.1016/j.pedn.2017.07.004. Epub 2017 Jul 18. PMID: 28733128; PMCID: PMC5681394.

Schwartz, Gary. Hippocrates revisited. Ethical commentary. Einstein J Biol Med 2004;21:33-34.

Schwingshackl L, Hoffmann G. Adherence to Mediterranean diet and risk of cancer: an updated systematic review and meta-analysis of observational studies. Cancer Med. 2015 Dec;4(12):1933-47. doi: 10.1002/cam4.539. Epub 2015 Oct 16. PMID: 26471010; PMCID: PMC5123783.

Scoditti E, Calabriso N, Massaro M, et al. Mediterranean diet polyphenols reduce inflammatory angiogenesis through MMP-9 and COX-2 inhibition in human vascular endothelial cells: a potentially protective mechanism in atherosclerotic vascular disease and cancer. Arch Biochem Biophys. 2012 Nov 15;527(2):81-9. PMID: 22634015.

Scontre VA, Martins JC, de Melo Sette CV, et al. Curcuma longa (turmeric) for prevention of capecitabine-induced hand-foot syndrome: a pilot study. J Diet Suppl. 2018 Sep 3;15(5):606-612. doi: 10.1080/19390211.2017.1366387. Epub 2017 Nov 2. PMID: 29095653.

Scott EC, Baines AC, Gong Y, et al. Trends in the approval of cancer therapies by the FDA in the twenty-first century. Nat Rev Drug Discov. 2023 Aug;22(8):625-640. doi: 10.1038/s41573-023-00723-4. Epub 2023 June 21. PMID: 37344568. [Documents the shift away from chemotherapy and towards targeted therapies and immunotherapies.]

Seeram NP. Berry fruits for cancer prevention: current status and future prospects. J Agric Food Chem. 2008 Feb 13;56(3):630-5. doi: 10.1021/jf072504n. Epub 2008 Jan 23. PMID: 18211019.

Sellam LS, Zappasodi R, Chettibi F, et al. Silibinin down-regulates PD-L1 expression in nasopharyngeal carcinoma by interfering with tumor cell glycolytic metabolism. Arch Biochem Biophys. 2020 Sep 15;690:108479. doi: 10.1016/j.abb.2020.108479. Epub 2020 Jul 15. PMID: 32679194; PMCID: PMC8507490.

Semov A, Iourtchenco L, Liu LF, et al. Diindolilmethane (DIM) selectively inhibits cancer stem cells. Biochem Biophys Res Commun. 2012 Jul 20;424(1):45-51. doi: 10.1016/j.bbrc.2012.06.062. Epub 2012 Jun 19. PMID: 22727906.

Sengupta M, Lendon JP, Caffrey C, et al. Post-acute and long-term care providers and services users in the United States, 2017–2018. National Center for Health Statistics. Vital Health Stat 3(47). 2022. Accessed February 28, 2024.

Sengupta S, Nagalingam A, Muniraj N, et al. Activation of tumor suppressor LKB1 by honokiol abrogates cancer stem-like phenotype in breast cancer via inhibition of oncogenic Stat3. Oncogene. 2017 Oct 12;36(41):5709-5721. doi: 10.1038/onc.2017.164. Epub 2017 June 5. PMID: 28581518; PMCID: PMC5793218.

Sen S, Hess K, Hong DS, et al. Development of a prognostic scoring system for patients with advanced cancer enrolled in immune checkpoint inhibitor phase 1 clinical trials. Br J Cancer. 2018 Mar 20;118(6):763-769. doi: 10.1038/bjc.2017.480. Epub 2018 Feb 20. PMID: 29462132; PMCID: PMC5886120.

Seyfried, TN. Cancer As A Metabolic Disease. ISBN-12: 978-0-470-58492-7. Hoboken: John Wiley & Sons, 2012. [In this book, and over 150 journal articles, Seyfried has demonstrated the central role of metabolism in the cancer process.]

Seyfried TN, Chinopoulos C. Can the mitochondrial metabolic theory explain better the origin and management of cancer than can the somatic mutation theory? Metabolites. 2021 Aug 25;11(9):572. doi: 10.3390/metabo11090572. PMID: 34564387; PMCID: PMC8467939.

Seyfried TN, Flores RE, Poff AM, et al Cancer as a metabolic disease: implications for novel therapeutics. Carcinogenesis. 2014 Mar;35(3):515-27. doi: 10.1093/carcin/bgt480. Epub 2013 Dec 16. PMID: 24343361; PMCID: PMC3941741.

Seyfried TN, Shelton LM. Cancer as a metabolic disease. Nutr Metab (Lond). 2010 Jan 27;7:7. doi: 10.1186/1743-7075-7-7. PMID: 20181022; PMCID: PMC2845135.

Shah D, Challagundla N, Dave V, et al. Berberine mediates tumor cell death by skewing tumor-associated immunosuppressive macrophages to inflammatory macrophages. Phytomedicine. 2022 May;99:153904. doi: 10.1016/j.phymed.2021.153904. Epub 2021 Dec 22. PMID: 35231825.

Shaito A, Posadino AM, Younes N, et al. Potential adverse effects of resveratrol: a literature review. Int J Mol Sci. 2020 Mar 18;21(6):2084. doi: 10.3390/ijms21062084. PMID: 32197410; PMCID: PMC7139620.

Sha J, Li J, Wang W, et al. Curcumin induces G0/G1 arrest and apoptosis in hormone independent prostate cancer DU-145 cells by down regulating Notch signaling. Biomed Pharmacother. 2016 Dec;84:177-184. doi: 10.1016/j.biopha.2016.09.037. Epub 2016 Sep 19. PMID: 27657825.

Shammas MA, Neri P, Koley H, et al. Specific killing of multiple myeloma cells by (-)-epigallocatechin-3-gallate extracted from green tea: biologic activity and therapeutic implications. Blood. 2006 Oct 15;108(8):2804-10. doi: 10.1182/blood-2006-05-022814. Epub 2006 Jun 29. PMID: 16809610; PMCID: PMC1895573.

Shanafelt TD, Call TG, Zent CS, et al. Phase 2 trial of daily, oral Polyphenon E in patients with asymptomatic, Rai stage 0 to II chronic lymphocytic leukemia. Cancer. 2013 Jan 15;119(2):363-70. doi: 10.1002/cncr.27719. Epub 2012 Jul 3. PMID: 22760587; PMCID: PMC3902473.

Shankar S, Nall D, Tang SN, et al. Resveratrol inhibits pancreatic cancer stem cell characteristics in human and KrasG12D transgenic mice by inhibiting pluripotency maintaining factors and epithelial-mesenchymal transition. PLoS One. 2011 Jan 31;6(1):e16530. doi: 10.1371/journal.pone.0016530. PMID: 21304978; PMCID: PMC3031576.

Sharma P, Wagner K, Wolchok JD, et al. Novel cancer immunotherapy agents with survival benefit: recent successes and next steps. Nat Rev Cancer. 2011 Oct 24;11(11):805-12. doi: 10.1038/nrc3153. PMID: 22020206; PMCID: PMC3426440.

Sharma R, Kumari M, Kumari A, et al. Diet supplemented with phytochemical epigallocatechin gallate and probiotic Lactobacillus fermentum confers second generation synbiotic effects by modulating cellular immune responses and antioxidant capacity in aging mice. Eur J Nutr. 2019 Oct;58(7):2943-2957. doi: 10.1007/s00394-018-01890-6. Epub 2019 Jan 3. Erratum in: Eur J Nutr. 2019 June 28; PMID: 30607562.

Shoaib A, Tabish M, Ali S, et al. Dietary phytochemicals in cancer signaling pathways: role of miRNA targeting. Curr Med Chem. 2021;28(39):8036-8067. doi: 10.2174/0929867328666210420101605. PMID: 33881968.

Shoaib S, Khan FB, Alsharif MA, et al. Reviewing the prospective pharmacological potential of isothiocyanates in the fight against female-specific cancers. Cancers (Basel). 2023 Apr 20;15(8):2390. doi: 10.3390/cancers15082390. PMID: 37190316; PMCID: PMC10137050.)

Shoba G, Joy D, Joseph T, et al. Influence of piperine on the pharmacokinetics of curcumin in animals and human volunteers. Planta Med. 1998 May;64(4):353-6. doi: 10.1055/s-2006-957450. PMID: 9619120.

Shumway BS, Kresty LA, Larsen PE, et al. Effects of a topically applied bioadhesive berry gel on loss of heterozygosity indices in premalignant oral lesions. Clin Cancer Res. 2008 Apr 15;14(8):2421-30. doi: 10.1158/1078-0432.CCR-07-4096. PMID: 18413833; PMCID: PMC3498466.

Simon D, Köhrle J, Schmutzler C, et al. Redifferentiation therapy of differentiated thyroid carcinoma with retinoic acid: basics and first clinical results. Exp Clin Endocrinol Diabetes. 1996;104 Suppl 4:13-5. doi: 10.1055/s-0029-1211692. PMID: 8980992.

Singh A, Kamath A. Attitude of medical students and doctors towards complementary, alternative and integrative medicine: a single-center, questionnaire-based study. J Pharmacopuncture. 2021 June 30;24(2):84-90. doi: 10.3831/KPI.2021.24.2.84. PMID: 34249399; PMCID: PMC8220508.

Singh RS, Kaur HP, Kanwar JR. Mushroom lectins as promising anticancer substances. Curr Protein Pept Sci. 2016;17(8):797-807. doi: 10.2174/1389203717666160226144741. PMID: 26916164.

Singh S, Chitkara D, Mehrazin R, et al. Chemoresistance in prostate cancer cells is regulated by miRNAs and Hedgehog pathway. PLoS One. 2012;7(6):e40021. doi: 10.1371/journal.pone.0040021. Epub 2012 Jun 29. PMID: 22768203; PMCID: PMC3386918.

Singh S, Sahadevan R, Roy R, et al. Structure-based design and synthesis of a novel long-chain 4"-alkyl ether derivative of EGCG as potent EGFR inhibitor: in vitro and in silico studies. RSC Adv. 2022 Jun 16;12(28):17821-17836. doi: 10.1039/d2ra01919a. PMID: 35765335; PMCID: PMC9201511.

Singh SK, Hawkins C, Clarke ID, et al. Identification of human brain tumor initiating cells. Nature. 2004 Nov 18;432(7015):396-401. doi: 10.1038/nature03128. PMID: 15549107.

Singh SV, Warin R, Xiao D, et al. Sulforaphane inhibits prostate carcinogenesis and pulmonary metastasis in TRAMP mice in association with increased cytotoxicity of natural killer cells. Cancer Res. 2009 Mar 1;69(5):2117-25. doi: 10.1158/0008-5472.CAN-08-3502. Epub 2009 Feb 17. PMID: 19223537; PMCID: PMC2683380.

Singh Tuli H, Rath P, Chauhan A, et al. Luteolin, a potent anticancer compound: from chemistry to cellular interactions and synergetic perspectives. Cancers (Basel). 2022 Oct 31;14(21):5373. doi: 10.3390/cancers14215373. PMID: 36358791; PMCID: PMC9658186.

Slamon D, Pegram M. Rationale for trastuzumab (Herceptin) in adjuvant breast cancer trials. Semin Oncol. 2001 Feb;28(1 Suppl 3):13-9. doi: 10.1016/s0093-7754(01)90188-5. PMID: 11301370.

Slider L, Erwin S, Ownby S, et al. A novel combination of sulforaphane and maitake extract induces phase II enzymes. The FASEB Journal, 2015[29:250.2.

Smyth, M. Lloyd John Old 1933–2011. Nat Immunol. 2012;13:103.

So JY, Suh N. Targeting cancer stem cells in solid tumors by vitamin D. J Steroid Biochem Mol Biol. 2015 Apr;148:79-85. doi: 10.1016/j.jsbmb.2014.10.007. Epub 2014 Oct 16. PMID: 25460302; PMCID: PMC4361233.

Somers-Edgar TJ, Scandlyn MJ, Stuart EC, et al. The combination of epigallocatechin gallate and curcumin suppresses ER alpha-breast cancer cell growth in vitro and in vivo. Int J Cancer. 2008 May 1;122(9):1966-71. doi: 10.1002/ijc.23328. PMID: 18098290.

Sonnenschein C, Soto AM. The aging of the 2000 and 2011 Hallmarks of Cancer reviews: a critique. J Biosci. 2013 Sep;38(3):651-63. doi: 10.1007/s12038-013-9335-6. PMID: 23938395; PMCID: PMC3882065. [Two researchers at Tufts University who have challenged the exclusive focus on genetics of cancer.]

Sonnenschein C, Soto AM. The Society of Cells: Cancer and Control of Cell Proliferation. London and New York: Taylor & Francis, 1999.

Spencer CN, Gopalakrishnan V, McQuade J,et al. The gut microbiome (GM) and immunotherapy response are influenced by host lifestyle factors. Cancer Res 1 July 2019; 79 (13_Supplement): 2838.

Spencer CN, McQuade JL, Gopalakrishnan V, et al. Dietary fiber and probiotics influence the gut microbiome and melanoma immunotherapy response. Science. 2021 Dec 24;374(6575):1632-1640. doi: 10.1126/science.aaz7015. Epub 2021 Dec 23. PMID: 34941392; PMCID: PMC8970537.

Srivastava NS, Srivastava RAK. Curcumin and quercetin synergistically inhibit cancer cell proliferation in multiple cancer cells and modulate Wnt/β-catenin signaling and apoptotic pathways in A375 cells. Phytomedicine. 2019 Jan;52:117-128. doi: 10.1016/j.phymed.2018.09.224. Epub 2018 Sep 28. PMID: 30599890.

Stampfer MJ, Colditz GA, Willett WC, et al. A prospective study of moderate alcohol consumption and the risk of coronary disease and stroke in women. N Engl J Med. 1988 Aug 4;319(5):267-73. doi: 10.1056/NEJM198808043190503. PMID: 3393181.

Steffen LM, Folsom AR, Cushman M, et al. Greater fish, fruit, and vegetable intakes are related to lower incidence of venous thromboembolism: the Longitudinal Investigation of Thromboembolism Etiology. Circulation. 2007 Jan 16;115(2):188-95. doi: 10.1161/CIRCULATIONAHA.106.641688. Epub 2006 Dec 18. PMID: 17179018.

Steinberg FM, Bearden MM, Keen CL. Cocoa and chocolate flavonoids: implications for cardiovascular health. J Am Diet Assoc. 2003 Feb;103(2):215-23. doi: 10.1053/jada.2003.50028. PMID: 12589329.

Stenner-Liewen F, Liewen H, Cathomas R, et al. Daily pomegranate intake has no impact on PSA levels in patients with advanced prostate cancer - Results of a phase IIb randomized controlled trial. J Cancer. 2013 Aug 29;4(7):597-605. doi: 10.7150/jca.7123. PMID: 24069070; PMCID: PMC3781990.

Stoner GD, Chen T, Kresty LA, et al. Protection against esophageal cancer in rodents with lyophilized berries: Potential mechanisms. Nutr Cancer. 2006;54(1):33-46. doi: 10.1207/s15327914nc5401_5. PMID: 16800771; PMCID: PMC3015107.

Sugiura K, Benedict SR. The influence of insufficient diets upon tumor recurrence and growth in rats and mice. The Journal of Cancer Research 1926;10:309–318. [One of the earliest papers on calorie restriction as an anticancer strategy; Sugiura was my friend and mentor at Sloan-Kettering.]

Sun DW, Zhang HD, Mao L, et al. Luteolin inhibits breast cancer development and progression in vitro and in vivo by suppressing notch signaling and regulating MiRNAs. Cell Physiol Biochem. 2015;37(5):1693-711. doi: 10.1159/000438535. Epub 2015 Nov 9. PMID: 26545287.

Sun ML, Yao W, Wang XY, et al. Intermittent fasting and health outcomes: an umbrella review of systematic reviews and meta-analyses of randomized controlled trials. EClinicalMedicine. 2024 Mar 11;70:102519. doi: 10.1016/j.eclinm.2024.102519. PMID: 38500840; PMCID: PMC10945168.

Sun X, Song J, Li E, et al. (-)Epigallocatechin-3-gallate inhibits bladder cancer stem cells via suppression of Sonic Hedgehog pathway. Oncol Rep. 2019 Jul;42(1):425-435. doi: 10.3892/or.2019.7170. Epub 2019 May 24. PMID: 31180522.

Suolinna EM, Lang DR, Racker E. Quercetin, an artificial regulator of the high aerobic glycolysis of tumor cells. J Natl Cancer Inst. 1974 Nov;53(5):1515-9. doi: 10.1093/jnci/53.5.1515. PMID: 4279302.

Su X, Tamimi RM, Collins LC, et al. Intake of fiber and nuts during adolescence and incidence of proliferative benign breast disease. Cancer Causes Control. 2010 Aug;21(8):1033-46. doi: 10.1007/s10552-010-9532-7. PMID: 20383576; PMCID: PMC2902733.

Suzuki I, Itani T, Ohno N, et al. Antitumor activity of a polysaccharide fraction extracted from cultured fruiting bodies of Grifola frondosa. J Pharmacobiodyn. 1984 Jul;7(7):492-500. doi: 10.1248/bpb1978.7.492. PMID: 6491867.

Swamy MV, Citineni B, Patlolla JM, et al. Prevention and treatment of pancreatic cancer by curcumin in combination with omega-3 fatty acids. Nutr Cancer. 2008;60 Suppl 1:81-9. doi: 10.1080/01635580802416703. PMID: 19003584.

Swift DL, Johannsen NM, Lavie CJ, et al. The role of exercise and physical activity in weight loss and maintenance. Prog Cardiovasc Dis. 2014 Jan-Feb;56(4):441-7. doi: 10.1016/j.pcad.2013.09.012. Epub 2013 Oct 11. PMID: 24438736; PMCID: PMC3925973.

Sztiller-Sikorska M, Czyz M. Parthenolide as cooperating agent for anti-cancer treatment of various malignancies. Pharmaceuticals (Basel). 2020 Aug 14;13(8):194. doi: 10.3390/ph13080194. PMID: 32823992; PMCID: PMC7466132.

Szychowski KA, Skóra B, Pomianek T, et al. Inonotus obliquus—from folk medicine to clinical use. J Tradit Complement Med. 2020 Aug 22;11(4):293-302. doi: 10.1016/j.jtcme.2020.08.003. PMID: 34195023; PMCID: PMC8240111.

Tang J, Feng Y, Tsao S, et al. Berberine and coptidis rhizoma as novel antineoplastic agents: a review of traditional use and biomedical investigations. J Ethnopharmacol. 2009 Oct 29;126(1):5-17. doi: 10.1016/j.jep.2009.08.009. Epub 2009 Aug 15. PMID: 19686830.

Tang SN, Fu J, Shankar S, et al. EGCG enhances the therapeutic potential of gemcitabine and CP690550 by inhibiting STAT3 signaling pathway in human pancreatic cancer. PLoS One. 2012;7(2):e31067. doi: 10.1371/journal.pone.0031067. Epub 2012 Feb 13. PMID: 22348037; PMCID: PMC3278426.

Tang SN, Singh C, Nall D, et al. The dietary bioflavonoid quercetin synergizes with epigallocathechin gallate (EGCG) to inhibit prostate cancer stem cell characteristics, invasion, migration and epithelial-mesenchymal transition. J Mol Signal. 2010 Aug 18;5:14. doi: 10.1186/1750-2187-5-14. PMID: 20718984; PMCID: PMC2933702.

Tang X, Ding H, Liang M, et al. Curcumin induces ferroptosis in non-small-cell lung cancer via activating autophagy. Thoracic Cancer. 2021 Apr;12(8):1219-1230. doi: 10.1111/1759-7714.13904. Epub 2021 Mar 3. Erratum in: Thoracic Cancer. 2024 Apr 5;: PMID: 33656766; PMCID: PMC8046146.

Tang Y, Cao Y. Curcumin inhibits the growth and metastasis of melanoma via miR-222-3p/SOX10/Notch axis. Dis Markers. 2022 May 9;2022:3129781. doi: 10.1155/2022/3129781. PMID: 35585935; PMCID: PMC9110126.

Tannenbaum A, Silverstone H. Failure to inhibit the formation of mammary carcinoma in mice by intermittent fasting. Cancer Res. 1950 Sep;10(9):577-9. PMID: 14772734.

Tannenbaum A, Silverstone H. Nutrition in relation to cancer. Adv Cancer Res. 1953;1:451-501. doi: 10.1016/s0065-230x(08)60009-3. PMID: 13057710. [Summary of the work of two Manhattan Project scientists who kept the diet-cancer link alive after WWII.]

Taubes, Gary. What If It's All Been a Big Fat Lie? New York Times, July 2, 2002. [An enjoyable diatribe: "The unrepentant [Dr.] Atkins was right all along."]

Terry P, Lichtenstein P, Feychting M, et al. Fatty fish consumption and risk of prostate cancer. Lancet. 2001 Jun 2;357(9270):1764-6. doi: 10.1016/S0140-6736(00)04889-3. PMID: 11403817.

Thomas L. Discussion of cellular and humoral aspects of hypersensitive states. In: Lawrence HS [editor]. Cellular and Humoral Aspects of the Hypersensitive States: a Symposium Held at the New York Academy of Medicine. New York, Hoeber-Harper: 1959, pp. 529-532. Accessed February 18, 2024.

Thomas R, Williams M, Sharma H, et al. A double-blind, placebo-controlled randomized trial evaluating the effect of a polyphenol-rich whole food supplement on PSA progression in men with prostate cancer--the U.K. NCRN Pomi-T study. Prostate Cancer Prostatic Dis. 2014 June;17(2):180-6. doi: 10.1038/pcan.2014.6. Epub 2014 Mar 11. PMID: 24614693; PMCID: PMC4020278.

Till JE, McCulloch EA. A direct measurement of the radiation sensitivity of normal mouse bone marrow cells. Radiat Res. 1961 Feb;14:213-22. PMID: 13776896.

Toledo E, Salas-Salvadó J, Donat-Vargas C, et al. Mediterranean diet and invasive breast cancer risk among women at high cardiovascular risk in the PREDIMED Trial: a randomized clinical trial. JAMA Intern Med. 2015 Nov;175(11):1752-1760. doi: 10.1001/jamainternmed.2015.4838. Erratum in: JAMA Intern Med. 2018 Dec 1;178(12):1731-1732. PMID: 26365989.

Tong Y, Liu Y, Zheng H, et al. Artemisinin and its derivatives can significantly inhibit lung tumorigenesis and tumor metastasis through Wnt/β-catenin signaling. Oncotarget. 2016 May 24;7(21):31413-28. doi: 10.18632/oncotarget.8920. PMID: 27119499; PMCID: PMC5058767.

Travis RC, Perez-Cornago A, Appleby PN, et al. A collaborative analysis of individual participant data from 19 prospective studies assesses circulating vitamin D and prostate cancer risk. Cancer Res. 2019 Jan 1;79(1):274-285. doi: 10.1158/0008-5472.CAN-18-2318. Epub 2018 Nov 13. PMID: 30425058; PMCID: PMC6330070.

Trichopoulou A, Bamia C, Lagiou P, et al. Mediterranean diet and survival among patients with coronary heart disease in Greece. Arch Intern Med. 2005;165(8):929-935.

Trichopoulou A, Costacou T, Bamia C, et al. Adherence to a Mediterranean diet and survival in a Greek population. N Engl J Med. 2003;348:2599-2608.

Trichopoulou A, Martínez-González MA, Tong TY, et al. Definitions and potential health benefits of the Mediterranean diet: views from experts around the world. BMC Med. 2014 Jul 24;12:112. doi: 10.1186/1741-7015-12-112. PMID: 25055810; PMCID: PMC4222885.

Trichopoulou A. Mediterranean diet: the past and the present. Nutr Metab Cardiovasc Dis. 2001 Aug;11(4 Suppl):1-4. PMID: 11894739.

Trinchieri, Giorgio. Microbiome and cancer, chapter 4. DeVita, Jr. VT, Rosenberg S, Lawrence T. [Editors]. DeVita, Hellman, and Rosenberg's Cancer. 11th Edition. Philadelphia: Wolters Kluwer Health, 2019. Accessed February 1, 2024. [Subscription required.]

Tsai PH, Cheng CH, Lin CY, et al. Dietary flavonoids luteolin and quercetin suppressed cancer stem cell properties and metastatic potential of isolated prostate cancer cells. Anticancer Res. 2016 Dec;36(12):6367-6380. doi: 10.21873/anticanres.11234. PMID: 27919958.

Ujiki MB, Ding XZ, Salabat MR, et al. Apigenin inhibits pancreatic cancer cell proliferation through G2/M cell cycle arrest. Mol Cancer. 2006 Dec 29;5:76. doi: 10.1186/1476-4598-5-76. PMID: 17196098; PMCID: PMC1779363.

UNESCO [United Nations Educational, Scientific and Cultural Organization]. Mediterranean diet. 2003. Accessed October 14, 2023.

UNESCO [United Nations Educational, Scientific and Cultural Organization]. The United Nations World Water Development Report 2022: Groundwater: Making the Invisible Visible. Accessed April 13, 2024.

United States Department of Agriculture [USDA], Economic Research Service. Definitions of food security, October 25, 2023. Accessed April 6, 2024.

United States Department of Agriculture [USDA] and U.S. Department of Health and Human Services (DHHS). Dietary Guidelines for Americans, 2020-2025. 9th Edition. December 2020. Accessed February 27, 2024.

United States House of Representatives, Committee on Science, Subcommittee on Environment, Technology, and Standards. Hearing before the Subcommittee on Environment, Technology, and Standards, 2005 Jun 28; Washington. 109th Congress, 1st Session; Serial No. 109-20. Accessed December 22, 2023.

Vadhwana B, Tarazi M, Boshier PR, et al. Evaluation of the oesophagogastric cancer-associated microbiome: a systematic review and quality assessment. Cancers (Basel). 2023 May 9;15(10):2668. doi: 10.3390/cancers15102668. PMID: 37345006; PMCID: PMC10216300.

Vahedi Larijani L, Ghasemi M, Abedian Kenari S, et al. Evaluating the effect of four extracts of avocado fruit on esophageal squamous carcinoma and colon adenocarcinoma cell lines in comparison with peripheral blood mononuclear cells. Acta Med Iran. 2014;52(3):201-5. PMID: 24901722.

Vatankhah MA, Panahizadeh R, Nejati-Koshki K, et al. Curcumin upregulates miR-148a to increase the chemosensitivity of CD44-positive prostate cancer stem cells to paclitaxel through targeting the MSK1/IRS1 axis. Drug Res (Stuttg). 2022 Oct;72(8):457-465. doi: 10.1055/a-1867-4805. Epub 2022 Jul 22. PMID: 35868335.

Vaux DL. In defense of the somatic mutation theory of cancer. Bioessays. 2011 May;33(5):341-3. doi: 10.1002/bies.201100022. PMID: 21503936.

Vetizou M, Trinchieri G. Anti-PD1 in the wonder-gut-land. Cell Res. 2018 Mar;28(3):263-264. doi: 10.1038/cr.2018.12. Epub 2018 Jan 16. PMID: 29336431; PMCID: PMC5835771.

Vira D, Basak SK, Veena MS, et al. Cancer stem cells, microRNAs, and therapeutic strategies including natural products. Cancer Metastasis Rev. 2012 Dec;31(3-4):733-51. doi: 10.1007/s10555-012-9382-8. PMID: 22752409.

Virchow, Rudolph. *Cellular Pathology. As Based Upon Physiological and Pathological Histology. Twenty Lectures Delivered in the Pathological Institute of Berlin During the Months of February, March and April, 1858.* Translated from German by Frank Chance. London: John Churchill, 1860. Accessed January 17, 2024.

Wade N. Laetrile at Sloan-Kettering: a question of ambiguity. Science. 1977 Dec 23;198(4323):1231-4. doi: 10.1126/science.198.4323.1231. PMID: 17741690.

Wang D, Kong X, Li Y, et al. Curcumin inhibits bladder cancer stem cells by suppressing Sonic Hedgehog pathway. Biochem Biophys Res Commun. 2017 Nov 4;493(1):521-527. doi: 10.1016/j.bbrc.2017.08.158. Epub 2017 Sep 4. PMID: 28870814.

Wang H, Olivero W, Wang D, et al. Cold as a therapeutic agent. Acta Neurochir (Wien). 2006 May;148(5):565-70; discussion 569-70. doi: 10.1007/s00701-006-0747-z. Epub 2006 Feb 17. PMID: 16489500.

Wang J, Wang C, Bu G. Curcumin inhibits the growth of liver cancer stem cells through the phosphatidylinositol 3-kinase/protein kinase B/mammalian target of rapamycin signaling pathway. Exp Ther Med. 2018 Apr;15(4):3650-3658. doi: 10.3892/etm.2018.5805. Epub 2018 Jan 29. PMID: 29545895; PMCID: PMC5840955.

Wang J, Xie Y, Feng Y, et al. (-)-Epigallocatechingallate induces apoptosis in B lymphoma cells via caspase-dependent pathway and Bcl-2 family protein modulation. Int J Oncol. 2015 Apr;46(4):1507-15. doi: 10.3892/ijo.2015.2869. Epub 2015 Feb 3. PMID: 25647297; PMCID: PMC4356505.

Wang J, Zhang H, Sun Y. [Phase III clinical trial of elemenum emulsion in the management of malignant pleural and peritoneal effusions]. Zhonghua Zhong Liu Za Zhi. 1996 Nov;18(6):464-7. Chinese. PMID: 9387305.

Wang J-Q, Fu Y-Q, Granato D, et al. Study on the color effects of (-)-epigallocatechin-3-gallate under different pH and temperatures in a model beverage system. Food Control. 2022;139: 109112.

Wang K, Zhang C, Bao J, et al. Synergistic chemopreventive effects of curcumin and berberine on human breast cancer cells through induction of apoptosis and autophagic cell death. Sci Rep. 2016 Jun 6;6:26064. doi: 10.1038/srep26064. PMID: 27263652; PMCID: PMC4893614.

Wang L, Du M, Cudhea F, et al. Disparities in health and economic burdens of cancer attributable to suboptimal diet in the United States, 2015–2018. Am J Public Health. 2021 Nov;111(11):2008-2018. doi: 10.2105/AJPH.2021.306475. Epub 2021 Oct 14. PMID: 34648383; PMCID: PMC8630501.

Wang L, Jiang G, Jing N, et al. Bilberry anthocyanin extracts enhance anti-PD-L1 efficiency by modulating gut microbiota. Food Funct. 2020 Apr 30;11(4):3180-3190. doi: 10.1039/d0fo00255k. PMID: 32211663.

Wang L, Liu H, Liu Y, et al. Potential markers of cancer stem-like cells in ESCC: a review of the current knowledge. Front Oncol. 2024 Jan 4;13:1324819. doi: 10.3389/fonc.2023.1324819. PMID: 38239657; PMCID: PMC10795532.

Wang M, Tang L, Chen S, et al. ZNF217-activated Notch signaling mediates sulforaphane-suppressed stem cell properties in colorectal cancer. J Nutr Biochem. 2024 Mar;125:109551. doi: 10.1016/j.jnutbio.2023.109551. Epub 2023 Dec 20. PMID: 38134973.

Wang MC, Jiao M, Wu T, et al. Polycomb complex protein BMI-1 promotes invasion and metastasis of pancreatic cancer stem cells by activating PI3K/AKT signaling, an ex vivo, in vitro, and in vivo study. Oncotarget. 2016 Feb 23;7(8):9586-99. doi: 10.18632/oncotarget.7078. PMID: 26840020; PMCID: PMC4891062.

Wang N, Wang Q, Tang H, et al. Direct inhibition of ACTN4 by ellagic acid limits breast cancer metastasis via regulation of β-catenin stabilization in cancer stem cells. J Exp Clin Cancer Res. 2017 Dec 2;36(1):172. doi: 10.1186/s13046-017-0635-9. Erratum in: J Exp Clin Cancer Res. 2022 Mar 31;41(1):118. PMID: 29197410; PMCID: PMC5712102.

Wang P, Henning SM, Heber D, et al. Sensitization to docetaxel in prostate cancer cells by green tea and quercetin. J Nutr Biochem. 2015 Apr;26(4):408-15. doi: 10.1016/j.jnutbio.2014.11.017. Epub 2015 Jan 15. PMID: 25655047; PMCID: PMC4375039.

Wang Q, Li J, Gu J, et al. Potentiation of (-)-epigallocatechin-3-gallate-induced apoptosis by bortezomib in multiple myeloma cells. Acta Biochim Biophys Sin (Shanghai). 2009 Dec;41(12):1018-26. doi: 10.1093/abbs/gmp094. PMID: 20011976.

Wang SY, Eberly LA, Roberto CA, et al. Food insecurity and cardiovascular mortality for nonelderly adults in the United States From 2011 to 2017: a county-level longitudinal analysis. Circ Cardiovasc Qual Outcomes. 2021 Jan;14(1):e007473. doi: 10.1161/CIRCOUTCOMES.120.007473. Epub 2020 Nov 9. PMID: 33164557; PMCID: PMC7855295.

Wang W, Yang M, Kenfield SA, et al. Nut consumption and prostate cancer risk and mortality. Br J Cancer. 2016 Jul 26;115(3):371-4. doi: 10.1038/bjc.2016.181. Epub 2016 Jun 9. PMID: 27280637; PMCID: PMC4973153.

Wang W, Zhao C, Jou D, et al. Ursolic acid inhibits the growth of colon cancer-initiating cells by targeting STAT3. Anticancer Res. 2013 Oct;33(10):4279-84. PMID: 24122993.

Wang X, Chan YS, Wong K, et al. Mechanism-driven and clinically focused development of botanical foods as multitarget anticancer medicine: collective perspectives and insights from preclinical studies, IND applications and early-phase clinical trials. Cancers (Basel). 2023 Jan 23;15(3):701. doi: 10.3390/cancers15030701. PMID: 36765659; PMCID: PMC9913787.

Wang X, Ouyang YY, Liu J, et al. Flavonoid intake and risk of CVD: a systematic review and meta-analysis of prospective cohort studies. Br J Nutr. 2014 Jan 14;111(1):1-11. doi: 10.1017/S000711451300278X. Epub 2013 Aug 16. PMID: 23953879.

Wang Y, Shen X, Liao W, et al. A heteropolysaccharide, L-fuco-D-manno-1,6-α-D-galactan extracted from Grifola frondosa and antiangiogenic activity of its sulfated derivative. Carbohydr Polym. 2014 Jan 30;101:631-41. doi: 10.1016/j.carbpol.2013.09.085. Epub 2013 Oct 4. PMID: 24299820.

Warburg, Otto Heinrich; Frank Dickens (editor). On Metabolism of Tumors. London: Constable, London, 1930. (A translation and expansion of Warburg's 1924 and 1927 articles.) **[A great classic of cancer research that has had enormous repercussions for 100 years.]**

Warburg O, Burk D. The maximum efficiency of photosynthesis. Arch Biochem. 1950 Feb;25(2):410-43. PMID: 15404831.

Warburg O. On the origin of cancer cells. Science. 1956 Feb 24;123(3191):309-14. doi: 10.1126/science.123.3191.309. PMID: 13298683. **[Warburg's most condense statement of his basic philosophy and argument for English-speaking readers.]**

Warburg O, Posener K, Negelein KE. Über den Stoffwechsel der Tumoren [About the metabolism of tumors]. Biochemische Zeitschrift. 1924;152:319-344. German.

Warburg O, Wind F, Negelein E. The metabolism of tumors in the body. J Gen Physiol. 1927 Mar 7;8(6):519-30. doi: 10.1085/jgp.8.6.519. PMID: 19872213; PMCID: PMC2140820.

Ward ZJ, Bleich SN, Cradock AL, et al. Projected U.S. state-level prevalence of adult obesity and severe obesity. N Engl J Med. 2019 Dec 19;381(25):2440-2450. doi: 10.1056/NEJMsa1909301. PMID: 31851800.

Warrell RP Jr, Frankel SR, Miller WH Jr, et al. Differentiation therapy of acute promyelocytic leukemia with tretinoin (all-trans-retinoic acid). N Engl J Med. 1991 May 16;324(20):1385-93. doi: 10.1056/NEJM199105163242002. PMID: 1850498.

Wasta, Vanessa. Paul Talalay, Hopkins researcher famed for finding cancer-preventing compounds in broccoli, dies. Johns Hopkins Medicine News Release. March 14, 2019. Accessed February 19, 2024.

Watson JD, Crick FH. Molecular structure of nucleic acids; a structure for deoxyribose nucleic acid. Nature. 1953 Apr 25;171(4356):737-8. doi: 10.1038/171737a0. PMID: 13054692. **[One of the most influential papers of all time, proving the double helix structure of DNA.]**

Watson JD. To fight cancer, know the enemy. New York Times, August 9, 2009. Accessed December 22, 2023. [Requires subscription.] **[A takedown of the somatic mutation theory from the man who co-discovered DNA's "double helix."]**

Webb MJ, Kukard C. A review of natural therapies potentially relevant in triple negative breast cancer aimed at targeting cancer cell vulnerabilities. Integrative Cancer Therapies.

2020;19. doi:10.1177/1534735420975861. [**An attempt to solve one individual's breast cancer diagnosis by targeting specific cancer stem cells.**]

Weinberg, Robert A. _The Biology of Cancer_, Third Edition. New York: Garland Science. 2013. [**The fullest exposition of Hanahan and Weinberg's hallmarks of cancer concept.**]

Weinhouse S. The Warburg hypothesis fifty years later. Z Krebsforsch Klin Onkol Cancer Res Clin Oncol. 1976;87(2):115-26. doi: 10.1007/BF00284370. PMID: 136820. [**A summary of the work of the Philadelphia researcher whose own work undermined the influence of Warburg's theories.**]

Welch DR, Hurst DR. Defining the hallmarks of metastasis. Cancer Res. 2019 Jun 15;79(12):3011-3027. doi: 10.1158/0008-5472.CAN-19-0458. Epub 2019 May 3. PMID: 31053634; PMCID: PMC6571042.

Wesa KM, Cunningham-Rundles S, Klimek VM, et al. Maitake mushroom extract in myelodysplastic syndromes (MDS): a phase II study. Cancer Immunol Immunother. 2015 Feb;64(2):237-47. doi: 10.1007/s00262-014-1628-6. Epub 2014 Oct 29. PMID: 25351719; PMCID: PMC4317517. [**Positive study of maitake mushrooms from Memorial Sloan-Kettering.**]

Wolf S, Herrenkohl RC, Lasker J, et al. Roseto, Pennsylvania 25 years later--Highlights of a medical and sociological survey. Trans Am Clin Climatol Assoc. 1989;100:57-67. PMID: 3269103; PMCID: PMC2376462.

Wong CH, Siah KW, Lo AW. Estimation of clinical trial success rates and related parameters. Biostatistics. 2019 Apr 1;20(2):273-286. doi: 10.1093/biostatistics/kxx069. Erratum in: Biostatistics. 2019 Apr 1;20(2):366. PMID: 29394327; PMCID: PMC6409418.

Wong CP, Hsu A, Buchanan A, et al. Effects of sulforaphane and 3,3'-diindolylmethane on genome-wide promoter methylation in normal prostate epithelial cells and prostate cancer cells. PLoS One. 2014 Jan 22;9(1):e86787. doi: 10.1371/journal.pone.0086787. PMID: 24466240; PMCID: PMC3899342.

Wong VW, Ekstedt M, Wong GL, et al. Changing epidemiology, global trends and implications for outcomes of NAFLD. J Hepatol. 2023 Sep;79(3):842-852. doi: 10.1016/j.jhep.2023.04.036. Epub 2023 May 9. PMID: 37169151.

World Bank. GDP [Gross Domestic Product], Current US$. World Bank national accounts data, and OECD National Accounts data files, 2022. Accessed February 18, 2024.

World Health Organization [WHO]. _The European Health Report 2021._ Taking stock of the health-related sustainable development goals in the COVID-19 era with a focus on leaving no one behind. ISBN: 978-92-890-5754-7, 2022.

Wu AT, Yeh YC, Huang YJ, et al. Gamma-mangostin isolated from garcinia mangostana suppresses colon carcinogenesis and stemness by downregulating the GSK3β/β-catenin/CDK6 cancer stem pathway. Phytomedicine. 2022 Jan;95:153797. doi: 10.1016/j.phymed.2021.153797. Epub 2021 Oct 21. PMID: 34802869.

Wu D, Liu Z, Li J, et al. Epigallocatechin-3-gallate inhibits the growth and increases the apoptosis of human thyroid carcinoma cells through suppression of EGFR/RAS/RAF/MEK/ERK signaling pathway. Cancer Cell Int. 2019 Feb 28;19:43. doi: 10.1186/s12935-019-0762-9. PMID: 30858760; PMCID: PMC6394055.

Wu K, Ning Z, Zeng J, et al. Silibinin inhibits β-catenin/ZEB1 signaling and suppresses bladder cancer metastasis via dual-blocking epithelial-mesenchymal transition and stemness. Cell Signal. 2013 Dec;25(12):2625-33. doi: 10.1016/j.cellsig.2013.08.028. Epub 2013 Sep 4. PMID: 24012496.

Wu LY, De Luca T, Watanabe T, et al. Metabolite modulation of HeLa cell response to ENOX2 inhibitors EGCG and phenoxodiol. Biochim Biophys Acta. 2011 Aug;1810(8):784-9. doi: 10.1016/j.bbagen.2011.04.011. Epub 2011 May 5. PMID: 21571040.

Xie Z, Sun Y, Ye Y, et al. Randomized controlled trial for time-restricted eating in healthy volunteers without obesity. Nat Commun. 2022 Feb 22;13(1):1003. doi: 10.1038/s41467-022-28662-5. PMID: 35194047; PMCID: PMC8864028.

Xing Z, Su A, Mi L, et al. Withaferin A: a dietary supplement with promising potential as an anti-tumor therapeutic for cancer treatment - pharmacology and mechanisms. Drug Des Devel Ther. 2023 Sep 21;17:2909-2929. doi: 10.2147/DDDT.S422512. PMID: 37753228; PMCID: PMC10519218.

Xu L, Zhang Y, Tian K, et al. Apigenin suppresses PD-L1 expression in melanoma and host dendritic cells to elicit synergistic therapeutic effects. J Exp Clin Cancer Res. 2018 Oct 29;37(1):261. doi: 10.1186/s13046-018-0929-6. PMID: 30373602; PMCID: PMC6206930.

Xu M, Wang S, Song YU, et al. Apigenin suppresses colorectal cancer cell proliferation, migration and invasion via inhibition of the Wnt/β-catenin signaling pathway. Oncol Lett. 2016 May;11(5):3075-3080. doi: 10.3892/ol.2016.4331. Epub 2016 Mar 16. PMID: 27123066; PMCID: PMC4840993.

Yadav MK, Kumari I, Singh B, et al. Probiotics, prebiotics and synbiotics: safe options for next-generation therapeutics. Appl Microbiol Biotechnol. 2022 Jan;106(2):505-521. doi: 10.1007/s00253-021-11646-8. Epub 2022 Jan 11. PMID: 35015145; PMCID: PMC8749913.

Yang YM, Hong P, Xu WW, et al. Advances in targeted therapy for esophageal cancer. Signal Transduct Target Ther. 2020 Oct 7;5(1):229. doi: 10.1038/s41392-020-00323-3. PMID: 33028804; PMCID: PMC7542465.

Yan M, Zhang Y, He B, et al. IKKalpha restoration via EZH2 suppression induces nasopharyngeal carcinoma differentiation. Nat Commun. 2014;5:3661.

Yao CJ, Chang CL, Hu MH, et al. Drastic synergy of lovastatin and Antrodia camphorata extract combination against PC3 androgen-refractory prostate cancer cells. Accompanied by

AXL and stemness molecules inhibition. Nutrients. 2023 Oct 24;15(21):4493. doi: 10.3390/nu15214493. PMID: 37960146; PMCID: PMC10647293.

Yılmaz İ, Dolar ME, Özpınar H. Effect of administering kefir on the changes in fecal microbiota and symptoms of inflammatory bowel disease: a randomized controlled trial. Turk J Gastroenterol. 2019 Mar;30(3):242-253. doi: 10.5152/tjg.2018.18227. PMID: 30662004; PMCID: PMC6428516.

Yu H, Pan C, Zhao S, et al. Resveratrol inhibits tumor necrosis factor-alpha-mediated matrix metalloproteinase-9 expression and invasion of human hepatocellular carcinoma cells. Biomed Pharmacother. 2008 Jul-Aug;62(6):366-72. doi: 10.1016/j.biopha.2007.09.006. Epub 2007 Oct 22. PMID: 17988825.

Yu X, Bao Z, Zou J, et al. Coffee consumption and risk of cancers: a meta-analysis of cohort studies. BMC Cancer. 2011 Mar 15;11:96. doi: 10.1186/1471-2407-11-96. PMID: 21406107; PMCID: PMC3066123.

Yu Y, Kanwar SS, Patel BB, et al. Elimination of colon cancer stem-like cells by the combination of curcumin and FOLFOX. Transl Oncol. 2009 Dec;2(4):321-8. doi: 10.1593/tlo.09193. PMID: 19956394; PMCID: PMC2781082.

Zborowski, Mark and Herzog, Elizabeth. *Life is With People: The Culture of the Shtetl.* New York: Schocken, 1962.

Zhai K, Mazurakova A, Koklesova L, et al. Flavonoids synergistically enhance the anti-glioblastoma effects of chemotherapeutic drugs. Biomolecules. 2021 Dec 7;11(12):1841. doi: 10.3390/biom11121841. PMID: 34944485; PMCID: PMC8699565.

Zhang L, Chen W, Liu S, et al. Targeting breast cancer stem cells. Int J Biol Sci. 2023 Jan 1;19(2):552-570. doi: 10.7150/ijbs.76187. PMID: 36632469; PMCID: PMC9830502.

Zhang L, Li L, Jiao M, et al. Genistein inhibits the stemness properties of prostate cancer cells through targeting Hedgehog-Gli1 pathway. Cancer Lett. 2012 Oct 1;323(1):48-57. doi: 10.1016/j.canlet.2012.03.037. Epub 2012 Apr 3. PMID: 22484470.

Zhang L, Virgous C, Si H. Synergistic anti-inflammatory effects and mechanisms of combined phytochemicals. J Nutr Biochem. 2019 Jul;69:19-30. doi: 10.1016/j.jnutbio.2019.03.009. Epub 2019 Mar 31. PMID: 31048206.

Zhang L, Yang G, Zhang R, et al. Curcumin inhibits cell proliferation and motility via suppression of TROP2 in bladder cancer cells. Int J Oncol. 2018 Aug;53(2):515-526. doi: 10.3892/ijo.2018.4423. Epub 2018 May 30. PMID: 29901071; PMCID: PMC6017220.

Zhang M, Zhao R, Wang D, et al. Ginger (Zingiber officinale Rosc.) and its bioactive components are potential resources for health beneficial agents. Phytother Res. 2021 Feb;35(2):711-742. doi: 10.1002/ptr.6858. Epub 2020 Sep 20. PMID: 32954562.

Zhang Y, Li X, Zou D, et al. Treatment of type 2 diabetes and dyslipidemia with the natural plant alkaloid berberine. J Clin Endocrinol Metab. 2008 Jul;93(7):2559-65. doi: 10.1210/jc.2007-2404. Epub 2008 Apr 8. PMID: 18397984.

Zhang Y, Talalay P, Cho CG, et al. A major inducer of anticarcinogenic protective enzymes from broccoli: isolation and elucidation of structure. Proc Natl Acad Sci U S A. 1992 Mar 15;89(6):2399-403. doi: 10.1073/pnas.89.6.2399. PMID: 1549603; PMCID: PMC48665.

Zhao L, Zhang X, Coday M, et al. Sugar-sweetened and artificially sweetened beverages and risk of liver cancer and chronic liver disease mortality. JAMA. 2023 Aug 8;330(6):537-546. doi: 10.1001/jama.2023.12618. PMID: 37552302; PMCID: PMC10410478.

Zhao Z, Zeng J, Guo Q, et al. Berberine suppresses stemness and tumorigenicity of colorectal cancer stem-like cells by inhibiting m6a methylation. Front Oncol. 2021 Nov 15;11:775418. doi: 10.3389/fonc.2021.775418. PMID: 34869024; PMCID: PMC8634032.

Zheng JS, Hu XJ, Zhao YM, Yet al. Intake of fish and marine n-3 polyunsaturated fatty acids and risk of breast cancer: meta-analysis of data from 21 independent prospective cohort studies. BMJ. 2013 Jun 27;346:f3706. doi: 10.1136/bmj.f3706. PMID: 23814120.

Zheng Y, Sun Y, Liu Y, et al. The miR-31-SOX10 axis regulates tumor growth and chemotherapy resistance of melanoma via PI3K/AKT pathway. Biochem Biophys Res Commun. 2018 Sep 18;503(4):2451-2458. doi: 10.1016/j.bbrc.2018.06.175. Epub 2018 July 3. PMID: 29969627.

Zhou DH, Wang X, Yang M, et al. Combination of low concentration of (-)-epigallocatechin gallate (EGCG) and curcumin strongly suppresses the growth of non-small cell lung cancer in vitro and in vivo through causing cell cycle arrest. Int J Mol Sci. 2013 June 5;14(6):12023-36. doi: 10.3390/ijms140612023. PMID: 23739680; PMCID: PMC3709771.

Zhou W, Yang Y, Gu Z, et al. ALDH1 activity identifies tumor-initiating cells and links to chromosomal instability signatures in multiple myeloma. Leukemia. 2014 May;28(5):1155-8. doi: 10.1038/leu.2013.383. Epub 2013 Dec 24. PMID: 24365790; PMCID: PMC4018236.

Zhou X, Afzal S, Wohlmuth H, et al. Synergistic anti-inflammatory activity of ginger and turmeric extracts in inhibiting lipopolysaccharide and interferon-γ-induced proinflammatory mediators. Molecules. 2022 Jun 16;27(12):3877. doi: 10.3390/molecules27123877. PMID: 35745000; PMCID: PMC9229778.

Zhu A, Lee D, Shim H. Metabolic positron emission tomography imaging in cancer detection and therapy response. Semin Oncol. 2011 Feb;38(1):55-69. doi: 10.1053/j.seminoncol.2010.11.012. PMID: 21362516; PMCID: PMC3075495.

Zhuang W, Long L, Zheng B, et al. Curcumin promotes differentiation of glioma-initiating cells by inducing autophagy. Cancer Sci. 2012 Apr;103(4):684-90. doi: 10.1111/j.1349-7006.2011.02198.x. Epub 2012 Jan 30. PMID: 22192169; PMCID: PMC7659256.

Zhu J, Jiang Y, Yang X, et al. Wnt/β-catenin pathway mediates (-)-Epigallocatechin-3-gallate (EGCG) inhibition of lung cancer stem cells. Biochem Biophys Res Commun. 2017 Jan 1;482(1):15-21. doi: 10.1016/j.bbrc.2016.11.038. Epub 2016 Nov 9. PMID: 27836540.

Zhuo Y, Chen Q, Chen B, et al. Berberine promotes antiproliferative effects of epirubicin in T24 bladder cancer cells by enhancing apoptosis and cell cycle arrest . Int J Clin Pharmacol Ther. 2017 Jan;55(1):32-40. doi: 10.5414/CP202534. PMID: 27719740.

Zhu Y, Mao Y, Chen H, et al. Apigenin promotes apoptosis, inhibits invasion and induces cell cycle arrest of T24 human bladder cancer cells. Cancer Cell Int. 2013 Jun 1;13(1):54. doi: 10.1186/1475-2867-13-54. PMID: 23724790; PMCID: PMC3674905.

Zucchi A, Claps F, Pastore AL, et al. Focus on the use of resveratrol in bladder cancer. Int J Mol Sci. 2023 Feb 26;24(5):4562. doi: 10.3390/ijms24054562. PMID: 36901993; PMCID: PMC10003096.

Zuniga KE, Parma DL, Muñoz E, et al. Dietary intervention among breast cancer survivors increased adherence to a Mediterranean-style, anti-inflammatory dietary pattern: the Rx for Better Breast Health Randomized Controlled Trial. Breast Cancer Res Treat. 2019 Jan;173(1):145-154. doi: 10.1007/s10549-018-4982-9. Epub 2018 Sep 26. PMID: 30259284; PMCID: PMC6387648.

Zwolak I. Epigallocatechin gallate for management of heavy metal-induced oxidative stress: mechanisms of action, efficacy, and concerns. Int J Mol Sci. 2021 Apr 14;22(8):4027. doi: 10.3390/ijms22084027. PMID: 33919748; PMCID: PMC8070748.

###

INDEX

A

B

C

T

U

V

X

Y

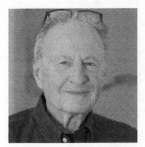

Ralph W. Moss, Ph.D.

Ralph W. Moss, Ph.D., is a prominent author and researcher in the field of cancer treatment and prevention, having authored twelve books and produced three documentaries on cancer research and treatment. Moss holds a BA cum laude from New York University (Phi Beta Kappa, 1965) and an MA (1973) and Ph.D. (1974) in Classics from Stanford University. In the same year, he began his career as a science writer and assistant director of public affairs at Memorial Sloan-Kettering Cancer Center (MSKCC) in New York City.

For the past fifty years, Moss has dedicated himself to independently evaluating both mainstream and non-conventional cancer treatments. His mission is to uncover and share the most advanced, yet least toxic, cancer treatments and prevention strategies, advocating a more holistic and gentle approach to healing from cancer.

Moss's notable works include *The Cancer Industry, Questioning Chemotherapy, Herbs Against Cancer, Antioxidants Against Cancer, Cancer Therapy, Doctored Results,* and *Cancer, Incorporated.* He was also a key participant in the award-winning PBS documentary, *The Cancer War, Second Opinion,* and *Immunotherapy: The Battle Within.* Currently, he co-directs *The Moss Report,* a website offering news and insights on cancer treatments. His YouTube channel, curated with his son Benjamin Moss, has garnered millions of views. His personal experiences with type 2 diabetes and prostate cancer have deepened his understanding of the link between diet, lifestyle, and disease, and has led to the development of The Moss Method.

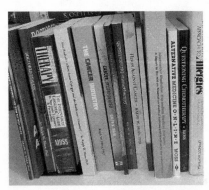

Some of Ralph Moss's book since 1980. Source: Author's collection.

412

Made in the USA
Columbia, SC
14 July 2024

d695786f-3919-43d2-bb85-949534bd17f8R01